Stroke Medicine

Dedication

This book is dedicated to Sue, Philippa, Susan and our children, who tolerated the many hours we spent working on the book without complaint.

Stroke Medicine

Martin M Brown MD FRCP
Professor of Stroke Medicine
Institute of Neurology, University College London
and Consultant Neurologist at the National Hospital,
Queen Square, London, UK

Hugh Markus DM FRCP
Professor of Neurology
St George's University of London
and Consultant Neurologist at St George's Hospital, London, UK

Stephen Oppenheimer DM FRCP FACP
Formerly Director, Cerebrovascular Program
Associate Professor of Neurology and Medicine (Cardiology)
The Johns Hopkins University School of Medicine
Baltimore, Maryland
and Professor of Neuroscience, NJ Neuroscience Institute
John F Kennedy Medical Center, Edison, New Jersey, USA

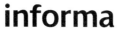

informa
healthcare

New York London

Contents

Preface

Stroke causes over 4.3 million deaths world-wide per annum and is second only to ischaemic heart disease as the major cause of mortality throughout the world, according to the WHO Global Burden of Disease Study. However, the burden of the disease is much more than just mortality, because two-thirds of patients survive their first stroke and half of these remain disabled. About one in six people will have a stroke at some time in their lives. Despite its importance, stroke has been neglected until recently.

Recent advances are transforming stroke management. Perhaps the most exciting development has been the introduction of intravenous thrombolysis for appropriate patients admitted within 3 hours of onset of ischaemic stroke. Patients with subarachnoid haemorrhage or intracerebral haemorrhage, particularly those with cerebellar haematoma, may require urgent neurosurgery or interventional radiology. For all types of stroke, there is good evidence that early admission to a stroke unit with care given by a specialised team has significant benefits in terms of survival and reduction in long-term disability. These advances have been instrumental in the development of the new and exciting discipline of stroke medicine. Stroke medicine is a fascinating specialty, which provides constant interest in terms of diagnosis, while the frequency of death and disability caused by stroke remains a challenge to effective stroke management. Treatment and rehabilitation require that the underlying pathology, aetiology and risk factors have been

identified, and an assessment made of the patient's impairment, functional disability, prognosis and social circumstances. Patients with stroke require active and enthusiastic management. Prevention of recurrence should start as soon as the patient has been diagnosed, and requires identification of the pathology, aetiology and risk factors. Rehabilitation should also start as soon as possible and may need to be continued for many months. The long-term management of the patient may require hospital- or community-based outpatient review and therapy, and is likely to involve the family doctor in continued risk factor control to prevent recurrence. The effective management of stroke therefore requires a coordinated approach between medical, radiological, surgical, nursing and therapy staff.

Our aim has been to produce an easily readable, informative text that describes this clinical approach to stroke, including succinct descriptions of the underlying pathophysiology of stroke and clearly expressed advice regarding clinical diagnosis and management. We have provided as many illustrations as we could fit in. We are grateful to our colleagues who helped provide some of these, especially Dr J Jarosz and Dr R Jäger. We have tried to avoid interrupting the flow of the text with too many source references, but have included key citations in the text of references listed at the end of each chapter. These papers have been individually selected by the authors, usually because they establish an important clinical principle, an evidence-based therapeutic approach to treatment or an up-to-date comprehensive review of the subject. The references are listed under topics at the end of each chapter to facilitate independent searching for key references. We hope that our readers will find the text interesting and useful. Feedback to m.brown@ion.ucl.ac.uk is welcome.

Martin M Brown
Hugh Markus
Stephen Oppenheimer

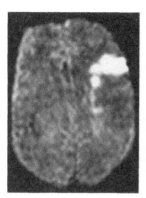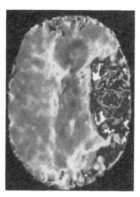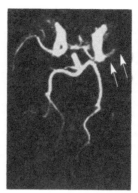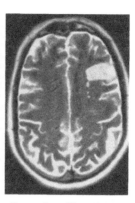

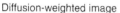

| Diffusion-weighted image | Perfusion-weighted image | Magnetic resonance angiogram | Conventional T$_2$-weighted MRI at 5 days (after thrombolysis with tPA) |

Colour Plate I   (Figure 3.4) Multimodal MRI scans in a patient with an acute middle cerebral artery territory infarct scanned within 6 hours of onset, showing perfusion–diffusion mismatch associated with left middle cerebral artery occlusion on MRA (arrows). From Jansen O *et al. Lancet* 1999;**353**:2036–2037.

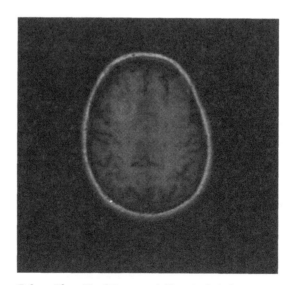

Colour Plate II   (Figure 3.9) Chemical shift imaging showing a focal area of high lactate concentration consistent with acute ischaemia. The lactate concentration calculated from the acquired spectra is shown superimposed on a baseline MRI using a colour scale (blue, absent to yellow, high).

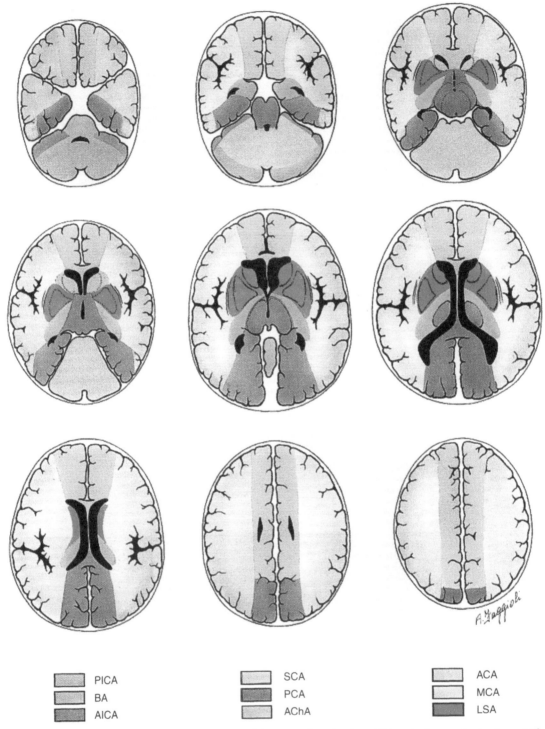

Colour Plate III (Figure 4.2) The distribution of the arterial territories: ACA, anterior cerebral artery; AChA, anterior choroidal artery; AICA, anterior inferior cerebellar artery; BA, basilar artery; LSA, lenticulostriate arteries; MCA, middle cerebral artery; PCA, posterior cerebral artery; PICA, posterior inferior cerebellar artery; SCA, superior cerebellar artery. From Damasio H. *Arch Neurol* 1983;**40**:138–142.

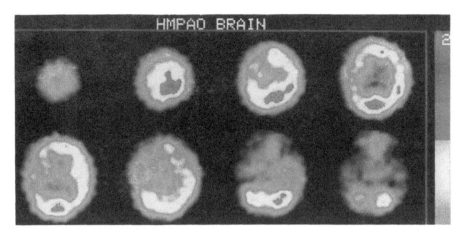

Colour Plate IV   (Figure 3.10) Single-photon emission computed tomography (SPECT) scan in acute stroke, showing the distribution of the blood flow ligand HMPAO. The axial images show high flow (yellow and red) in the normal cortex, with lower flow in the area of ischaemia in the right middle cerebral artery territory (green). Normal, much lower, flow is shown in the deep white matter (blue).

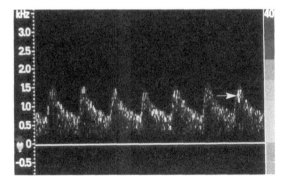

Colour Plate V   (Figure 3.12) Transcranial Doppler recording from the middle cerebral artery of a patient with atrial fibrillation, demonstrating a single high-intensity signal characteristic of micro-embolism (arrow).

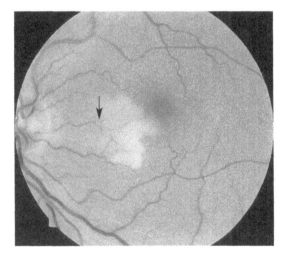

Colour Plate VI   (Figure 4.3) A cholesterol retinal embolus (arrow) with retinal infarction distal to the embolus.

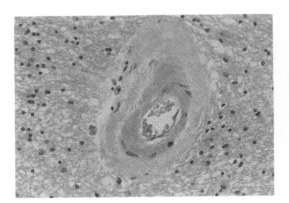

Colour Plate VII   (Figure 7.2) Microscopic cross-section of a perforating vessel showing the characteristic changes of lipohyalinosis.

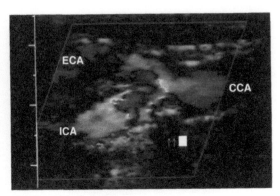

Colour Plate VIII   (Figure 15.13) Colour flow Doppler and duplex ultrasonography showing severe carotid stenosis. Arrows show a large echo-dense atheromatous plaque. Turbulent flow is indicated by colour variation beyond the stenosis. ECA, external carotid artery; ICA, internal carotid artery; CCA, common carotid artery.

Clinical Approach

CHAPTER 1

Classification

Cerebrovascular disease is an all-embracing term that includes any disease of the brain caused by an abnormality of the blood supply. Any part of the brain can be affected by an enormous variety of pathological processes, including almost any disease of blood vessels, diseases of the heart and abnormalities of the blood. This variety of causes, added to the complexity of the different functions of the brain, means that the manifestations of cerebrovascular disease are protean.

The description of the variety of pathological processes underlying cerebrovascular disease, the different clinical presentations and the wide range of severity and prognosis of stroke requires a number of different methods of classification. These are variously based on:

- Duration of symptoms
- Severity
- Anatomy and vascular territory
- Underlying pathology (haemorrhage or infarct)
- Cause
- Risk factors
- Neurological examination
- Functional outcome

None of these classifications is satisfactory alone, because of the wide variety of manifestations of cerebrovascular disease. A full description within each of the classifications is required to provide a complete picture of the patient. In clinical practice, the individual patient should have at least some assessment made within each of these categories, although a more detailed description within each category will only be necessary for certain purposes; for example, a functional outcome scale may be used to assess progress during rehabilitation. In research studies, particularly clinical trials, only one or two measures may be chosen in order to simplify data collection and analysis.

DURATION AND SEVERITY OF SYMPTOMS

Asymptomatic patients

These patients have some evidence of cerebrovascular disease, but have not had any symptoms that can be identified as a consequence of the disease. Examples include patients with asymptomatic carotid stenosis and patients who are found to have cerebral infarction or small vessel disease on computed tomography (CT) without an appropriate history. Of course, it is always possible that such findings were at some stage associated with symptoms but these have been neglected, forgotten or misinterpreted.

Symptomatic patients

The simplest classification of cerebrovascular disease divides symptomatic patients, according to the duration of symptoms, into transient ischaemic attack and stroke.

Transient ischaemic attack (TIA)

This is defined as an acute neurological deficit resulting from focal cerebrovascular disease from which the patient makes a full recovery within 24 hours. The definition is identical to that of stroke (see below), except for the duration of symptoms and the assumption that transient stroke-like symptoms are caused by ischaemia, not haemorrhage. The distinction from stroke and the cut-off period of 24 hours are entirely arbitrary. In practice, most TIAs last less than 30 minutes. If a severe deficit has not started to recover within 60 minutes, the majority of patients will still have a major deficit the next day. This is an important point, because new treatments for stroke, particularly thrombolysis, have to be given within a few hours of onset. It would clearly be undesirable, because of the hazards of treatment, to give thrombolysis to patients who were going to recover spontaneously. In fact, it is unlikely that a patient will be wrongly diagnosed as having had a stroke when in fact they have had a TIA if a major deficit is still present by the time the patient reaches an accident and emergency department.

The standard definition of TIA is based only on symptom duration and does not take into account imaging findings. However, a proportion of patients with TIA will be found to have had an acute infarct (and very occasionally haemorrhage) on CT or magnetic resonance imaging (MRI). The proportion increases in patients with longer-lasting TIAs. It has therefore been proposed recently that the definition of TIA should be changed so that the term is only used if brain imaging has excluded an infarct in a relevant area (Albers *et al.*, 2002). Patients with transient symptoms and relevant infarction would then be labelled as stroke patients, irrespective of the duration of symptoms. However, this suggestion has not received wide support to date. It has also been argued that the duration of TIA should be redefined as a much shorter period of up to 60 minutes, to allow for thrombolysis to be given to any patient with longer-lasting symptoms. One could even suggest that the distinction between TIA and stroke should be abolished, since from the patient's point of view there may be little difference between a TIA that recovers within a few hours and a stroke that recovers within a few days. However, one argument for retaining the distinction between TIA and stroke based only on duration is that the diagnosis of transient symptoms as being the result of ischaemia almost always depends entirely upon a description from the patient or a non-medical witness. The nature of the symptoms may have been ignored or distorted because of neglect, confusion, anxiety or misinterpretation at the time of the symptoms. In contrast, most patients with stroke are seen by a physician while they still have significant symptoms, allowing assessment of the history to be supplemented by clinical examination. In general, symptoms are recognised as being the result of a TIA only because they are very similar to the syndromes seen in stroke.

Investigations rarely contribute to the diagnosis of TIA and CT is usually normal, in contrast to stroke, which is much more likely to be confirmed by an abnormal scan. However, MRI is more likely to show a relevant abnormality in TIAs lasting more than an hour, which supports the idea of shortening the definition of TIA, but still keeping the distinction. Another reason for keeping the distinction is that there is a much wider differential diagnosis of TIA because there are several other neurological disorders that cause transient neurological symptoms and may be confused with TIA (e.g. epilepsy – see Chapter 2). A careful history is therefore essential to distinguish TIA from other non-specific transient neurological symptoms. The annual incidence of first-ever TIA in the UK population is about 0.4 per 1000, which is about one-fifth the incidence of stroke (Dennis *et al.*, 1989). However, there are at least as many patients with non-specific transient symptoms, and the diagnosis, investigation and management of TIAs is an important activity for the physician in an outpatient neurovascular clinic (Bots *et al.*, 1997). Even after thorough assessment, the diagnosis of TIA often remains less certain than the diagnosis of stroke.

The causes of TIA are identical to those of ischaemic stroke. Although cerebral haemorrhage rarely causes symptoms lasting less than 24 hours, small haemorrhages can cause transient symptoms indistinguishable from TIA. The diagnosis of TIA therefore has the same implications as those of stroke with regard to the risk of recurrence. Both require equally rigorous attention to history, examination and investigations in order to identify treatable causes and risk factors for recurrent stroke so that secondary prevention can be initiated. The term TIA therefore has the value of focusing attention on the importance of transient neurological symptoms. It is easy for the patient to dismiss such symptoms as unimportant, and in the past physicians also fell into this trap, assuming that TIAs were the result of 'spasm' of no great import. However, the fact that the patient with TIA may be at high risk of having a subsequent stroke requires the symptoms to be taken seriously by full investigation and appropriate preventive measures (Chapter 2). The expression '*mini-stroke*' can be used as an alternative to TIA when explaining the diagnosis to patients to emphasize the significance of the symptoms and the importance of secondary prevention.

Stroke

This can be briefly defined as an acute neurological deficit resulting from focal cerebrovascular disease that lasts for more than 24 hours. A longer definition has been recommended by the World Health Organization (WHO) (Table 1.1). Stroke is therefore a shorthand clinical description to describe a neurological event that has happened to the patient. The term therefore includes all the different varieties of cerebrovascular disease that involve focal areas of the brain and cause symptoms or signs lasting for more than 24 hours.

Most patients with stroke have a sudden onset of focal neurological deficit, e.g. dysphasia or hemiparesis resulting from occlusion, thrombosis or haemorrhage from arteries. In other cases, the symptoms or signs may be more generalized (e.g. coma in a brainstem stroke).

Table 1.1 WHO definition of stroke

Rapidly developing clinical signs of focal (or global) disturbance of cerebral function, with symptoms lasting 24 hours or longer, or leading to death, with no apparent cause other than of vascular origin

Subarachnoid haemorrhage is usually classified as one of the causes of stroke, even though the symptoms may be limited to the sudden onset of focal headache and neck stiffness, because subarachnoid bleeding may be followed by neuropsychological or focal ischaemic cerebral deficits secondary to vasospasm, and because the underlying causes (e.g. cerebral aneurysm) can also cause intracerebral haemorrhage.

Focal deficits resulting from cerebral venous thrombosis are also regarded as the result of a stroke, but the symptoms of raised intracranial pressure, if they occurred as the only symptoms of cerebral venous thrombosis, would not usually be classified as stroke.

Stroke and TIA are shorthand descriptions for the clinical event that has befallen the patient. Neither term is sufficient as a diagnosis alone, because the underlying pathology or aetiology is not specified. However, these terms have considerable clinical utility and serve to identify distinct syndromes. Most patients present in a similar way and stroke is usually fairly easily recognized as such, even by the lay person. The terms also have the value of identifying patients sharing related pathological processes, with similar underlying risk factors, and who benefit from a similar approach to investigation, treatment and rehabilitation. On the other hand, the common use of stroke as a diagnostic term disguises the fact that stroke may be caused by two opposing pathological processes associated with blood vessels, namely infarction and haemorrhage. There is therefore a danger that stroke will be used as a diagnosis without further inquiry into the underlying cause, despite the fact that haemorrhage and infarction have different causes, management and prognosis. Stroke should be thought of as a syndrome, caused by heterogeneous pathologies, rather than a specific disease.

Reversible ischaemic neurological deficit (RIND)

This term is used to describe symptoms of stroke that last more than 24 hours but then recover completely within a short time, variously defined by different authors as within 1, 2 or 3 weeks. Most experts do not use the term RIND because it has little utility. Other authors have used the term *minor stroke* for symptoms that recover within this length of time. However, the time to full recovery is less important to the patient than whether there is eventual full recovery or long-lasting disability. Clinicians often use the term minor stroke as an equivalent to a mild stroke – namely a patient who has made a good, but not necessarily complete, recovery, although minor stroke has been defined in terms of duration in research studies. In contrast, *major stroke* has been defined in research studies as one that persists for more than 1–4 weeks irrespective of disability, whereas the clinician usually intends the term to refer to any patient with severe residual disability.

Non-disabling, disabling and fatal stroke

One of the simplest methods of classifying the severity of stroke is to distinguish between non-disabling, disabling and fatal stroke. An arbitrary time point for the assessment needs to be chosen (e.g. 1 month after onset). In clinical trials comparing different treatments, the usual times for assessment have been 3 and 6 months after onset. Commonly, the distinction between disabling and non-disabling stroke has been made on the basis of the modified Rankin score (see below), with patients scoring 3 or more being classified as disabled.

One difficulty with any classification of cerebrovascular disease based on the duration of symptoms is that the assessment can only be done retrospectively and is of no use when the patient is first seen, unless they have recovered. Another difficulty is how to classify the patient whose symptoms have almost recovered completely, but is then left with minor problems such as fatigue, or the patient whose symptoms have recovered completely, but who is left with minor neurological signs (e.g. an extensor plantar response of no importance to the patient).

Other symptoms of cerebrovascular disease

Other manifestations of cerebrovascular disease not covered by the categories of TIA or stroke include vascular dementia, vascular epilepsy, raised intracranial pressure from cerebral venous thrombosis, giant aneurysms and vascular cranial neuropathies.

Exclusions to the definition of stroke

- Diffuse brain damage from ischaemia, hypoxia or cardiac arrest is not usually regarded as the result of a stroke, even though the mechanism of brain damage may be similar.
- Focal neurological deficit resulting directly from trauma, even if this causes intracerebral haemorrhage, is also not usually considered within the category of stroke. Thus cerebral contusions, subdural haematoma and extracranial haematoma are not considered by most authors to lie within the category of stroke. However, the distinction is arbitrary and the patient with a cerebral infarct secondary to traumatic carotid or intracranial artery dissection would certainly be regarded as having had a stroke.

Terms to avoid

The expressions 'cerebrovascular accident' and 'CVA' should be avoided. Stroke is not an accident, but has causes that should be identified. The term suggests an old-fashioned approach to stroke, with the misleading implication that nothing much can be done for the patient and the danger that the patient will be neglected in a corner of the ward. Modern specialists prefer the term stroke, which also has the advantage of being more familiar to the patient.

The use of the term stroke should be restricted to a description of the clinical event suffered by the patient. Appearances on a CT scan, MRI or pathological specimen should not be described as 'showing a stroke', but instead as 'showing cerebral infarction or haemorrhage'. Of course, the finding of cerebral infarction or haemorrhage on a scan confirms that the patient's symptoms can be properly described as resulting from a stroke, but the investigations demonstrate pathology not symptoms. One cannot have an asymptomatic stroke.

In describing the laterality of symptoms or signs, it is confusing to use the terminology 'left- or right-sided stroke', which is ambiguous with regard to whether the patient has weakness of that side or whether the observer is referring to the side of the brain involved, in which case the opposite side of the body is likely to be weak. It is much better to describe the stroke in more specific terms, for example, 'the patient has a left hemiparesis' or 'the patient has had a left-hemisphere infarct'.

ANATOMICAL CLASSIFICATION

The clinical presentation of stroke is determined by the site of the infarct or haemorrhage. The management of the patient may also be influenced significantly by the anatomical location of the symptoms. For example, if the patient's symptoms suggest an origin in the posterior fossa, urgent CT or MRI is indicated to exclude a cerebellar haematoma, because this may need neurosurgical evacuation to prevent death from brainstem compression. As another example, carotid endarterectomy is only indicated for symptomatic carotid stenosis if the patient's symptoms arise in the territory of the relevant carotid artery. Identification of the anatomical location of the symptoms is also important in interpreting the findings on imaging, so that the correct part of

a scan can be inspected carefully for the early changes of infarction, and so that abnormalities on the scan can be identified as relevant, or unrelated, to the patient's current symptoms. The site of infarction or intracerebral haematoma will be determined by the vascular territory of the affected blood vessel. The symptoms of stroke should therefore be compatible with impairment of the function of an area of the brain supplied by a single artery or a branch of the artery, e.g. the middle cerebral artery. If the symptoms are not consistent with an origin from a single artery, an alternative diagnosis should be considered, although it is possible that the patient has had multiple emboli to different territories or has an unusual cause of cerebral infarction (e.g. cerebral venous thrombosis).

Large vessel disease

The simplest anatomical classification divides the anatomical origin of stroke into the territories of the major vessels supplying the brain, namely the right and left carotid arteries and the vertebrobasilar system (Figure 1.1). Within the carotid territory, most strokes arise within the middle cerebral artery territory, but occasionally the anterior cerebral artery territory is involved. In carotid occlusion, both anterior and middle cerebral artery territories may be involved. Within the vertebrobasilar territory, common branches to be involved are the posterior inferior cerebellar artery and the posterior cerebral artery. Occlusion or haemorrhage from these major vessels causes characteristic clinical syndromes, which can be identified at the bedside and are described in detail in Chapter 4.

Small vessel disease (lacunar stroke)

Occlusion of small penetrating arteriolar branches of the major vessels in the subcortical white matter, internal capsule, basal ganglia or pons causes small infarcts known as lacunes. These are not necessarily symptomatic, but when they occur in eloquent areas, lacunes are associated with characteristic

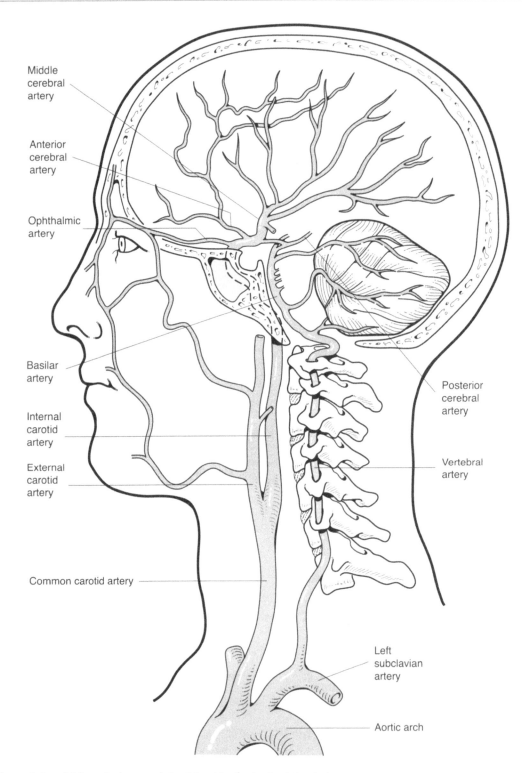

Middle
cerebral
artery

Anterior
cerebral
artery

Ophthalmic
artery

Basilar
artery

Internal
carotid
artery

External
carotid
artery

Common carotid artery

Posterior
cerebral
artery

Vertebral
artery

Left
subclavian
artery

Aortic arch

Figure 1.1a   Major arteries supplying blood to the brain: lateral view.

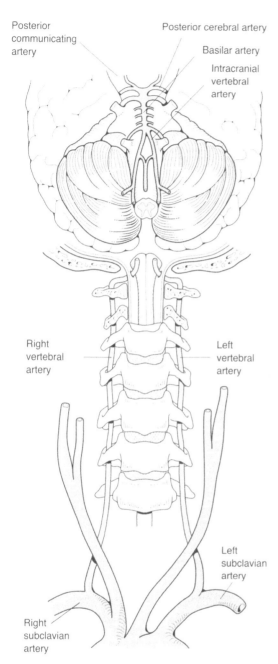

Posterior communicating artery

Posterior cerebral artery

Basilar artery

Intracranial vertebral artery

Right vertebral artery

Left vertebral artery

Left subclavian artery

Right subclavian artery

Figure 1.1b   Major arteries supplying blood to the brain: anterior–posterior view.

clinical symptoms and signs, known as the lacunar syndromes (Bamford and Warlow, 1988). These can often be identified from the history and clinical signs (Chapter 4).

Identification of the site of infarction also has implications concerning the aetiology of stroke. For example, lacunar stroke is more likely to be caused by hypertensive small vessel disease than by cardiac embolism. Conversely, cortical infarction, particularly occipital lobe infarction, is more likely to be caused by cardiac embolism (e.g. from atrial fibrillation).

CAUSES OF STROKE

The three main causes of stroke and their approximate frequency in the Oxfordshire Community Stroke Project were as follows (Bamford *et al.*, 1990):

- Cerebral infarction (85%)
- Primary intracerebral haemorrhage (10%)
- Subarachnoid haemorrhage (5%)

No diagnosis of stroke is sufficient unless this underlying pathology is specified, because infarction and haemorrhage are opposing pathological processes. Indeed, the effective modern management of stroke in terms of investigation, treatment and secondary prevention depends on making the distinction, as will be seen in the following chapters. Infarction or haemorrhage are the end-results (i.e. the final common pathway) of any cause of cerebrovascular disease. An adequate description of the cause of stroke requires the mechanism and aetiology of the infarct or haemorrhage to be determined in as much detail as possible so that treatment and prevention of recurrence can be targeted appropriately (Bogousslavsky *et al.*, 1988; Foulkes *et al.*, 1998). Part of the interest in caring for patients with stroke is to find out which of the large variety of possible underlying vascular and systemic conditions is responsible for the stroke. Table 1.2 lists the main causes according to the main mechanism. Common causes of ischaemic and haemorrhagic stroke are discussed in Chapters 7–9. Dissection and additional rarer causes are discussed in Chapters 10 and 11 (Table 11.1, p. 143). The individual conditions are discussed in more detail in the appropriate chapters.

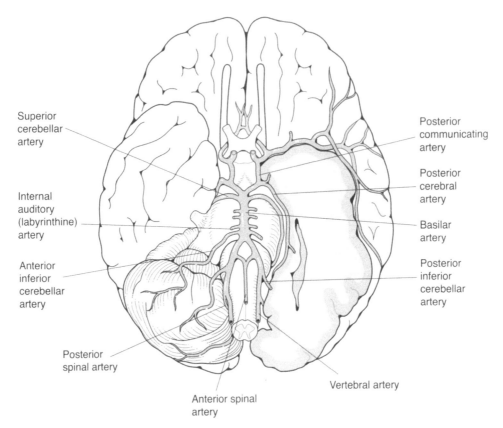

Figure 1.1c   Major arteries supplying blood to the brain: view of base of brain.

CLASSIFICATION OF STROKE TYPE

In research studies, it may be important to use a standard method of classifying stroke type using a combination of clinical features and the results of investigations. One widely used schemata was first developed for use in the Trial of Organon in Acute Stroke and is known as the TOAST classification (Adams *et al.*, 1993). This divides ischaemic stroke into atherothrombotic, cardio-embolic, small vessel occlusion, other determined cause, and undetermined cause. When only limited investigations are available, the Oxfordshire Community Stroke Project classification has been used. This divides stroke on clinical features alone into total anterior cerebral infarction (TACI, usually total middle cerebral artery territory infarction), partial anterior territory infarcts (PACI), lacunar infarcts (LACI) and posterior cerebral infarction (POCI). However, it should be noted that this classification only predicts the size of infarction on CT or MRI in about three-quarters of patients (Mead *et al.*, 2000).

RISK FACTORS

Risk factors are pre-existing medical conditions, social factors, or findings on examination and investigation, which predispose to stroke (Table 1.3). Our knowledge about these risk factors is based on epidemiological studies (Hajat *et al.*, 2001; Simmons *et al.*, 1998). The epidemiology of stroke is described in more detail in Chapter 5. Modification of risk factors is an important strategy in the primary and secondary prevention of stroke. Risk factors are not the direct cause of stroke, but contribute to the development of disease of the blood vessels (e.g. hypertension causing arteriosclerosis) or predispose to thrombosis or embolism (e.g.

Table 1.2 Classification of stroke by cause

Mechanism and source	*Underlying pathology*
Cerebral infarction	
Cerebral embolism	
• Extracranial arterial embolism	
Aorta	Atherosclerosis
Internal carotid artery	Dissection
Vertebral artery	Fibromuscular dysplasia
	Vasculitis
	Arterial trauma
• Cardiac embolism	
Left ventricle	Myocardial infarction
	Cardiac failure
	Cardiomyopathy
Aortic or mitral valves	Rheumatic heart disease
	Calcific valves
	Prosthetic valves
	Endocarditis
Left atrium	Atrial fibrillation
	Atrial myxoma
• Paradoxical embolism	Deep vein thrombosis with atrial septal defect
• Trauma	Fat emboli
	Air emboli
• Iatrogenic	Cardiac surgery
	Cardiac catheterization
	Cerebral angiography
Local intracranial arterial thrombosis	
• Major- or branch-vessel occlusion	
Middle cerebral artery	Atherosclerosis
Anterior cerebral artery	Vasculitis
Posterior cerebral artery	Dissection
Vertebral artery	Hypercoagulable states
Basilar artery	Sickle cell disease
Intracranial internal carotid	Moyamoya disease
• Small vessel occlusion	Hypertensive arteriosclerosis
(lacunar stroke)	Diabetes
	CADASIL
	Vasculitis
Vasospasm	Subarachnoid haemorrhage
Haemodynamic ischaemia	Internal carotid artery occlusion
	Tandem stenoses
	Bilateral vertebral artery occlusion
	Systemic hypotension
	Severe stenoses with poor collaterals
	Cardiac arrest

(Continued)

Table 1.2   (Continued)

Mechanism and source	Underlying pathology
Cerebral venous thrombosis	Hypercoagulable states
	Puerperium
	Intracranial sepsis
	Invasion by tumour
Intracranial haemorrhage[a]	
Subarachnoid haemorrhage	Aneurysm
	Arteriovenous malformation
	Bleeding disorders
	Vascular tumours
	Vasculitis
	Drug abuse
Intracerebral haemorrhage	Causes as for subarachnoid haemorrhage
	Cerebral amyloid angiopathy
	Cavernous angioma
	Hypertensive small vessel disease
	Cerebral venous thrombosis
	Venous anomalies

[a]Trauma also causes subarachnoid and intracerebral haemorrhage, but this is not usually considered as a stroke.

Table 1.3   Some of the major established risk factors for stroke[a]

Risk factor	Cerebral infarction	Intracerebral haemorrhage	Subarachnoid haemorrhage
Increasing age	++	++	+
Hypertension	++	++	+
Smoking	++	+	++
Ischaemic heart disease	++	0	0
Atrial fibrillation	++	0	0
Peripheral arterial disease	++	0	0
Raised haematocrit	+	0	0
High cholesterol	+	0	0
Low cholesterol	0	?	0
High plasma fibrinogen	+	0	0
Alcohol	–	++	++
Obesity	++	+	?
Transient ischaemic attack	++	0	0

++, strong association; +, moderate association; 0, no association; –, protective in moderation, ?, uncertain association.
[a]See also Chapter 5.

atrial fibrillation) (Oppenheimer, 1998; Sacco *et al.*, 1999). The main modifiable risk factor, which accounts for as much as 80% of the risk of stroke in the community, is hypertension, which increases the risk of both ischaemic and haemorrhagic stroke. Most other risk factors are associated with cerebral infarction and not cerebral haemorrhage, although only the more recent epidemiological studies have made this distinction (Woo *et al.*, 2002). Some risk factors (e.g. the presence of peripheral arterial disease) do not in themselves cause stroke, but identify patients at higher risk of stroke because of the association of atherosclerosis at one site with atherosclerosis elsewhere.

The identification of known risk factors in individual patients is usually relatively straightforward, partly because the measurements have to be sufficiently easy to establish from history or investigation to have been studied in large-scale epidemiological studies. There are clearly other predisposing causes that increase the risk of stroke in individual patients; an example is rheumatic heart disease, but because this condition is not common and not easily studied in large populations, it is not usually listed as a risk factor for stroke. There are almost certainly other important risk factors (e.g. specific genetic predispositions) that have not yet been identified (Sacco, 1999).

FUNCTIONAL OUTCOME

The description of stroke according to its effect on the patient in terms of impairment and disability provides a better measure of the severity of the stroke, particularly in those who have not recovered, than classifications based on the duration of symptoms alone. The effects or outcomes of stroke can be measured at several different levels. Any description of outcome must be qualified by a statement of the time at which the assessment was carried out. The severity of neurological disability on admission, and within the first week or so after onset, is a poor guide to eventual outcome, particularly in those with complete paralysis, posterior circulation strokes or cerebral haemorrhage. In those who survive, there is gradual neurological recovery, which is maximal in the first few weeks. However, functional gains (e.g. increased mobility) may be obtained with rehabilitation therapy, even after several months. It is therefore usual to assess functional outcome at standard times (e.g. on admission and discharge from a stroke unit) or in clinical trials at a fixed period (e.g. 3 or 6 months) after onset of the stroke.

Neurological rating scales

The neurological examination plays a dual role in the assessment of the patient with stroke. It has the primary aim of establishing the location of the neurological lesion, but also has a valuable role to play in determining impairment. For the latter function, it is essential that the neurological examination include assessments of cognitive function, language and communication skills, spatial skills, gait, limb function, and swallowing. Although the conventional neurological examination is a useful tool for diagnosis, it does not describe how the patient will function in the activities of daily life and it neglects aspects important in determining handicap (e.g. feeding and continence). The neurological examination is therefore not complete as a tool to assess disability. Moreover, the usual recording of the conventional neurological examination in medical records is not particularly sensitive to mild or even moderate changes in muscle strength or changes in spasticity. *Neurological rating scales* have therefore been developed to record the neurological examination in a standard manner that is more sensitive to the impairments of stroke (Brott *et al.*, 1989). Various components of the examination may be included, and individual components of the examination (e.g. limb strength) are scored according to the severity of the deficit. Neurological rating scales have the advantage that the measures bear a direct relationship to components of the physical examination that are routinely performed in patients with stroke and do not require any additional assessments. The scales are usually quite detailed and sensitive to changes in the neurological condition of the patient (Muir *et al.*, 1996). Two commonly used examples are the Scandinavian Stroke Scale and the National Institutes of Health Stroke Score (NIHSS).

The disadvantage of these scales is that they require a neurologically trained observer (usually a doctor) and are fairly time-consuming if the examination is only being carried out for research purposes. There is also the problem that two patients with very different deficits may receive the same score because a number of different aspects of the neurological examination are scored, while an improvement of one point may mean something quite different in different patients. Furthermore, it is not necessarily obvious what a particular difference in the score means in terms of functional outcome (De Haan *et al.*, 1993). Clinical signs may change without any obvious improvement or decline in function (e.g. an isolated change in reflexes). Conversely, in the later stages of recovery from stroke, the patient's functional capacity (e.g. walking distance) may improve without any significant alteration in the neurological examination. However, these scores have the advantage that the neurological examination is clearly related to the site and size of the cerebral lesion, in a way that is not obvious with the functional outcome scales, described below.

Functional outcome scales

Because the goal of rehabilitation is improvement in function and not an improvement in the neurological examination, a number of scales have been developed to record handicap in terms of activities relevant to daily life. The most widely used are the Barthel Index (Table 1.4) and the Modified Rankin Scale (Table 1.5). The Barthel Index is more orientated towards assessing the activities of daily living, and concentrates on motor handicaps, ignoring communication skills (Wade and Hewer, 1987). The Rankin Scale is orientated towards handicap, in terms of dependence on others, irrespective of the nature of the disability (van Swieten *et al.*, 1988). The Barthel Index requires the patient to be observed carrying out the activities recorded, but is easily performed by a nurse or therapist. It may appear to be more sensitive in that several different activities are assessed on a three-point scale, but may not be more discriminating because each item is heavily dependent on limb function and no measures of communication skills or cognitive function are included.

Table 1.4   The Barthel Index

Score	Factor
	Bowels
0	Incontinent (or needs to be given enemas)
1	Occasional accident (once/week)
2	Continent
	Bladder
0	Incontinent, or catheterized and unable to manage
1	Occasional accident (maximum once per 24 hours)
2	Continent (for over 7 days)
	Grooming
0	Needs help with personal care
1	Independent face/hair/teeth/shaving (implements provided)
	Toilet use
0	Dependent
1	Needs some help, but can do something alone
2	Independent (on and off, dressing, wiping)
	Feeding
0	Unable
1	Needs help cutting, spreading butter, etc.
2	Independent (food provided in reach)
	Transfer
0	Unable – no sitting balance
1	Major help (one or two people, physical), can sit
2	Minor help (verbal or physical)
3	Independent
	Mobility
0	Immobile
1	Wheelchair-independent including corners, etc.
2	Walks with help of one person (verbal or physical)
3	Independent (but may use any aid, e.g. stick)
	Dressing
0	Dependent
1	Needs help, but can do about half unaided
2	Independent (including buttons, zips, laces, etc.)
	Stairs
0	Unable
1	Needs help (verbal, physical, carrying aid)
2	Independent up and down
	Bathing
0	Dependent
1	Independent (or in shower)
Total (0–20)	

Table 1.5 The Modified Rankin Scale

Grade	Description
0	No symptoms at all
1	No significant disability despite symptoms: able to carry out all usual duties and activities
2	Slight disability: unable to carry out all previous activities but able to look after own affairs without assistance
3	Moderate disability: requires some help, but able to walk without assistance
4	Moderately severe disability: unable to walk without assistance, and unable to attend to own bodily needs without assistance
5	Severe disability: bedridden, incontinent, and requires constant nursing care and attention

In clinical trials, a grade of 6 is often added to record patients who have died

These relatively simple classifications have the advantage that they can be performed by non-medical staff. The Rankin Scale can even be collected by telephone interview, because it does not require an examination of the patient. However, these scales have a number of disadvantages:

- There may be disagreement between different observers.
- Disability resulting from coincidental disorders (e.g. arthritis) may be inappropriately attributed to the stroke.
- The scales are insensitive to anything other than a major change in function between each grade.
- The scales suffer from ceiling effects.
- No distinction is made between different types of disability (e.g. memory problems versus gait difficulty).
- Two very different patients (e.g. one with dysphasia and one without) may achieve identical scores.
- Although the scales produce a numerical score, these are not continuous variables or linear, and an increase in the score of one unit in a patient at one point of the scale does not imply the same degree of improvement in another patient from a different point.

Other disability scales assessing individual skills (e.g. speech or fine motor control) and more complex detailed assessment of the activities of daily living are available, but these require specialist training or considerable time, which make them unsuitable for routine use (van der Putten et al., 1999). Scales can also be used to assess the psychological and cognitive consequences of stroke and the presence of anxiety or depression.

All the measures of functional outcome discussed so far do not take into account the patient's own view of their illness and its consequences. There is therefore an increasing tendency in research studies to include a measure of the patient's (or their carer's) own assessment of their health status using specific questionnaires.

KEY REFERENCES

TIA

Albers GW, Caplan LR, Easton JD et al. Transient ischemic attack – proposal for a new definition. *N Eng J Med* 2002;**347**:1713–1716

Bots ML, van der Wilk EC, Koudstaal PJ et al. Transient neurological attacks in the general population. Prevalence, risk factors, and clinical relevance. *Stroke* 1997;**28**:768–773

Dennis MS, Bamford JM, Sandercock PA et al. Incidence of transient ischemic attacks in Oxfordshire, England. *Stroke* 1989;**20**:333–339

Causes of stroke

Bamford JM, Warlow CP. Evolution and testing of the lacunar hypothesis. *Stroke* 1988;**19**:1074–1082

Bamford J, Sandercock P, Dennis M et al. A prospective study of acute cerebrovascular disease in the community: the Oxfordshire Community Stroke Project – 1981–86. 2. Incidence, case fatality rates and overall outcome at one year after cerebral infarction, primary intracerebral and subarachnoid haemorrhage. *J Neurol Neurosurg Psychiatry* 1990;**53**:16–22

Bogousslavsky J, Van Melle G, Regli F. The Lausanne Stroke Registry: analysis of 1,000 consecutive patients with first stroke. *Stroke* 1988; **19**:1083–1092

Foulkes MA, Wolf PA, Price TR et al. The Stroke Data Bank: design, methods and baseline characteristics. *Stroke* 1998;**19**:547–554

Classification of stroke type

Adams HP, Bendixen BH, Kappelle LJ et al. Classification of subtype of acute ischemic stroke. Definitions for use in a multicenter clinical trial. *Stroke* 1993;**24**:35–41

Mead GE, Lewis SC, Wardlaw JM et al. How well does the Oxfordshire community stroke project classification predict the site and size of the infarct on brain imaging? *J Neurol Neurosurg Psychiatry* 2000;**68**:558–562

Risk factors

Hajat C, Dundas R, Stewart JA et al. Cerebrovascular risk factors and stroke subtypes: difference between ethnic groups. *Stroke* 2001;**32**:37–42

Oppenheimer SM, Lima J. Neurology and the heart. *J Neurol Neurosurg Psychiatry* 1998;**64**:289–297

Sacco RL. Newer risk factors for stroke. *Neurology* 2001;**57**(5 Suppl 2):S31–S34

Sacco RL, Wolf PA, Gorelick PB. Risk factors and their management for stroke prevention: outlook for 1999 and beyond. *Neurology* 1999;**53**(Suppl 4): S15–S24

Simmons LA, McCallum J, Friedlander Y et al. Risk factors for ischemic stroke: Dubbo Study of the elderly. *Stroke* 1998;**29**:1341–1346

Woo D, Sauerbeck LR, Kissela BM et al. Genetic and environmental risk factors for intracerebral hemorrhage: preliminary results of a population based study. *Stroke* 2002;**33**:1190–1195

Rating scales

Brott T, Adams HP, Olinger CP et al. Measurements of acute cerebral infarction: A clinical examination scale. *Stroke* 1989;**20**:864–870

De Haan R, Horn J, Limburg M et al. A comparison of five stroke scales with measures of disability, handicap, and quality of life. *Stroke* 1993;**24**: 1178–1181

Muir KW, Weir CJ, Murray GD et al. Comparison of neurological scales and scoring systems for acute stroke prognosis. *Stroke* 1996;**27**:1817–1820

van der Putten JJ, Hobart JC, Freeman JA et al. Measuring change in disability after inpatient rehabilitation. Comparison of the responsiveness of the Barthel index and the Functional Independence Measure. *J Neurol Neurosurg Psychiatry* 1999;**66**:480–484

van Swieten JC, Koudstaal PJ, Visser MC et al. Interobserver agreement for the assessment of handicap in stroke patients. *Stroke* 1988;**19**:604–607

Wade DT, Hewer RL. Functional abilities after stroke: measurement, natural history and prognosis. *J Neurol Neurosurg Psychiatry* 1987;**50**:177–182

CHAPTER 2

Clinical Evaluation

THE CLINICAL APPROACH TO STROKE

The aims of the clinical approach to a patient with stroke are outlined in Table 2.1. The initial structured evaluation discussed in this chapter is essential to guide treatment, rehabilitation and the prevention of recurrence. The evaluation follows a number of steps, which may overlap in time (Table 2.2). The diagnosis of stroke is not satisfactory unless all the questions in Table 2.2 have been answered as far as possible.

IS IT A STROKE?

The clinical approach to the patient with suspected stroke starts with a detailed history (Bamford, 2001). In most cases, it is possible to diagnose strokes clinically, but even the experienced clinician may misdiagnose another focal brain lesion as a stroke (Huff, 2002). Brain imaging is therefore recommended in all cases. Diagnostic certainty is frequently less good after transient ischaemic attacks. When diagnosing stroke, much of the relevant information comes from the history, and in patients who are unconscious, confused or aphasic, obtaining a history from relatives or observers is crucial. The first aim of the history is to establish the tempo, nature and location of the patient's neurological symptoms and whether there are any associated symptoms (e.g. head or neck ache).

Time course

The sudden onset of focal neurological symptoms is very characteristic of stroke. Most strokes reach their maximum deficit over seconds or minutes, but sometimes evolve over a few hours, before starting to improve. Patients with large infarcts or haemorrhage may remain stable for a day or two after the onset of a severe deficit, but then deteriorate further around the third day because of the development of cerebral oedema. The mass effect from the oedema compresses the brainstem, and this may lead to coma and death from respiratory depression. A small number of patients, almost always with subarachnoid haemorrhage or large intracerebral haemorrhages, die very suddenly or succumb rapidly within a few hours of onset. Overall, about 5% of sudden deaths are caused by haemorrhagic stroke. Alternative diagnoses (e.g. cerebral tumour or subdural haematoma) should be considered if the symptoms and signs progress for more than a few hours after onset, or if the symptoms do not improve after a few days. Occasionally, propagation of thrombus, particularly in patients with carotid or basilar artery occlusion, may cause the ischaemic stroke to progress in a stepwise fashion over several days. Lacunar stroke may also progress over several hours for reasons that are not understood. If the patient does not succumb, almost all strokes improve over the first few weeks, although this improvement may not start for several weeks in patients with cerebral

Table 2.1 The clinical approach to stroke

Aim	Procedure
Confirm diagnosis	History CT or MRI scan
Identify underlying pathology	CT or MRI scan LP if SAH suspected and scan normal
Identify anatomical location	History and examination CT or MRI scan
Identify aetiology	History, examination and investigation
Identify risk factors	History, examination and investigation
Establish impairment and disability	Examination
Treat acute stroke	Admission to stroke unit Medical therapy and early rehabilitation Neurosurgery for some haemorrhages
Prevent recurrence	Lifestyle changes Medical therapy Surgery or interventional radiology for aneurysm, AVM and carotid stenosis
Rehabilitation	Stroke unit care or outpatient therapy

AVM, arteriovenous malformation; CT, computed tomography; LP, lumbar puncture; MRI, magnetic resonance imaging; SAH, subarachnoid haemorrhage.

Table 2.2 Initial evaluation of stroke

- Is it a stroke?
- Where is the lesion (i.e. what part of the brain is affected)?
- Is it a haemorrhage or infarct?
- What pathological process has caused the stroke?
- What are the treatable risk factors?
- What are the functional consequences of the stroke?

haemorrhage. The improvement is maximal in the first 2 or 3 months, but may continue more slowly for 6 or 12 months after onset.

Clinical pattern

Stroke results in a neurological deficit that is focal, i.e. can be attributed to involvement of one localized part of the brain. An important consideration in evaluation of patients with suspected stroke is therefore to determine whether the pattern of neurological deficit fits within an arterial territory (see 'Where is the lesion?' below). Such clinical localization may be confirmed by neuroimaging and can help differentiate stroke from other organic neurological disorders and psychological presentations. The neurological deficit is usually negative (e.g. weakness or numbness) rather than positive (e.g. involuntary movements, jerking or tingling). However, very occasionally, haemodynamic ischaemia, particularly in patients with severe carotid artery disease, can result in positive retinal or hemispheric phenomena (Brown, 2001).

DIFFERENTIAL DIAGNOSIS

There are a number of conditions that may present in a similar manner and mimic acute stroke

Table 2.3 Differential diagnosis: conditions that may occasionally mimic stroke

- Subdural haematoma
- Cerebral tumour
- Arteriovenous malformation
- Epileptic seizure and post-ictal neurological deficit
- Head injury
- Multiple sclerosis
- Focal encephalitis
- Cerebral abscess
- Hypoglycaemia
- Metabolic encephalopathy
- Toxic encephalopathy
- Hypertensive encephalopathy
- Familial periodic paralyses
- Central pontine myelinolysis
- Acute polyneuropathy
- Myasthenia gravis
- Motor neurone disease
- Porphyria
- Mitochondrial encephalopathy
- Functional disorder

(Table 2.3). About 5% of patients presenting with stroke-like symptoms have a subdural haematoma, tumour or cerebral abscess. Brain tumours may present as an acute neurological event mimicking stroke, because of sudden haemorrhage into the tumour, post-ictal weakness (Todd's paresis) associated with a seizure, or rapid onset of oedema or compression of the intracerebral microcirculation resulting in ischaemia. The distinction from stroke is usually readily made on computed tomography (CT) or magnetic resonance imaging (MRI). If there is any doubt, repeating the scan after 6 weeks will usually resolve the diagnosis. Occasionally, a cerebral biopsy is required.

Diagnostic confusion is also especially common if the patient is unconscious or if an adequate history cannot be obtained. For example, patients with post-ictal hemiparesis and confusion may well be diagnosed as having suffered a stroke if the ictal activity was subtle, silent or unobserved. Similarly, non-convulsive status may mimic a vascular disorder. Patients with hypoglycaemia secondary to diabetic treatment,

insulinoma or retroperitoneal sarcoma may well present with focal neurological findings, often involving the brainstem. These may reverse completely on prompt elevation of blood sugar.

Multiple sclerosis may present with hemiparesis, sensory impairment or brainstem symptoms that mimic stroke. Usually, the symptoms come on gradually over a few days. Abnormal visual evoked potentials, characteristic MRI appearances and oligoclonal immunoglobulin in the cerebrospinal fluid (CSF) may elucidate the diagnosis. Familial periodic paralyses may also present with an acute quadraparesis, or paraparesis of metabolic cause. Hyponatraemia may be associated with similar focal neurological findings. In the hospital setting, rapid correction of hyponatraemia may be associated with central pontine myelinolysis, a condition in which rapidly advancing tetraplegia and pseudobulbar and bulbar paresis occur. The unwary may find this very difficult to distinguish from an acute stroke.

Acute paralysis may occur in a number of conditions, and may again be confused with stroke if no adequate history can be taken. Acute peripheral polyneuropathy (e.g. Guillain–Barré syndrome) can in rare cases produce paralysis over a very short time indeed (an hour or two). This is usually symmetrical and associated with absent reflexes, but can resemble a brainstem stroke, particularly when there is also dysarthria, ophthalmoplegia and ataxia in the Miller–Fisher variant of this syndrome. Patients with acute intermittent porphyria may be rendered completely quadriplegic on exposure to a precipitating agent (e.g. a barbiturate). Myasthenia gravis may present acutely with focal opthalmoplegia, bulbar palsy or limb weakness. Motor neurone disease may be diagnosed as stroke if the history of progressive onset of bulbar palsy or spasticity is not obtained. Functional disorders (e.g. hysteria or somatization) should be considered if there is marked fluctuation and signs inconsistent with organic disease.

Confusional states may be caused by stroke, especially if the confusion is the result of dysphasia or amnesia. Confusion may occur as an

Table 2.4 Investigations in acute stroke to differentiate metabolic causes
<ul><li>Full blood picture (infections, blood dyscrasias)</li><li>Blood glucose (diabetes, insulinoma, sarcoma)</li><li>Blood gases (where appropriate)</li><li>Electrolytes (periodic paralyses, hyponatraemia)</li><li>Liver and renal function tests</li><li>Electroencephalogram (hepatic coma, other metabolic encephalopathies, ictal and post-ictal states and non-convulsive status)</li><li>Electrocardiogram (hyperkalaemia, hypokalaemia, hypercalcaemia, heart block, myocardial infarction, arrhythmias)</li><li>Blood and urinary drug screening (drug abuse)</li><li>Cardiac monitoring (arrhythmias)</li></ul>

Table 2.5 Differential diagnoses of transient ischaemic attack (TIA)
<ul><li>Migraine aura (with or without headache)</li><li>Partial epileptic seizures</li><li>Todd's paresis</li><li>Labyrinthine disorders</li><li>Transient global amnesia</li><li>Paroxysmal symptoms of multiple sclerosis</li><li>Hypoglycaemia</li><li>Other metabolic disorders</li><li>Cerebral tumours, especially meningioma</li><li>Arteriovenous malformation</li><li>Functional disorders</li></ul>

isolated feature in stroke without other focal signs, especially in non-dominant parietal infarcts, but is more often caused by post-ictal state, infection or metabolic derangements.

A careful history, examination and appropriate investigations, including imaging (Chapter 3) and blood tests (Table 2.4), should elucidate the diagnosis.

The diagnosis of transient ischaemic attack (TIA) relies upon history alone, unless by chance the patient happens to have been examined during an attack. Most TIAs last from minutes to 2 hours at the most, and therefore when the patient is seen they have almost always recovered. Again it is important to determine whether the onset was sudden, whether the neurological deficit was maximal at onset, and whether the deficit was focal and was consistent with being in a single cerebral arterial territory. The diagnosis of TIA can be difficult because neurological examination and neuroimaging are frequently normal by the time the patient is seen (Brown, 2001). The common differential diagnoses of TIA are shown in Table 2.5. There are a number of clinical symptoms that are frequently wrongly diagnosed as TIA but that are rarely caused by cerebral ischaemia. These include non-focal symptoms (e.g. loss of consciousness, presyncopal episodes and dizziness). Occasionally, true vertigo can be caused by a TIA, although one should be cautious about making the diagnosis if vertigo is an isolated symptom without other brainstem symptoms or signs.

WHERE IS THE LESION? (I.E. WHAT PART OF THE BRAIN IS AFFECTED)

Localization of the site of the lesion is important for a number of reasons:

- Establishing that the clinical picture can be accounted for by a lesion in the territory of one cerebral artery supports the suspicion of stroke.
- Localization may provide important information relating to the underlying cause; for example, subcortical stroke is likely to be the result of small vessel disease.
- Determining the territory of infarct or haemorrhage may have a direct impact on treatment; for example, a patient with symptoms in the carotid territory associated with an ipsilateral tightly stenosed carotid artery should have endarterectomy, while, in contrast, the benefit of operating on a similarly stenosed carotid artery in the presence of vertebrobasilar symptoms is very much less.

Localization depends upon a knowledge of the intracerebral circulation and the arterial distributions. This is covered in detail later in Chapter 4. Localization may be confirmed by imaging (Chapter 3).

IS IT A HAEMORRHAGE OR INFARCT?

Primary subarachnoid haemorrhage is usually easy to diagnose. Typically, the patient presents with sudden onset of very severe headache, which is of maximum intensity at onset, accompanied by signs typical of meningism (neck stiffness, vomiting and photophobia). Occasionally, there are accompanying focal neurological signs (Chapter 9). In contrast, the differentiation of cerebral infarction from intracerebral haemorrhage depends upon neuroimaging. Although there are a number of clinical pointers to intracerebral haemorrhage, and clinical scores have been devised to try to exploit these, the scores are unreliable. Drowsiness or coma, vomiting, severe headache, and also progression of neurological deficit after onset may point towards haemorrhage, but even these features are found in cerebral infarction. However, if secondary leakage of blood into the subarachnoid space occurs in an individual with a large intracerebral haemorrhage, this may result in the typical signs of meningism with neck stiffness and photophobia. The combination of sudden onset of a focal deficit (e.g. hemiparesis) with signs of meningism therefore provides strong evidence of an intracerebral haemorrhage, but could also be the result of cerebral infarction secondary to meningitis. Small or moderately sized intracerebral haemorrhages will not produce these signs or symptoms and can only be differentiated by scanning.

CT or MRI scanning is therefore an essential investigation in all patients with stroke to determine whether the symptoms are the result of haemorrhage or infarction (Jager, 2000). The scan also serves to confirm the diagnosis, if abnormal, and excludes the main conditions entering the differential diagnosis of stroke, particularly cerebral tumours and subdural haematoma. CT scan is normal in about 30% of cases of ischaemic stroke, but is always abnormal within the first few days in intracerebral haemorrhage. CT invariably shows high signal intensity from blood in a haematoma within a few minutes of onset, but the high signal on CT only persists variably between 4 days and 3–4 weeks. It is therefore important that patients be scanned as early as possible to distinguish between infarction and haemorrhage. Very early MRI may be difficult to interpret in acute haemorrhage unless special sequences are used, but gradient echo sequences may show previous haemorrhage indefinitely. In patients in whom the CT scan is normal, MRI should be considered because it is much more sensitive to the changes of ischaemia. In suspected subarachnoid haemorrhage, CT may show evidence of subarachnoid blood or a visible aneurysm or arteriovenous malformation. However, CT is normal in about 50% of cases of subarachnoid haemorrhage, and in these cases a lumbar puncture is indicated to examine for uniform blood staining and xanthochromia of the CSF. MRI is rarely helpful in showing subarachnoid haemorrhage that has not been shown by CT. Lumbar puncture is unnecessary in any other variety of stroke, unless infection or vasculitis is suspected. In all cases of stroke, lumbar puncture may be hazardous if there is significant cerebral oedema. The appearances of haemorrhage and infarction on CT and MRI change with time and are discussed in more detail in the Chapter 3.

WHAT PATHOLOGICAL PROCESS HAS CAUSED THE STROKE?

Stroke is a syndrome rather than a specific diagnosis, and both cerebral haemorrhage and cerebral infarction can be caused by a number of different pathologies (see Chapter 1, especially Table 1.2). Both the mechanism (e.g. embolism or local thrombosis) and the underlying aetiology (e.g. atherosclerosis) should be described. Identifying the pathophysiology requires a careful history, supplemented by investigations. For example, in a patient in whom CT shows a wedge-shaped cortical infarct, the history may identify ischaemic heart disease and

Table 2.6 Common screening investigations for stroke and TIA[a]

	Routine investigation	*Selected patients*
All strokes	Brain CT or MRI Full blood count Platelet count ESR Electrolytes Renal and liver function tests	
Cerebral infarction	Fasting blood sugar Fasting lipids ECG Neck-vessel ultrasound or MRA or CTA	Thrombophilia screen Sickle screen Autoantibody screen Echocardiography Syphilis serology Cerebral angiography Drug screen Homocysteine levels 24 h ECG recording
Intracranial haemorrhage	Clotting screen	Sickle screen Cerebral angiography Drug screen
Subarachnoid haemorrhage	Clotting screen Cerebral angiography	Drug screen Sickle screen

CT, computed tomography; CTA, CT angiography; ECG, electrocardiogram; ESR, erythrocyte sedimentation rate; MRA, magnetic resonance angiography; MRI, magnetic resonance imaging.
[a]Other investigations will be needed in occasional patients, e.g. lactate in suspected MELAS (Chapter 11).

the examination may reveal atrial fibrillation, which is confirmed on electrocardiogram (ECG). The combination strongly suggests cerebral infarction secondary to cardiac embolism from left-atrial thrombus as the likely cause for the stroke, if there are no other relevant findings. Symptoms associated with the stroke may also suggest possible aetiological factors – for example, neck pain suggests carotid or vertebral artery dissection.

Specific investigations are necessary to identify the mechanism and aetiology of stroke in most patients. A standard sequence of investigations is therefore required (Table 2.6). The investigations required are different for cerebral haemorrhage and infarction – another important reason for scanning early. In general,

young stroke patients will require more elaborate investigation because the cause of stroke is less likely to be due to simple embolization from a high-grade atherosclerotic lesion in the extracranial vasculature. Cardiac, haematological or a non-atheromatous structural lesion of the vasculature (e.g. dissection) are more likely causes. Thorough investigation will establish the mechanism of stroke in the majority of cases (Figure 2.1). Clearly, appropriate investigation should be tailored to each individual case and circumstance. For example, catheter angiography is rarely necessary in acute stroke, but if intervention with direct intra-arterial thrombolytic therapy is contemplated then imaging of the involved vessel with conventional X-ray angiography will

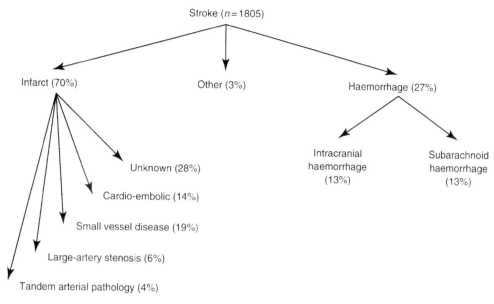

Stroke (*n* = 1805)

Infarct (70%)   Other (3%)   Haemorrhage (27%)

Unknown (28%)

Cardio-embolic (14%)

Small vessel disease (19%)

Large-artery stenosis (6%)

Tandem arterial pathology (4%)

Intracranial haemorrhage (13%)   Subarachnoid haemorrhage (13%)

Figure 2.1   Relative proportions of different identified causes of stroke in the NINDS Stroke Data Bank (1983–1986). Values are taken from Foulkes MA *et al. Stroke* 1988;**19**:547–554.

be required to ensure that the vessel is still occluded. If intravenous thrombolytic therapy is to be given then MRI and magnetic resonance angiography (MRA) might prove effective screening tools, although this remains to be fully evaluated in this circumstance (Chapter 3).

Blood tests

A full blood count, including platelet count and white cell count, is essential to detect polycythaemia, platelet disorders and a raised leukocyte count suggestive of infection. The erythrocyte sedimentation rate (ESR) test may be helpful, because a raised ESR suggests infection, systemic vasculitis or carcinoma and should lead to further investigations (e.g. autoantibody screen or chest X-ray). It is essential to measure fasting blood sugar levels to detect diabetes mellitus and fasting lipids to detect hyperlipidaemia (except perhaps in the very elderly, in whom hyperlipidaemia may not be relevant). Cholesterol levels drop slightly after acute stroke, and if an initial cholesterol level is borderline then the test should be repeated a

month or two after the stroke. Investigation of blood clotting is needed in intracerebral and subarachnoid haemorrhage, while a thrombophilia screen should be performed for anticardiolipin antibodies, protein C, protein S and antithrombin III levels, and activated protein C resistance (or the factor V Leiden gene polymorphism) in patients with cerebral venous thrombosis and in patients under the age of 60 years with otherwise unexplained TIA or ischaemic stroke. Syphilis serology should be investigated in patients at risk of the infection because the diagnosis may not otherwise be suspected. Blood cultures are indicated if bacterial endocarditis is suspected.

Cardiac investigations

These are orientated towards detecting sources of cardiac embolism. An ECG should be performed in every patient. A rhythm strip should be included to detect atrial fibrillation. If there is any suggestion of cardiac arrhythmia, 24-hour monitoring should be performed if the initial ECG is not revealing. Ideally, every patient should have echocardiography to identify cardiac sources of cerebral embolism, but where facilities are limited, echocardiography is indicated in patients under 60 years or in older patients with significant cardiac abnormalities or recurrent unexplained stroke. If transthoracic echocardiography shows no abnormality, transoesophageal echocardiography (TOE) should be considered because it is more likely to identify an atrial abnormality or a patent foramen ovale (Palazzuoli *et al.*, 2000). An intravenous injection of agitated saline can be given to detect right-to-left shunting of blood, which is visualized by the passage of air bubbles across the patent foramen from the right atrium to the left atrium during a Valsalva manoeuvre. TOE may also identify ulcerated aortic atherosclerosis or dissection.

Carotid ultrasound

Duplex ultrasound with imaging and colour-coded Doppler measurement of blood flow velocity should be performed in patients with TIA and stroke in the carotid territories, in order to identify internal carotid artery stenosis, occlusion or dissection. Magnetic resonance angiography (MRA) and CT angiography (CTA) provide alternative non-invasive techniques for identifying large-artery pathology. Auscultation for a carotid bruit is an unreliable indicator of carotid stenosis and will not identify all patients with significant internal carotid artery stenosis. These techniques are discussed in more detail in Chapter 3.

Cerebral angiography

This may be required in selected patients – particularly those with cerebral haemorrhage – in order to identify underlying aneurysm or arteriovenous malformation. Angiographic techniques, including non-invasive MRA and catheter angiography, are discussed in more detail in Chapters 3 and 15.

Idiopathic stroke

In perhaps a quarter to a third of cases of infarct or haemorrhage, it is not possible to make a firm diagnosis as to the underlying mechanism, even after extensive investigations, although patients with idiopathic stroke will often have vascular risk factors such as smoking. Nevertheless, it is important to attempt a pathophysiological diagnosis, as this may have a direct bearing on treatment. Specific causes may require specific treatments – for example clipping for intracranial aneurysm, interventional treatment for arteriovenous malformation, endarterectomy for symptomatic carotid stenosis, antibiotics for infective endocarditis and immunosuppressive regimens for cerebral vasculitis. Establishing the pathophysiology allows a logical approach to be taken in the implementation of secondary preventative measures and allows useful information to be given on the prognosis for recurrence.

WHAT ARE THE TREATABLE RISK FACTORS?

The vascular risk factors are identified from the past medical history, the social history, sometimes the drug history and investigations. Not infrequently, examination or investigation may detect a previously unrecognised risk factor (e.g. hypertension or diabetes mellitus).

WHAT ARE THE FUNCTIONAL CONSEQUENCES OF STROKE?

The functional consequences of stroke may have profound implications for both patients and carers. They also determine patients' rehabilitation needs and the input required from nursing and therapy staff. The effects of the stroke on the patient's neurological, cognitive and psychological functions and their ability to carry out the activities of daily living should also be assessed on admission. The assessments may need to be repeated at regular intervals to guide therapy and assess progress. Some of the functional outcome scales (e.g. the Barthel Index) used as tools to assist this process are described in Chapter 1.

USE OF A DETAILED PROFORMA

The management of patients with stroke, which needs to include the sequence of detailed history taking, examination, recording of disability and investigation described above, is very much aided by the use of a standardized clerking proforma. Although completing the proforma takes a little more time than the standard clerking, the extra time is well used to systematically record important aspects of the patient's history (e.g. risk factors and premorbid disability) and examination (e.g. conscious level and current disability), which are often missed out from routine clerking. The use of a check list of investigations ensures that no relevant tests are omitted. The proforma also improves communication between the many different medical, nursing and therapy professionals often involved in the care of the patient. Integrated care pathways have a similar role.

KEY REFERENCES

Diagnosis of stroke

Bamford J. Assessment and investigation of stroke and transient ischaemic attack. *J Neurol Neurosurg Psychiatry* 2001;**70**(Suppl 1):13–16

Brown MM. Identification and management of difficult stroke and TIA syndromes. *J Neurol Neurosurg Psychiatry* 2001;**70**(Suppl 1):117–122

Foulkes MA, Wolf PA, Price TR et al. The stroke Data Bank: design, methods, and baseline characteristics. *Stroke* 1988;**19**:547–554

Huff JS. Stroke mimics and chameleons. *Emerg Med Clin North Am* 2002;**20**:583–595

Jager HR. Diagnosis of stroke with advanced CT and MR imaging. *Br Med Bull* 2000;**56**:318–333

Cardiac investigations

Palazzuoli A, Ricci D, Lenzi J et al. Transesophageal echocardiography for identifying potential cardiac sources of embolism in patients with stroke. *Neurol Sci* 2000;**21**:195–202

CHAPTER 3

Imaging

This chapter reviews the main imaging techniques available to investigate stroke (Table 3.1). Structural imaging of the brain is an essential investigation, and cranial computed tomography (CT) or magnetic resonance imaging (MRI) is required in all patients with stroke to:

- Confirm the diagnosis (if positive)
- Exclude conditions mimicking stroke (e.g. subdural haematoma)
- Establish the pathological diagnosis (e.g. infarction or haemorrhage)
- Indicate the arterial territory or territories involved
- Guide investigations
- Guide treatment

The distinction of haemorrhage from infarction by CT or MRI is important to facilitate appropriate management. This is of paramount importance in the hyperacute stroke if thrombolytic therapy is being considered, because thrombolysis clearly must not be given to patients with intracerebral haemorrhage. But the distinction is equally important in other patients because aspirin or, in some cases, anticoagulant therapy may be indicated in patients with cerebral infarction, but are contraindicated in intracranial haemorrhage. The site of infarction or haemorrhage can be identified and may give clues to the pathogenesis (e.g. borderzone infarction suggests a haemodynamic origin, multiple cortical infarcts in different territories suggest a cardiac source of emboli, and

superficial lobar haemorrhage suggests cerebral amyloid angiopathy). In suspected subarachnoid haemorrhage, scanning is used to show subarachnoid blood and may therefore avoid the need for a lumbar puncture.

Every patient with suspected stroke should therefore have a scan – preferably as soon as possible and certainly within 24 hours of onset. If imaging facilities are limited, early scanning is indicated in every patient in whom active management (i.e. thrombolysis, surgery, anticoagulation or antiplatelet therapy) is contemplated. An urgent scan is required to exclude surgically treatable conditions (e.g. subarachnoid haemorrhage, cerebellar haematoma, tumour and cerebral abscess) if the patient with suspected stroke:

- Has progressive or fluctuating symptoms
- Is drowsy or in coma
- Has brainstem symptoms or signs
- Has papilloedema, neck stiffness or fever
- Has severe headache
- Deteriorates unexpectedly

Urgent scanning is also necessary if thrombolysis or early anticoagulation is contemplated.

COMPUTED TOMOGRAPHY

Established infarction shows on CT as a well-defined area of reduced attenuation. However, the earliest changes can be very subtle. In middle cerebral artery territory infarction, the

Table 3.1 Imaging modalities available for the investigation of stroke

Structural brain imaging

Computed tomography (CT)
Magnetic resonance imaging (MRI)
Diffusion-weighted imaging (DWI)

Blood vessel imaging

Magnetic resonance angiography (MRA)
Contrast-enhanced MRA
CT angiography
Carotid and vertebral ultrasound
Transoesophageal echocardiography (TOE)
(images ascending aorta)

Blood flow imaging

Magnetic resonance perfusion imaging
Transcranial Doppler (TCD)
Positron emission tomography (PET)
Single-photon emission computed tomography (SPECT)

Metabolic imaging

Magnetic resonance spectroscopy (MRS)
PET

Emboli detection

TCD

Cardiac imaging

Transthoracic echocardiography
TOE

early changes on CT include blurring of the clarity of the internal capsule, loss of distinction of the insular ribbon cortex, loss of cortical definition between grey and white matter, and effacement of the sulci (Beauchamp *et al.*, 1999). These appearances gradually evolve into those of a clear area of low attenuation over the first 24 hours. Over the next few weeks, the lesion becomes more clearly demarcated (Figure 3.1). However, CT is completely normal in as many as 50% of cases at 6 hours and remains normal even if the scan is repeated later in about 30% of all cases. This is usually because the infarct is too small to be seen (particularly in lacunar syndrome), missed because

of the CT slice placement or obscured by artefact. However, even patients with large cortical infarcts may have a negative CT scan within the first 24 hours because the initial ischaemia is not severe enough to cause the changes of established complete infarction. Because of the relatively low resolution and the effect of image degradation due to adjacent bone, CT is especially likely to miss infarction within the posterior fossa, cerebellum or brain stem. Infarction is occasionally missed if the scan is performed on about day 7, because the infarct may go through a stage of being isodense with normal brain ('CT fogging').

Early CT may occasionally show increased attenuation of an artery indicating acute thrombosis ('dense middle cerebral artery sign', Figure 3.2) at a time when the remainder of the CT is normal or shows only early subtle signs of infarction. This finding can therefore help in early cases to establish the diagnosis. It is also a poor prognostic sign.

Haemorrhage is much more easily visualized than infarction and can be seen on CT within a few minutes as an area of increased attenuation. Intracerebral haemorrhage sufficient to cause symptoms will nearly always be visible on early CT, but subarachnoid bleeding is only seen in about 50% of cases. However, after a few weeks, haemorrhage becomes cystic and of low attenuation, so that if CT is not performed within 1 week, it may not be possible to distinguish between infarct and haemorrhage.

Thus, a normal early CT excludes primary intracerebral haemorrhage and is compatible with the diagnosis of ischaemic stroke, but does not exclude subarachnoid haemorrhage or conditions mimicking stroke (e.g. hypoglycaemia).

MAGNETIC RESONANCE IMAGING

MRI has a number of advantages over CT for imaging stroke (Beauchamp *et al.*, 1999). Its resolution is greater and it is less susceptible to bony artefact, meaning that smaller infarcts (e.g. lacunes) and lesions in the posterior fossa are more visible. MRI is more sensitive to early

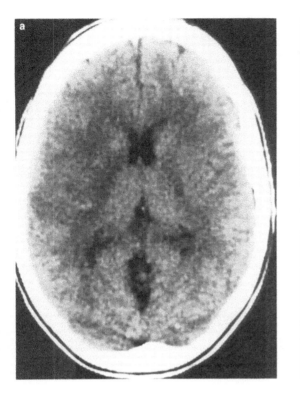

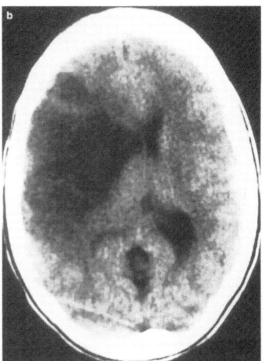

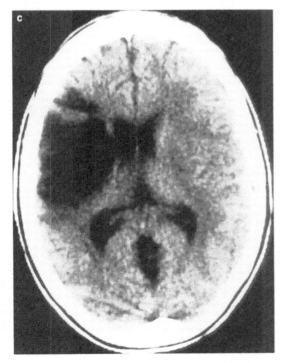

Figure 3.1 Evolution of the changes of cerebral infarction on CT: (a) 4 hours after onset showing early changes within the right middle cerebral artery territory (see text); (b) 48 hours after onset; (c) 1 month after onset.

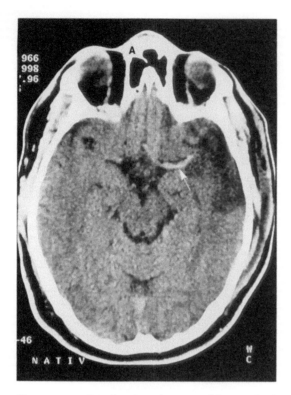

Figure 3.2 CT showing dense middle cerebral artery sign (arrow).

ischaemia and is particularly helpful if the first scan is performed more than a few weeks after onset, because MRI, particularly gradient echo sequences (T_2^*), can detect the traces of old haemorrhage, haemosiderin deposits, indefinitely. On the other hand, the appearances, particularly of haemorrhage, may be more difficult for inexperienced physicians to interpret, and MRI is contraindicated or poorly tolerated in a small percentage of patients. MRI is also not so widely available and is more expensive than CT.

The earliest changes of ischaemia on conventional MRI sequences are seen on T_2-weighted images, with an increase in signal intensity. T_2-weighted images may become abnormal within 4–6 hours of onset, but the latency is greater than 6 hours in many cases, with increasing signal intensity up to 12 hours. It is generally accepted that the visibly abnormal T_2 signal represents irreversible infarction,

although, as in CT, fogging of the image may result in pseudonormalization at about day 7. T_1-weighted images show a reduction in signal intensity in areas of ischaemia and are useful for delineating the anatomy. A fluid attenuation inversion recovery (FLAIR) scan, which is essentially a T_2-weighted scan with an inversion recovery sequence, suppresses signal from free water, primarily the cerebrospinal fluid (CSF) in the ventricles and the subarachnoid space. It shows white matter lesions (e.g. small vessel ischaemic disease) and small cortical lesions adjacent to the sulci particularly well. FLAIR is also particularly sensitive to the changes of gliosis, which develop as a result of chronic scarring after brain injury. Marked signal change on FLAIR imaging around an infarct can therefore help to establish that the lesion is at least several months old.

MRI may also contribute to the diagnosis by showing flow void in patent blood vessels. Conversely, lack of flow void where one would be expected implies vessel occlusion. High intensity in the wall of the carotid or vertebral artery on cross-sectional MRI suggests dissection (Chapter 10). This may only be noted if appropriate fat-suppressed images are requested to include the extracranial internal carotid and vertebral arteries.

The MRI appearances of acute haemorrhage are described in Chapter 8.

There are several new MRI sequences that are even more sensitive to ischaemia than conventional MRI techniques and that provide additional information about the stroke and its metabolic consequences. These require the latest generation of very fast echo planar scanners, but in units where this technology is available, MRI is replacing CT as the investigation of choice in acute stroke.

Diffusion-weighted imaging (DWI)

This employs a sequence of MRI pulses that are very sensitive to restriction in the diffusion of water associated with early intracellular oedema. Normally, mobile molecules acquire phase shifts, resulting in alterations of the MRI signal. Acute ischaemia results in failure of ionic membrane pumps, swelling of the ischaemic cells and compression of the extracellular space. This results in restriction of the space available for free diffusion of water and a change in the phase shift of the MRI signal. Changes in the diffusion-weighted signal intensity resulting from ischaemia can be seen in animals within minutes of stroke onset. In humans, DWI is usually abnormal within 2 hours of stroke onset but may occasionally be normal up to 3 hours. The use of DWI increases the diagnostic yield of imaging in acute stroke substantially compared with CT (Fiebach *et al.*, 2002).

In most cases, significant early changes in diffusion are only seen in areas of critical ischaemia that are destined to infarct (Crisostomo *et al.*, 2003). Ischaemic brain tissue with restricted diffusion is shown on DWI as intensely bright increases in signal intensity ('light bulb' sign), which are very easy to see (Figure 3.3). Because DWI is abnormal in the first few hours after onset, the sequences are particularly useful in acute stroke imaged within the first few hours when conventional T_2-weighted MRI is often normal. Between about 7 and 14 days after onset, the diffusion of water returns to normal and then increases, presumably because of cell lysis. Infarcts older than 14 days therefore show a reduction in signal intensity on DWI, although between 7 and 14 days there may be a pseudonormalization of the signal intensity, which may make an infarct less visible on DWI. Thus, DWI can be used to distinguish between new and old infarcts. However, a number of artefacts may be seen on DWI, particularly at air–bone interfaces and in the posterior fossa, which may hinder interpretation. Established infarcts with an intense increase in the T_2 signal may appear bright on DWI, giving the false impression on the DWI films that the lesion is acute (T_2 shine-through). In such cases, it is helpful to examine MRI films, known as apparent diffusion coefficient (ADC) maps, which more directly image the change in diffusion in the brain. Acute infarction is seen as a reduction

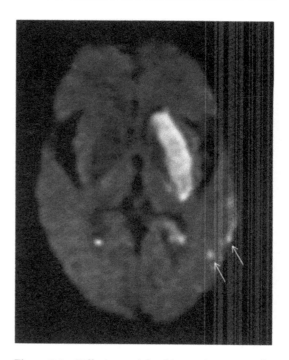

Figure 3.3 Diffusion-weighted image in acute stroke showing bright signal in the area of infarction. This is the same patient as shown in Figure 3.5. Note that, in addition to the large striatocapsular infarct, there are additional small peripherally located areas of infarction (arrows) indicative of distal clot embolism, which were not seen on the T_2-weighted MRI.

in signal on ADC maps – the opposite convention to DWI.

Perfusion MRI

This measures the distribution and transit time of intravenously injected MRI contrast to provide an image of cerebral blood volume and transit time. A series of T_2^*-weighted gradient echo images are performed at 1 s intervals immediately after the rapid intravenous bolus injection of the MRI contrast agent. The passage of the contrast medium through the microvasculature produces a transient loss in MRI signal characteristics (susceptibility artefact), which is proportional to the local blood flow. This allows mean transit time and cerebral blood volume to be measured, from which

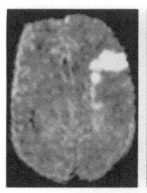
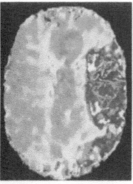
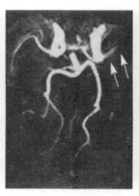
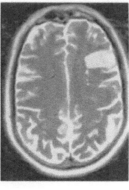

| Diffusion-weighted image | Perfusion-weighted image | Magnetic resonance angiogram | Conventional T$_2$-weighted MRI at 5 days (after thrombolysis with tPA) |

Figure 3.4　(See also Colour Plate I, p. ix). Multimodal MRI scans in a patient with an acute middle cerebral artery territory infarct scanned within 6 hours of onset, showing perfusion–diffusion mismatch associated with left middle cerebral artery occlusion on MRA (arrows). From Jansen O *et al. Lancet* 1999;**353**:2036–2037.

maps of regional cerebral blood flow can be derived. Other MRI methods for obtaining quantitative measures of cerebral blood flow are being developed that do not require the injection of contrast. These make a number of assumptions and require further evaluation.

Perfusion imaging allows areas of impaired blood supply to be imaged, which may be particularly useful if an area of impaired perfusion is identified without associated infarction (Figure 3.4). It has been suggested in a number of small studies that a mismatch between a larger area of perfusion defect and a smaller area of abnormal DWI (*perfusion–diffusion mismatch*) may indicate the presence of salvageable penumbra (Chapter 13) in the region of impaired perfusion without DWI changes (Jansen *et al.*, 1999). There is evidence from case series that such regions can progress to infarction in some patients unless saved by early thrombolysis or spontaneous reperfusion. However, this suggestion needs to be confirmed by larger studies. Caution must be used when interpreting perfusion MRI in patients with carotid artery stenosis or occlusion, because this may result in increased transit time in the absence of acute ischaemia.

Magnetic resonance angiography (MRA)

This allows non-invasive imaging of the extracranial carotid and vertebral arteries and, using different coils, the circle of Willis and second-order bifurcation of the middle cerebral arteries. The main use of extracranial MRA is for the identification of stenosis or occlusion of the carotid or vertebral arteries, which is discussed in more detail in Chapter 15. A potential problem is the differentiation of tight stenosis from occlusion due to signal dropout at regions of very low flow. Intracranial MRA can be used to demonstrate larger aneurysms, arteriovenous malformations, and major intracranial vessel occlusion or severe stenosis (Figure 3.5), but does not currently have sufficient resolution to exclude smaller lesions, which still requires conventional catheter angiography. However, the introduction of contrast-enhanced MRA (CEMRA) with improved, faster scanners is improving the resolution considerably, obviating the need for catheter angiography in many cases. Intracranial MRA may be particularly useful in the future in assessing the presence or absence of middle cerebral artery occlusion in acute stroke.

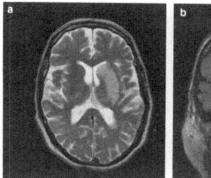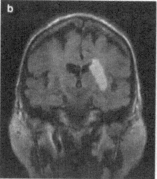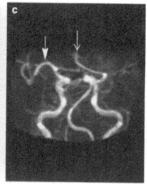

Figure 3.5 (a) Axial T$_2$-weighted MRI, (b) coronal FLAIR and (c) intracranial MRA in a patient with striato-capsular infarction associated with left middle cerebral artery occlusion. (Note the absence of left middle cerebral artery flow on MRA with patent right middle (solid arrow head) and left anterior cerebral arteries (open arrow head)).

Multimodal MRI

This refers to the use of a combination of DWI, perfusion MRI and MRA in an acute stroke patient to identify vessel occlusion and its consequences in terms of reduction in blood flow, tissue infarction and, hopefully, residual penumbra. In the future, these techniques may allow treatment to be targeted at those patients who are most likely to benefit; for example, thrombolysis might only be appropriate if there is both vessel occlusion on MRA and perfusion–diffusion mismatch (Figure 3.4).

Functional MRI (fMRI)

This refers to the use of MRI to measure changes in the focal activity of the brain during specific tasks. Functional imaging techniques are based on the finding that localized neuronal activity is associated with an increase in the metabolic requirements of the neurones, which is closely coupled to a co-localized increase in regional cerebral blood flow. The increase in cerebral blood flow can be measured by a number of MRI methods, including blood oxygen level-dependent imaging (BOLD). This relies on the phenomenon that the local increase in blood flow associated with neuronal activation is greater than the increase in oxygen requirements, so that only a small

proportion of the extra oxygen delivered to the tissues is used. There is therefore a net increase in the tissue concentration of oxy-haemoglobin and a net reduction in the concentration of deoxyhaemoglobin. This results in an increase in signal intensity on gradient echo (T$_2^*$) images. In studying stroke patients with this technique, it has to be assumed that the coupling between blood flow and neuronal activity has not been significantly affected by ischaemia. In stroke, fMRI has primarily been used as a research tool to investigate the reorganization of cortical activity (cerebral plasticity) underlying recovery from focal motor weakness or aphasia.

SPIRAL CT

Spiral CT scanning provides a very fast technique for imaging the brain. Scans of the whole head can be acquired in 15 seconds. *CT angiography* (CTA) provides an alternative to MRA, with an equivalent resolution of the extracranial and intracranial vasculature (Figure 3.6). An intravenous contrast agent is injected by rapid bolus and then the CT device rapidly rotates in a spiral fashion around the head or neck, tracking the contrast as it progresses cranially (Verro *et al.*, 2002). This technique is particularly suitable for the non-invasive screening of patients who are unable

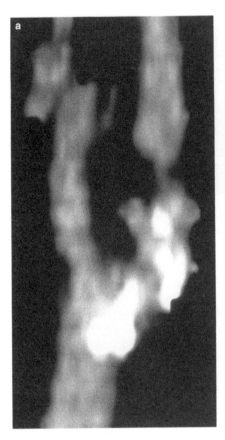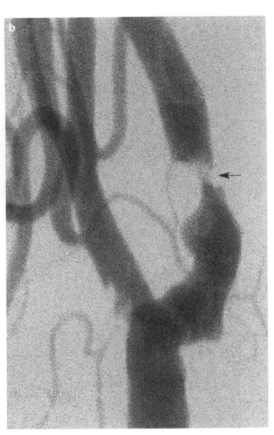

Figure 3.6   Spiral CT angiography (CTA): (a) reconstructed CTA showing carotid artery stenosis; (b) conventional digital subtraction angiography of the same artery showing the stenosis (arrow).

to tolerate MRI either because of implants (e.g. pacemakers) or claustrophobia. However, artefact may obscure the severity of carotid stenosis in patients with highly calcified atherosclerotic plaque. Perfusion CT is currently being developed, and may prove more practical than perfusion MRI in the future (Eastwood *et al.*, 2003).

XENON-CT

Xenon-CT is a method of imaging cerebral blood flow in a CT scanner using stable inhaled xenon gas as an inert tracer (Kilpatrick *et al.*, 2001). During inhalation, the xenon diffuses into the brain substance, causing an increase in the attenuation of the tissues to X-rays, which is measured on serial CT scans. Local cerebral blood flow can be calculated on a pixel-to-pixel basis according to the degree of enhancement

(Figure 3.7). Xenon-CT may in the future provide an alternative to perfusion MRI as a method of identifying salvageable penumbra, and in subarachnoid haemorrhage it can be used to identify areas of vasospasm and predict prognosis. However, xenon inhalation is not tolerated by all patients because of side-effects and the calculation of blood flow is very sensitive to the slightest movement, which invalidates the results. Thus, its use remains to be clearly defined in acute stroke.

MAGNETIC RESONANCE SPECTROSCOPY (MRS)

Proton magnetic resonance spectroscopy (^{1}H-MRS) acquires signals from resonating protons to give information about cerebral metabolism. This technique has been used to identify

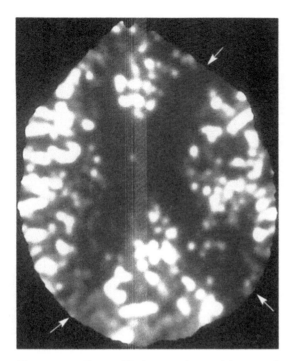

Figure 3.7 Xenon-CT in a patient with several cortical infarcts (arrows), which are shown as areas of markedly reduced flow (the brightness of each pixel is proportional to the local blood flow).

the ischaemic penumbra in humans, but is currently mainly a research tool (Barker *et al.*, 1994; Lanfermann *et al.*, 1995). Signals can be acquired from a number of important compounds and are displayed in a spectrum (Figure 3.8). The spectrum is acquired from a region of interest (single-voxel spectroscopy). The height of the peaks is proportional to the concentration of the compound producing the peak. One of the highest peaks in normal brain is produced by *N*-acetylaspartate (NAA). This is found exclusively within neurones in the central nervous system, but its role in neuronal metabolism is unclear. It is thought to be a constituent of central myelin, and to act as a possible metabolic precursor of excitatory amino acids acting as neurotransmitters within the brain. The value of NAA in MRS is that it serves as a marker of neuronal function and its concentration declines after ischaemia (Saunders *et al.*, 1995). Lactate is another substance that produces a striking peak on

MRS, but is not normally found in the brain in sufficient quantities to be visualized. In conditions of acute ischaemia, the concentration of intracerebral lactate rises markedly and may be detected by spectroscopy. The centres of infarcts may show a complete absence of NAA, which is thought to correspond to dead tissue (the core of the infarct), surrounded by an area of tissue where NAA is present, but reduced compared with normal brain, and lactate is detected. This may represent penumbra. Also of interest is the fact that these changes can be detected within the very early stages of infarction before T_2-weighted MRI has shown the presence of an infarct. The concentration of NAA within an area of infarction declines with time over the first 7 days, but may recover in areas surrounding the infarct. Within the core of the infarct, the concentration of NAA appears to correlate with prognosis, particularly in smaller infarcts (Pereira *et al.*, 1999).

MRS can also be used to measure intracerebral pH and energy metabolism (ATP and ADP concentrations) using resonances from phosphorus compounds (^{31}P-MRS). Both MRS techniques have been used in the diagnosis of the MELAS syndrome (mitochondrial myopathy, encephalopathy with lactic acidosis, and stroke-like episodes; Chapter 11). In this rare condition, which may mimic stroke, lactate can be elevated without much change in NAA, while ATP levels may also be reduced.

Techniques have been developed to display the results of spectroscopy in multiple voxels as an image showing the concentrations of individual compounds in different areas of the brain (chemical shift imaging; Figure 3.9). Spectroscopy is time-consuming and requires supervision from experienced physicists for optimum results. It is therefore unlikely to be widely applied for some time.

POSITRON EMISSION TOMOGRAPHY

In general, positron emission tomography (PET) is impracticable in the routine investigation of stroke. It is, however, a useful research tool to investigate the pathophysiology of stroke (Heiss

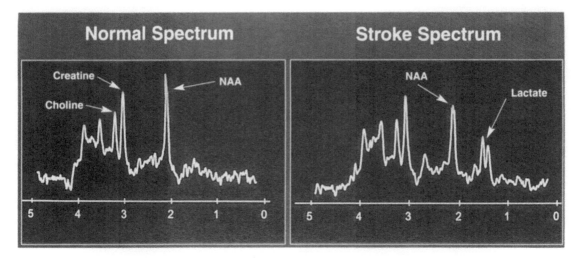

Figure 3.8   Proton magnetic resonance spectroscopy (^{1}H-MRS) in acute stroke, showing lactate and reduced N-acetylaspartate (NAA) concentrations in an infarct (right-hand side of figure) compared with the spectrum from the normal hemisphere of the same patient (left-hand side of the figure).

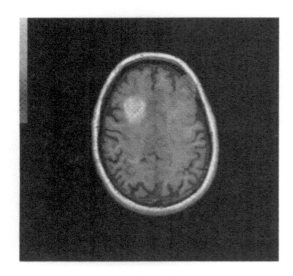

Figure 3.9   (See also Colour Plate II, p. ix). Chemical shift imaging showing a focal area of high lactate concentration consistent with acute ischaemia. The lactate concentration calculated from the acquired spectra is shown superimposed on a baseline MRI using a colour scale (blue, absent to yellow, high).

and Podreka, 1993; Baron, 2001). PET uses the injection and inhalation of a variety of radioactive isotopes with very short half-lives. The decay of these isotopes yields photons that can be tracked by a collimator and amplified using a tomographic technique in sequential axial planes, thus providing localizing information. PET provides information about cerebral blood flow, the metabolic demand of a region (by studying glucose metabolism and oxygen extraction) and its pH. The images obtained lack the resolution of structural CT and MRI scans, although the newer machines are improving in this regard. PET can also be used for functional imaging (see fMRI above). Because PET requires on-site isotope preparation and appropriate staffing, it is often impossible to arrange for urgent PET scanning of stroke patients, making the procedure impracticable in the very early phases of acute stroke except in research settings. Very few PET facilities are available, because of their expensive operational costs and the requirement for a cyclotron unit close to the scanner.

SINGLE-PHOTON EMISSION COMPUTED TOMOGRAPHY

Single-photon emission computed tomography (SPECT) is based on a similar priniciple to PET, but uses radiosotopes emitting single photons with longer decay times than those used in PET. SPECT is therefore cheaper and more widely available than PET, but does not have as good specificity or sensitivity. The main use of

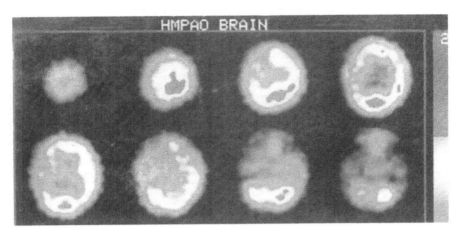

Figure 3.10 (See also Colour Plate IV, p. xi). Single-photon emission computed tomography (SPECT) scan in acute stroke, showing the distribution of the blood flow ligand HMPAO. The axial images show high flow (yellow and red) in the normal cortex, with lower flow in the area of ischaemia in the right middle cerebral artery territory (green). Normal, much lower, flow is shown in the deep white matter (blue).

SPECT in the investigation of stroke has been to produce images of blood flow distribution using technetium-99 bound to hexamethylpropyleneamine oxime (^{99m}Tc-HMPAO) (Figure 3.10). These images allow blood flow to be compared in different regions of the brain, but have not been widely used in clinical practice.

DIGITAL SUBTRACTION ANGIOGRAPHY (DSA)

Catheter angiography is the definitive method for imaging the cerebral circulation (Figure 3.11). However, it carries a significant risk of stroke – varying from 0.5% to as high as 5%, depending on the indication. DSA should therefore only be performed by experienced radiologists for specific indications, preferably after non-invasive imaging (Table 3.2). Catheter angiography is discussed in more detail in Chapter 15.

DUPLEX ULTRASOUND

Duplex ultrasound combines structural B-mode ultrasound imaging with flow information obtained from Doppler measurements. Modern colour-coded machines display the velocity information as a colour map, with red indicating

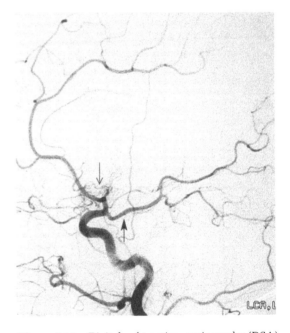

Figure 3.11 Digital subtraction angiography (DSA) of the cerebral circulation, showing occlusion of the middle cerebral artery close to its origin (open arrow head). This patient has a prominent posterior communicating artery (closed arrow head) supplying the posterior cerebral artery.

forward flow and blue reverse flow, and the speed of flow being indicated by the colour intensity. Duplex ultrasound is primarily used

Table 3.2 Indications for catheter cerebral angiography (digital subtraction angiography, DSA)

- To confirm severe carotid stenosis if there is doubt after non-invasive imaging
- To image the carotid and vertebral arteries origins not visualized well non-invasively
- To image the distal carotid and vertebral arteries not visualized well non-invasively
- To confirm arterial occlusion or dissection if the patient is suitable for anticoagulation
- To confirm cerebral venous thrombosis if non-invasive investigations are inconclusive
- To confirm intracranial artery occlusion if the patient is a candidate for arterial thrombolysis
- To diagnose the source of bleeding in subarachnoid and intracranial haemorrhage
- To plan treatment of cerebral aneurysm or arteriovenous malformation
- To support the diagnosis of vasculitis
- To investigate recurrent or unexplained symptoms in younger patients

to identify internal carotid artery stenosis or occlusion, and the patency and direction of flow in the vertebral arteries (Sidhu, 2000). It allows direct visualization of carotid atherosclerosis and the detection of increased velocity and turbulent flow through stenotic regions. It has the advantage of being non-invasive and relatively cheap, but a skilled operator is required to obtain reliable ultrasound results, even in the carotid arteries. In experienced hands, ultrasound may also be useful to identify carotid dissection close to the carotid bifurcation, although it may miss dissection arising in the more distal internal carotid artery. Intravenous ultrasound contrast agents have been developed, and these improve the differentiation of tight carotid stenoses from occlusion. Ultrasound has limited applicability to vertebral artery disease, because only a limited portion of the artery can be insonated, but certain features may suggest more proximal or distal disease of the vertebral artery, and the detection of a reversed direction of flow in one vertebral artery can confirm suspicion of subclavian steal.

TRANSCRANIAL DOPPLER (TCD)

TCD can be used to measure blood flow velocity in the major intracranial arteries (Markus, 2000). A low-frequency (2 MHz) transducer is used to allow penetration of the ultrasound through the bone, and insonation is through natural foramina or regions where the bone is thinnest, primarily the temporal bone. Despite this, an adequate window cannot be obtained in 10% of stroke patients. Conventional TCD utilises pulsed Doppler alone and allows flow velocity in the middle, anterior and posterior cerebral arteries and the carotid siphon to be determined. Stenoses or spasm of the intracranial arteries can be identified by focal segments of increased velocity. Vessel occlusion, particularly in the middle cerebral artery, and the direction and presence of flow in the collateral pathways (primarily the posterior communicating artery and the ophthalmic artery) can be easily determined.

The identification of middle cerebral artery occlusion on TCD may be useful in monitoring the effectiveness of thrombolysis, and possibly in selecting patients suitable for thrombolysis, although this remains to be proven (Baracchini *et al.*, 2000). There is some evidence that continuous application of TCD ultrasound to the site of intracranial occlusion may enhance the effectiveness of intravenous thrombolysis, and randomized trials testing this hypothesis are in progress (Alexandrov *et al.*, 2004).

TCD is increasingly being used in children with sickle cell disease to identify asymptomatic middle cerebral and distal internal carotid artery stenoses (Chapter 11). The presence of these predicts stroke risk, and the technique allows identification of a group of patients who may benefit from regular exchange transfusion. Increased flow velocities may also be seen in vasospasm after subarachnoid haemorrhage (Chapter 9). Improvements in technology allow intracranial structures to be imaged, although the resolution is limited by the low frequencies of ultrasound required for skull transmission. Transcranial colour-coded TCD utilises these B-mode images as well as colour flow mapping of intracranial vessel velocities. Power Doppler and the use of intravenous contrast agents increases the

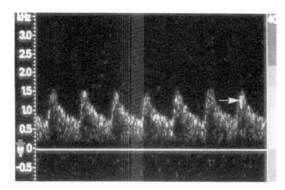

Figure 3.12 (See also Colour Plate V, p. xi). Transcranial Doppler recording from the middle cerebral artery of a patient with atrial fibrillation, demonstrating a single high-intensity signal characteristic of microembolism (arrow).

proportion of individuals in whom the basal cranial arteries can be well visualized.

TCD can also be used to detect microembolism (Markus, 2000). Microembolic particles of insufficient size to obstruct flow cause characteristic high-intensity, transient signals (HITS) on TCD recordings (Figure 3.12). These emboli are usually asymptomatic. Microembolic signals can frequently be detected in patients with potential sources of embolism (e.g. carotid stenosis), especially if they have had recent symptoms. Monitoring of middle cerebral artery blood flow for periods as short as 30 minutes may be sufficient to identify one or more microemboli. There is some evidence that the occurrence of microembolic signals predicts subsequent stroke, particularly in patients with carotid stenosis, and if these findings are confirmed in larger studies then TCD monitoring may have a role to play in risk assessment and selection of patients for particular treatments (e.g. carotid surgery in asymptomatic stenosis). TCD is also used in some units to monitor middle cerebral artery blood flow during carotid surgery and stenting or other interventional procedures. It is important to remember that TCD measures flow velocity, not flow, and any change in middle cerebral artery velocity will only reflect a change in flow if the vessel diameter remains constant.

ECHOCARDIOGRAPHY

This is discussed in Chapter 2.

KEY REFERENCES

CT and MRI in acute stroke

Beauchamp N, Barker P, Wang P et al. Imaging of acute cerebral ischaemia. *Radiology* 1999;**212**: 307–324

Crisostomo RA, Madelleine BS, Garcia M et al. Detection of diffusion-weighted MRI abnormalities in patients with transient ischemic attack. Correlation with clinical characteristics. *Stroke* 2003;**34**:932–937

Fiebach JB, Schellinger PD, Jansen O et al. CT and diffusion-weighted MR imaging in randomised order: diffusion-weighted imaging results in higher accuracy and lower interrater variability in the diagnosis of hyperacute ischemic stroke. *Stroke* 2002;**33**:2206–2210

Jansen O, Schellinger P, Fiebach J et al. Early recanalisation in acute ischaemic stroke saves tissue at risk defined by MRI. *Lancet* 1999;**353**:2036–2037

Spiral CT

Eastwood JD, Lev MH, Provenzale JM. Perfusion CT with iodinated contrast material. *Am J Roentgenol* 2003;**180**:3–12

Verro P, Tanenbaum LN, Borden NM et al. CT angiography in acute ischemic stroke: preliminary results. *Stroke* 2002;**33**:276–278

Xenon CT and SPECT

Kilpatrick MM, Yonas H, Goldstein S et al. CT-based assessment of acute stroke: CT, CT angiography, and xenon-enhanced CT cerebral blood flow. *Stroke* 2001;**32**:2543–2549

Magnetic resonance spectroscopy

Barker PB, Gillard JH, Van Zijl P et al. Acute stroke: evaluation with serial proton MR spectroscopic imaging. *Radiology* 1994;**192**:723–732

Lanfermann H, Kugel H, Heindel W et al. Metabolic changes in acute and subcortical cerebral infarctions: findings at proton MR spectroscopic imaging. *Radiology* 1995;**196**:203–210

Pereira AC, Saunders DE, Doyle VL et al. Measurement of initial *N*-acetyl aspartate concentration by magnetic resonance spectroscopy and initial infarct volume by MRI predicts outcome in patients with cerebral artery territory infarction. *Stroke* 1999;**30**:1577–1582

Saunders DE, Howe FA, van den Boogaart A et al. Continuing ischemic damage after acute middle cerebral artery infarction in humans demonstrated by short-echo proton spectroscopy. *Stroke* 1995; **26**:1007–1013

Positron emission tomography and single-photon emission computed tomography

Baron JC. Mapping the ischaemic penumbra with PET: a new approach. *Brain* 2001;**124**:2–4

Heiss WD, Podreka I. Role of PET and SPECT in the assessment of ischaemic cerebrovascular disease. *Cerebrovasc Brain Metab Rev* 1993;**5**:235–263

Duplex ultrasound and transcranial Doppler

Alexandrov AV, Molina CA, Grotta JC et al. Ultrasound-enhanced systemic thrombolysis for acute ischemic stroke. *N Engl J Med* 2004;**351**: 2170–2178

Baracchini C, Manara R, Ermani M et al. The quest of early predictors of stroke evolution: Can TCD be a guiding light? *Stroke* 2000;**31**:2942–2947

Markus HS. Transcranial Doppler ultrasound. *Br Med Bull* 2000;**56**:378–388

Sidhu PS. Ultrasound of the carotid and vertebral arteries. *Br Med Bull* 2000;**56**:346–366

CHAPTER 4

Clinical Anatomy

Diagnosis and management of the patient is facilitated if their physician is familiar with the relationships between the clinical signs of stroke, the underlying vascular anatomy and the corresponding changes on brain imaging (Damasio, 1983). Localizing the site of stroke depends on knowledge of both the anatomy of the brain's blood supply and the localization of neurological function within the brain. Cerebral vascular anatomy can be considered as two systems: the carotid or anterior system and the vertebrobasilar or posterior system. Within each system there are three main components: the extracranial arteries, the main intracranial arteries, and the smaller superficial and deep perforating arteries. The superficial perforating arteries arising from the pial surface and the small deep perforating arteries (e.g. the lenticulostriate arteries) are predominantly end-arteries. Therefore disruption of their supply will result in a small area of infarction. There is a rich anastomotic network between the arteries over the surface and back of the brain, including connections between the extracranial and intracranial circulations, connections between the basal intracranial arteries through the circle of Willis, and distal intracranial connections through meningeal and pial anastomoses over the cortical and cerebellar surfaces. The degree of this collateral supply varies greatly between individuals and with arterial disease. In particular, the completeness of the circle of Willis will have a great influence on the clinical consequences of an internal carotid occlusion. When the circle of Willis is complete, this may be asymptomatic, while if the collateral supply via the circle of Willis and pial collaterals is poor, carotid occlusion will result in a major hemispheric stroke.

THE CAROTID (ANTERIOR) SYSTEM

The anatomy of the major extracranial and intracranial arteries is shown in Figure 1.1 (page 8). The left common carotid artery usually arises directly from the aortic arch, while the right common carotid artery arises from the brachiocephalic (innominate) artery. The common carotid arteries ascend through the neck, each dividing into an internal carotid artery (ICA) and an external carotid artery at the level of the thyroid cartilage. The carotid bifurcation is one of the most common sites at which atherosclerosis causes severe stenosis. The external carotid artery has a number of branches in its proximal portion; these allow it to be distinguished from the ICA on an angiogram (Figure 4.1). These branches supply the pharynx, thyroid, tongue, face and scalp. They may be of clinical importance in patients with disease due to the potential for anastomoses with branches of the intracranial ICA, which may occur when there is occlusion or tight stenosis of the ICA.

The ICA does not give off any branches in the neck, and enters the cranium through the carotid canal. Each ICA divides into four main portions:

- The *cervical* portion runs from the bifurcation to the entrance to the carotid canal.

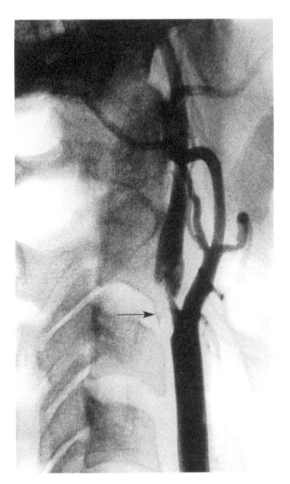

Figure 4.1 Carotid angiogram showing a stenosis at the origin of the internal carotid artery (arrow). The external carotid artery is identified by its numerous branches. The internal carotid artery does not branch in the neck.

- The *petrous* portion continues into the carotid canal of the petrous bone to pierce the dura at the foramen lacerum.
- The *cavernous* portion runs from the foramen lacerum and cavernous sinus entrance to just medial to the anterior clinoid process.
- The *supraclinoid* portion enters the intracranial space at the anterior clinoid after passing between the second and third cranial nerves. This continues to its termination into the middle and anterior cerebral arteries after giving off the ophthalmic, superior hypophyseal, posterior communicating and anterior choroidal arteries.

The carotid siphon is the term used to describe the S-shaped portion of carotid artery that lies within the venous plexus of the cavernous sinus and makes up part of both the cavernous and supraclinoid sections of the ICA. Here the artery lies adjacent to the cranial nerves III, IV, V (segments i and ii) and VI. These nerves run in the lateral wall of the cavernous sinus. Atheroma may affect the ICA in the siphon.

CLINICALLY IMPORTANT BRANCHES OF THE INTERNAL CAROTID ARTERY

Ophthalmic artery

This arises from the supraclinoid ICA. It is important because amaurosis fugax, or transient monocular blindness, is a frequent symptom of carotid stenosis, which itself most commonly occurs at the carotid bifurcation. The majority of cases of amaurosis fugax are caused by embolization, and sometimes emboli can be seen in the retinal circulation on fundoscopy. Occasionally, the symptom of amaurosis results from haemodynamic ischaemia in patients with severe carotid stenosis or occlusion, or other causes – for example, prothrombotic states, including the anticardiolipin syndrome, may be responsible. In patients with tight carotid stenosis or occlusion, the ophthalmic artery is also important because its branches form potential anastomotic links with the external carotid artery, which may allow retrograde filling of the ICA via the ophthalmic artery.

Anterior choroidal artery

The anterior choroidal artery arises from the ICA just before its bifurcation into the anterior cerebral and middle cerebral arteries. In addition to the choroid plexus, this supplies the optic tract, the inferior portion of the posterior limb of the internal capsule, the medial portion of the globus pallidus, the pyriform cortex and the uncus of the temporal lobe, the hippocampal and dentate gyri, the tail of the caudate nucleus, the middle third of the cerebral peduncle, the substantia nigra, parts of the red nucleus, a portion of the subthalamus, and the lateral geniculate body.

Potential anastomotic channels with the external carotid artery

A number of branches arise from the ICA, including the tympanic and pterygoid branches from the petrous portion, branches from the cavernous portion (including the meningohypophyseal trunk), and the ophthalmic artery and superior hypophyseal artery from the supraclinoid section. All of these may provide anastomotic channels with the external carotid artery; such channels may be important in maintaining blood supply in the presence of ICA occlusion or stenosis.

Posterior communicating artery

The posterior communicating artery (PCoA) usually arises just before the anterior choroidal artery and tracks back to join the posterior cerebral artery. It may give off small branches that contribute to the blood supply of the basal ganglia, and it forms an important collateral channel as part of the circle of Willis.

A common variant of the PCoA occurs in about 5% of subjects in which the fetal pattern persists so that the artery remains large and the posterior cerebral territory is then supplied by the ICA rather than the basilar artery. In such cases, embolism from the carotid artery may result in posterior cerebral artery infarction.

Other important anatomical features of the ICA

The common and internal carotid arteries are intimately associated with sympathetic fibres, which ascend around the carotid arteries. Therefore carotid artery lesions, particularly trauma and dissection, may result in an ipsilateral Horner's syndrome. The relationship of the ICA to the transverse process of C1/2 may result in carotid artery damage and dissection when the neck is hyperextended and/or rotated and therefore stretched over this transverse process. The superior laryngeal and hypoglossal nerves are close to the origin of the ICA and may be damaged during surgical procedures (e.g. carotid endarterectomy).

Middle cerebral artery

The middle cerebral artery (MCA) is the largest branch of the ICA and appears almost as its direct continuation. It begins as a single trunk or stem (M1 segment), which then passes into the Sylvian fissure, where it usually bifurcates to give superior and inferior divisions. The superior division usually gives rise to the orbitofrontal, prefrontal, pre-Rolandic, Rolandic, anterior parietal and posterior parietal branches, while the inferior division usually gives rise to the angular, temporo-occipital, posterior temporal, middle temporal, anterior temporal, and temporopolar branches. However, there are many variations on this pattern, and therefore defining clinical pictures to specific arterial territories can be difficult in practice. The portion of the cerebral hemispheres supplied by the MCA are shown in Figure 4.2. From the main MCA stem, a variable number of lenticulostriate perforating arteries originate at right-angles to the main vessels. These may supply the lentiform nucleus, the anterior limb of the internal capsule, the lateral head of the caudate nucleus, most of the globus pallidus, and the superior portion of the posterior limb of the internal capsule. Occlusion of a single perforating artery results in a lacunar syndrome. The superficial medullary perforating arteries arise from the cortical arteries on the pial surface of the hemispheres. These are usually about 20–50 mm in length and descend to supply the subcortical white matter in the centrum semi-ovale. These are also end-arteries, and therefore isolated infarcts in their territories result in small lacunar infarcts and usually cause clinical lacunar syndromes if the infarct is symptomatic (see below).

Anterior cerebral artery

The anterior cerebral artery (ACA) begins as a medial branch of the ICA. The proximal part of the ACA is known as the A1 segment up to the

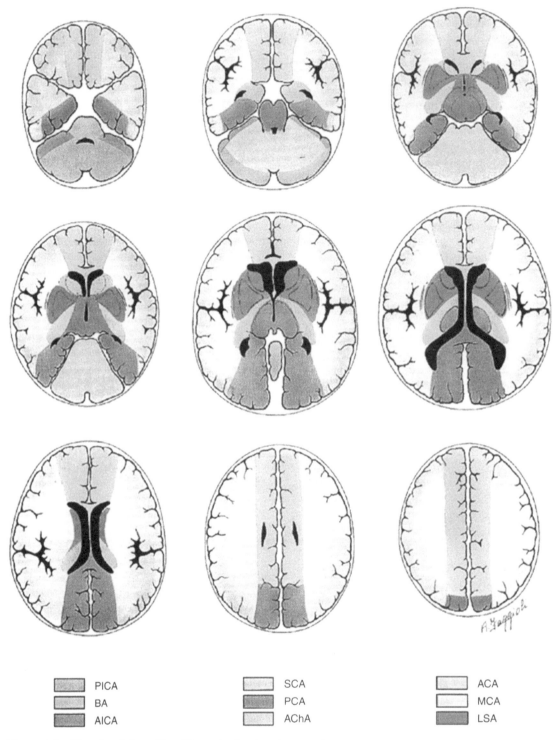

	PICA		SCA		ACA
	BA		PCA		MCA
	AICA		AChA		LSA

Figure 4.2 (See also Colour Plate III, p. x). The distribution of the arterial territories: ACA, anterior cerebral artery; AChA, anterior choroidal artery; AICA, anterior inferior cerebellar artery; BA, basilar artery; LSA, lenticulostriate arteries; MCA, middle cerebral artery; PCA, posterior cerebral artery; PICA, posterior inferior cerebellar artery; SCA, superior cerebellar artery. From Damasio H. *Arch Neurol* 1983;**40**:138–142.

junction with the anterior communicating artery, beyond which it continues as the A2 (distal) segment. Perforating arteries arise from the A1 and A2 segments to supply the para-olfactory structures, the medial anterior commissure, the anterior–inferior portions of the globus pallidus, the caudate nucleus, the putamen, the anterior hypothalamus, part of the anterior limb of the internal capsule and sometimes part of the anterior thalamus. However, the portions of these basal structures supplied by perforators from the MCA and ACA territories show individual variations. The distribution of ACA supply to the hemispheres is shown in Figure 4.2. The recurrent artery of Heubner is an inconstant branch of the ACA, which usually arises around the level of the anterior communicating artery and may supply the head of the caudate nucleus, the inferior portion of the anterior limb of the internal capsule, and the hypothalamus.

VERTEBROBASILAR (POSTERIOR) CIRCULATION

The extracranial right vertebral artery arises as the first branch of the right subclavian artery, which itself arises from the innominate artery, while the left vertebral artery arises as the first branch of the left subclavian artery, which itself arises directly from the aortic arch (Figure 1.1b and 1.1c, pp. 9 and 10). It is commonly divided into four segments:

- The *prevertebral* segment runs from its origin to the transverse foraminal entrance at the level of the sixth cervical vertebral body.
- The *cervical* segment passes through the transverse foramina.
- The *atlantic* segment exits from the transverse foramen of C2.
- The *intracranial* segment pierces the dura and enters the cranial cavity to join the contralateral vertebral artery and form the basilar artery.

The anterior and posterior meningeal branches originate at the upper end of the cervical and atlantic sections. The posterior spinal artery, posterior inferior cerebellar artery (PICA) and anterior spinal arteries originate from the intracranial section. There are a number of small perforating vessels to the medulla.

The basilar artery

The basilar artery is formed from the confluence of both vertebral arteries, usually at the level of the pontomedullary junction. It gives rise to the anterior inferior cerebellar artery (AICA) and the superior cerebellar arteries. It then terminates by dividing into the two posterior cerebral arteries. Along its course, the basilar artery also gives rise to perforating endarteries, which supply the pons, the inferior portion of the midbrain and the ventrolateral aspect of the cerebellar cortex. The internal auditory (labyrinthine) artery arises either directly from the basilar artery or from the AICA to supply the cochlea, the labyrinth and a portion of the facial nerve. The AICA supplies the middle cerebellar peduncle as well as the anterior–inferior aspect of the cerebellum. The superior cerebellar artery arises just proximal to the basilar termination; it usually supplies the dorsolateral midbrain and has branches to the superior cerebellar peduncle and the superior surfaces of the cerebellar hemispheres.

Posterior cerebral arteries

The basilar artery usually terminates by dividing into the right and left posterior cerebral arteries (PCAs). They are joined to the ICA by the PCoA. In 5–15% of people, the PCA on one side is a direct continuation of the PCoA (see Figure 3.11, p. 37). A number of penetrating arteries arise from the PoCA and the PCA to supply the hypothalamus, the dorsolateral midbrain, the lateral geniculate body and the thalamus. The PCA also gives rise to the medial and lateral posterior choroidal arteries, which supply the posterior portion of the thalamus and the choroid plexus. It then divides into the anterior division, which gives rise to the anterior and posterior temporal arteries, supplying the inferior surface of the temporal lobe, and the posterior division, which gives rise

Table 4.1 Differentiation of carotid from vertebrobasilar ischaemic symptoms

Symptom or sign	Likely arterial territory		
	Carotid	Vertebrobasilar	Either
Amaurosis fugax/retinal infarction	+		
Dysphasia	+		
Neglect	+		
Constructional dyspraxia	+		
Hemiparesis			+
Hemisensory loss			+
Hemianopia			+
Dysarthria			+
Dysphagia			+
Ataxia		+	(+)[a]
Diplopia		+	
Vertigo		+	
Bilateral weakness		+	
Bilateral sensory disturbance		+	
Crossed sensory/motor loss		+	
Complete visual loss		+	
Early coma		+	
Amnesia		+	

[a]Ataxia most commonly arises from posterior circulation ischaemia, but the ataxic hemiparesis lacunar syndrome can result from anterior circulation lacunar infarction (see 'Lacunar infarcts and syndromes').

to the posterior pericallosal, occipitoparietal, posterior parietal and calcarine branches. These supply the undersurface of the occipital lobe, including the lingual and fusiform gyrus and the medial surface of the occipital cortex. The portion of the cerebral hemisphere supplied by the PCA is shown in Figure 4.2.

CLINICAL SYNDROMES ASSOCIATED WITH SPECIFIC ARTERIAL OCCLUSIONS

The patterns of neurological symptoms and signs associated with carotid and vertebrobasilar territory ischaemia are shown in Table 4.1.

ANTERIOR (CAROTID) CIRCULATION SYNDROMES

Retinal symptoms

Unilateral amaurosis fugax ('fleeting blindness') or transient monocular blindness

results from temporary embolic obstruction of the ophthalmic artery. The classical presentation is with a black 'curtain' descending to completely obscure vision in one eye. Sometimes this may only affect the upper or lower part of the visual field, or the symptoms may be less typical, with merely a greying or blurring of vision. The attacks are usually brief, lasting only minutes and with full recovery of vision. Amaurosis fugax should always alert one to the possible presence of a carotid stenosis. Less commonly, positive retinal symptoms (e.g. flashing lights or 'white-out' of vision) may arise from haemodynamic compromise of the retinal circulation in the presence of very severe carotid stenosis or carotid occlusion.

More long-lasting, often permanent, acute visual loss usually indicates retinal infarction and can also result from carotid emboli. Retinal infarction from emboli is often partial because individual branch occlusion is frequent, but sometimes central retinal artery occlusion can

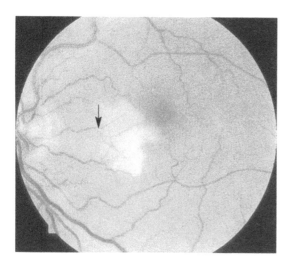

Figure 4.3 (See also Colour Plate VI, p. xi). A cholesterol retinal embolus (arrow) with retinal infarction distal to the embolus.

occur with complete loss of vision. Occlusion of the superior or inferior branches of the retinal artery may cause unilateral altitudinal field loss, involving the top or bottom half of the field of one eye. Emboli may be seen in the retinal circulation by fundoscopy both in patients with retinal infarction and in those with transient ischaemic attacks (TIAs). During or soon after the attacks, platelet–fibrin white–grey emboli may be seen and may break up and migrate through the retinal circulation. However, more frequently, cholesterol emboli are seen as brightly refractile objects within the retinal vessels (Figure 4.3). These may persist for a long time and therefore do not necessarily represent an acute episode.

Ischaemic retinopathy is a rare complication of carotid occlusion or very tight stenosis and may result in temporary visual loss caused by exposure to bright light. In addition, neovascularization of the iris may occur with secondary glaucoma, a condition known as rubeosis iridis.

Hemispheric symptoms – hemispheric transient ischaemic attacks

The most common features of carotid territory hemispheric TIA are contralateral weakness or sensory dysfunction, and/or dysphasia if the dominant hemisphere is involved. Less commonly, TIAs may include other cognitive dysfunction (e.g. neglect), but as the symptoms last only a short duration, they may not be noted by the patient. TIAs usually last minutes or occasionally a few hours. Neuroimaging studies have shown that the longer-duration TIAs lasting more than an hour are frequently accompanied by small areas of infarction. The distinction between a longer TIA and a brief stroke may be subtle. The definition of stroke as symptoms lasting more than 24 hours reflects an arbitrary, although useful, time point. In almost all cases, TIAs involve loss of function, but occasionally positive neurological phenomena can occur. Most commonly, these involve limb jerking in the absence of frank epileptiform activity. This usually occurs in patients with carotid artery occlusion or very severe stenosis and poor collateral supply via the circle of Willis, and in some cases revascularization has resulted in cessation of the attacks, suggesting that the mechanism is haemodynamic.

Rarely, both amaurosis fugax and hemispheric TIA occur together, and in such cases it is highly likely that the patient has an ipsilateral carotid stenosis.

Hemispheric infarction

The clinical consequences of hemispheric infarction vary according to infarct size and location. The size and location of the infarct will be determined by the site of vessel occlusion and also the collateral supply via the circle of Willis and pial anastomoses. Even in patients with complete carotid occlusion, the region of infarction may be much smaller than that of the carotid arterial distribution, and indeed, in many cases, there may be no infarction at all. Furthermore, due to interindividual variation in the anterior and middle cerebral artery territories, localization to particular arterial subterritories can be difficult. Nevertheless, there are a number of patterns of anterior circulation infarction that can be helpful in clinical practice.

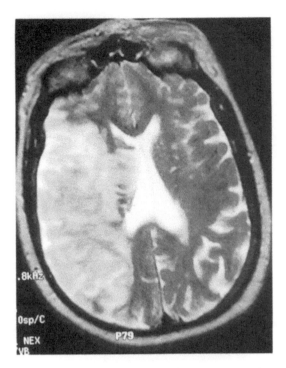

Figure 4.4   T$_2$-weighted MRI showing a complete MCA territory infarct.

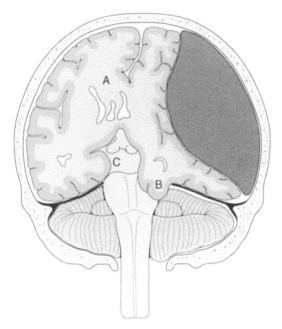

Figure 4.5   Herniation secondary to a large MCA infarct or haemorrhage. The cingulate gyrus (A) herniates under the falx, the temporal lobe uncus (B) herniates under the tentorium and the contralateral peduncle (C) becomes compressed. Adapted from Plum F, Posner JB. *The Diagnosis of Stupor and Coma*. Philadelphia: Davis FA Company, 1985.

Complete MCA infarction

Proximal MCA occlusion, before the origins of the lenticulostriate arteries, produces a maximal hemispheric deficit with contralateral hemiplegia, hemisensory loss and hemianopia (Figure 4.4). Global aphasia will occur if the dominant hemisphere is affected, while severe constructional dyspraxia and neglect of the whole left side will occur if the non-dominant hemisphere is affected. The large lesion may cause considerable oedema and hemispheric swelling, which may result in uncal, transtentorial, and cingulate herniation (Figure 4.5). This is sometimes referred to as *malignant middle cerebral artery infarction*. Cingulate herniation occurs when the cingulate gyrus is pushed under the falx cerebri and this compresses and displaces the ipsilateral ACA and the internal cerebral vein. This may lead to infarction in the territory of the ACA. Transtentorial herniation may occur, with compression and displacement of the diencephalon and adjoining brainstem

through the tentorial notch. This may lead to a hemiparesis on the side ipsilateral to the infarct, and caudal displacement of the midbrain may stretch the perforating arteries as they leave the basilar artery and result in brainstem infarction. Uncal herniation occurs due to downward pressure from the temporal lobe, which leads to its uncus herniating under the tentorium cerebelli. This may compress the ipsilateral oculomotor nerve, leading to a third-nerve palsy. Progressive brainstem compression may result in loss of consciousness and death.

If the occlusion of the MCA is more distal, occurring after the lenticulostriate arteries have arisen, the deep MCA territory is spared and infarction is limited to the cortex and underlying white matter. The cortex supplying the leg may then be spared due to supply from the ACA and some recovery of the leg may occur. In contrast, proximal MCA occlusion

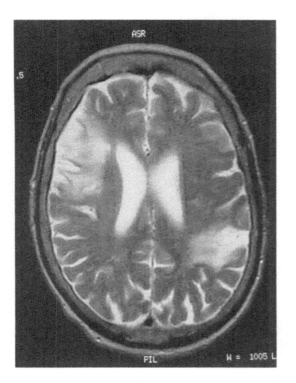

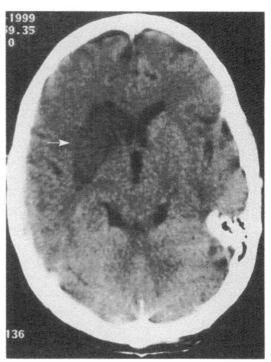

Figure 4.6 T$_2$-weighted MRI showing two partial MCA territory infarcts in opposite territories secondary to cardiac embolism from atrial fibrillation.

Figure 4.7 CT scan showing striatocapsular infarct (arrow).

with disruption of the corticospinal tract in the internal capsule is less likely to be accompanied by recovery of leg function.

ICA occlusion can cause identical patterns of infarction to that seen with MCA occlusion. This may be the result of embolism from the top of the occluded carotid or because of haemodynamic infarction with preservation of the ACA territory because of flow via the anterior communicating artery.

Partial MCA territory infarction (Figure 4.6)

More distal MCA occlusion may block either the superior or the inferior division. Superior division occlusion results in a contralateral hemiparesis and hemisensory loss affecting the face and arm to a greater extent than the leg. If the dominant hemisphere is affected predominantly, expressive aphasia or dysphasia occurs.

Hemianopia does not usually occur. If the inferior division of the MCA is occluded, there is usually little or no hemiparesis and the contralateral hemisensory loss rapidly resolves (Portera-Cailliau *et al.*, 2003). The predominant features are those of a contralateral homonymous hemianopia or upper quadrantanopia due to optic tract and radiation involvement, and a predominantly receptive aphasia as well as a dyspraxia or apraxia from parietal cortex involvement. Visual and sensory inattention may occur.

Striatocapsular infarction (Figure 4.7)

A discrete region of infarction affecting the striatocapsular region may occur from MCA stem occlusion. Studies have shown that in this pattern of infarction the MCA occlusion is frequently temporary. The occlusion leads to disruption of blood supply in the lenticulostriate arteries and therefore infarction in the striato-capsular region. Since these lenticulostriate arteries are end-arteries, they have no collateral supply and therefore infarction results rapidly. It is believed that the overlying cortex is spared due to good pial collateral supply, which allows it to survive until recanalization of the MCA occurs. Striatocapsular infarction is therefore more commonly seen in children and young adults. The identification of this pattern of infarction may be clinically useful because in the majority of cases an embolic source can be found, either carotid or cardiac in origin (see Figure 3.3, p. 31). The clinical picture is that of a contralateral hemiparesis and often sensory loss. Hemianopia is unusual. If the dominant hemisphere is affected, dysphasia may occur and other symptoms of cortical dysfunction have been reported, although these are usually mild (Weiller *et al.*, 1993). The origin of these 'cortical' symptoms has been debated but may include temporary but reversible cortical ischaemia, or disruption of cortical–subcortical connections and cortical deafferentation.

ACA infarction (Figure 4.8)

Anterior cerebral artery occlusions are relatively rare compared with MCA infarction. The clinical picture is variable, depending upon the extent of the ACA territory, but most commonly contralateral weakness, predominantly of the leg, is found. Contralateral sensory loss, again affecting the leg, may occur, but is usually mild. Other frontal lobe features, including incontinence, emotional lability, lack of motivation, and disinhibition, are more common with bilateral frontal ischaemic damage. If the dominant hemisphere is affected, speech disturbance can occur. This has been attributed to the supplementary motor area, with typically a loss of spontaneous output but preserved repetition.

Border-zone infarction (Figure 4.9)

A reduction in cerebral perfusion caused by severe hypotension or cardiac arrest (e.g.

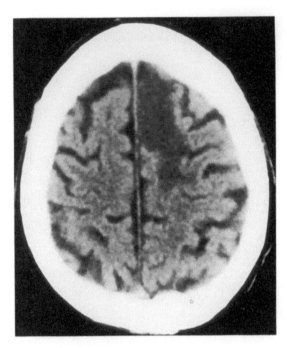

Figure 4.8   CT scan showing an old ACA territory infarct.

from cardiac arrhythmia or anti-hypertensive agents) may result in haemodynamic (low perfusion pressure) infarction, particularly in individuals with pre-existing stenotic or occlusive disease in the extracerebral or proximal intracerebral vessels. Classically, the site of infarction is in the border zones between the territories of the major intracerebral vessels (Mounier-Vehier *et al.*, 1995; Gandolfo *et al.*, 1998; Del Sette *et al.*, 2000). This is sometimes known as watershed infarction, but border-zone infarction is a more accurate term. A number of classical patterns have been reported, although it should be remembered that inter-individual variability in the arterial supply may make firm distinction between a haemodynamic border-zone infarct and an embolic territorial infarct difficult.

Anterior border-zone infarction   This occurs at the junction between the ACA and MCA territories. Infarction usually occurs in the superior frontal region, presenting with weakness; this may affect the arm, with the face and leg being relatively spared, or, if the ischaemic region is higher on the convexity, the leg may be involved.

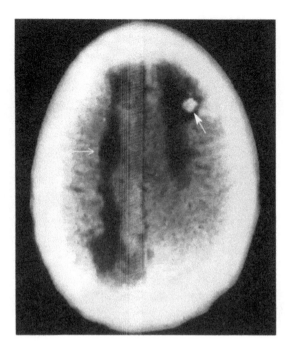

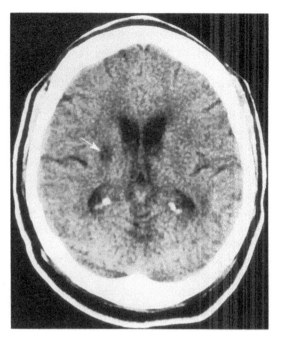

Figure 4.9 CT scan showing anterior border-zone infarction between the ACA and MCA territories in the right frontal lobe (solid arrow head) and extensive infarction in the left hemisphere involving the deep internal border zone (open arrow head) and the posterior border zone between the MCA, ACA and PCA territories.

Figure 4.10 Lacunar infarct in the left internal capsule (arrow).

Posterior border-zone infarction Hypoperfusion in the posterior border zone area between the MCA and PCA territories may result in a parieto-occipital infarct.

Internal border-zone infarction Hypoperfusion may result in infarction in the distal regions supplied by the deep perforating arteries in the deep white matter of the centrum semiovale.

Lacunar infarction in the MCA territory (Figure 4.10)

Occlusion of a single lenticulostriate artery results in a lacunar infarct due to the lack of anastomoses between the perforating arteries. Single lacunar infarcts may present with one of the classical lacunar syndromes, or occasionally with other syndromes including isolated movement disorders (e.g. chorea and hemiballismus), but the majority of lacunes do not have obvious clinical consequences and are found incidentally on neuroimaging. Lacunar syndromes may also occur from infarction in the posterior circulation, and therefore the classical lacunar syndromes are covered later in this chapter.

POSTERIOR (VERTEBROBASILAR) CIRCULATION SYNDROMES

A number of classical syndromes result from infarction in the territory of the individual arteries supplying the brainstem, which may allow accurate localization of the artery involved (Caplan, 2003). However, in practice, such classical syndromes are rare and a diagnosis of vertebrobasilar ischaemia is made on the basis of a constellation of symptoms or signs resulting from ischaemia in either the brainstem or occipital cortex. Many of the signs (e.g. hemiparesis) can also be caused by anterior circulation ischaemia. However, frequently localization to the posterior circulation is possible because of symptoms from involvement of cranial nerve nuclei or a pattern of bilateral symptoms (e.g. crossed sensory and motor loss). Such diagnostic syndromes include ipsilateral cranial nuclei involvement with contralateral motor or sensory deficit. This may affect only the arm and leg if infarction occurs below the facial nucleus and trigeminal nucleus respectively. Other classical syndromes include bilateral hemiparesis or sensory loss, with extraocular opthalmoplegia. Cerebellar signs point to posterior circulation ischaemia (Chaves *et al.*, 1994), although ataxia may occur with ipsilateral hemiparesis as part of the ataxic hemiparesis lacunar syndrome (see below). Hemianopia or bilateral blindness occurs from hypoperfusion in one or both posterior cerebral artery territories and usually indicates posterior circulation embolism (Brandt *et al.*, 2000). Bilateral limb weakness points to brainstem involvement. More frequently, posterior circulation ischaemia results in unilateral hemiparesis or hemisensory loss. Vertigo may be a presenting feature of brainstem ischaemia, but one should be wary of making this diagnosis in patients with isolated vertigo, in whom the origin is much more likely to be labyrinthine vestibular dysfunction. Vertigo and dizziness are overdiagnosed as resulting from vertebrobasilar ischaemia.

Lateral medullary syndrome

The classical picture of the lateral medullary syndrome (Wallenberg's syndrome) involves dorsolateral infarction of the medulla. This has been thought of as being synonymous with posterior inferior cerebellar artery occlusion, but it may also arise from occlusion of the vertebral artery and the perforating medullary arteries supplying the lateral medulla (Wityk *et al.*, 1998). The classical syndrome consists of:

- Ipsilateral Horner's syndrome (descending sympathetic fibres)
- Loss of pain and temperature sensation on the contralateral limbs and trunk (spinothalamic tract) and ipsilateral face (descending trigeminal tract)

- Vertigo, nausea and vomiting
- Nystagmus (lower vestibular nuclei)
- Ataxia on the side of the lesion (inferior cerebellar peduncle)
- Dysarthria, dysphagia and dysphonia resulting from ipsilateral paralysis of the palate, pharynx and larynx

This complete picture of Wallenberg's syndrome is rare, and partial syndromes are more common. Infarction in the territory of the PICA may occasionally present with isolated vertigo, or more commonly with a combination of vertigo, ataxia (both truncal and of the limbs) and nystagmus.

Basilar artery thrombosis (Figure 4.11)

The clinical consequences of basilar occlusion depend upon the location of the thrombus and in particular upon whether the origins of the perforating pontine arteries are affected (Glass *et al.*, 2002; Voetsch *et al.*, 2004). Collateral circulation can occur via the PICAs and anastomoses to the branches of the superior cerebellar artery and then the distal basilar artery and PCAs. Basilar thrombosis most commonly leads to infarction in the paramedian pontine region. If it extends to the distal segments and blocks the superior cerebellar artery origins, massive and usually fatal pontine and midbrain infarction occurs. The most common clinical findings in basilar thrombosis are bilateral limb paralysis with or without some ataxia. In some patients, this weakness may be asymmetrical, with hemiparesis on one side and only minor abnormalities (e.g. slight weakness or increased reflexes) on the other side. Involvement of the bulbar muscles causes dysarthria or anarthria, and dysphagia. Dysfunction of the vestibular and oculomotor systems in the pontine tegmentum may lead to diplopia and oscillopsia. Frequent manifestations include sixth-nerve palsy, conjugate gaze palsy ipsilateral or bilateral to the lesion, and unilateral or bilateral internuclear opthalmoplegia. Sensation is usually spared because the spinothalamic tract and descending tract of

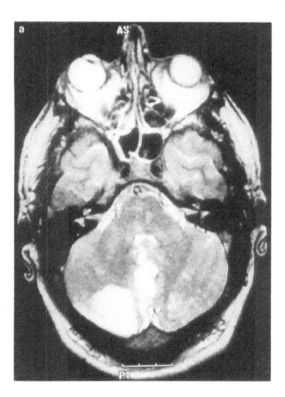

Figure 4.11 T$_2$-weighted MRI showing cerebellar and pontine infarction after basilar artery thrombosis.

the trigeminal nucleus are more laterally placed. If infarction extends to the paramedian pontine tegmentum bilaterally, patients may be comatose. This may also result in the *locked-in syndrome* in which patients are conscious and alert but unable to communicate except by signalling with their eyes. This is frequently misdiagnosed as a loss of consciousness, and in situations where it is suspected, it is important to specifically ask the patient to move their eyes in a particular direction.

Top of the basilar syndrome

The PCAs and perforating arteries to the paramedian midbrain and thalamus arise from the top of the basilar artery. Occlusion at this site, usually resulting from embolization, produces a characteristic clinical and neuroimaging picture. Midbrain, thalamic, and bilateral PCA territory infarction result in the complete syndrome. Infarction in the bilateral rostral

midbrain may result in a vertical gaze paresis, small and poorly reactive pupils, and disturbances of alertness, behaviour and memory. Patients may show reduced conscious level or hypersomnolence. When aroused, they may be confused and disorientated and may experience visual and tactile hallucinations. Memory dysfunction may result from infarction of the medial thalamus, the hippocampus and the adjacent medial temporal lobe structures. This is usually a Korsakoff-like syndrome with an inability to form new memories and amnesia for recent events. Complete cortical blindness may occur from infarction in both occipital lobes, but sometimes the infarction may be restricted to one occipital lobe with hemianopia.

Fusiform aneurysm of the basilar artery (Figure 4.12)

The basilar artery may become dilated and elongated in appearance – sometimes known as dolichoectasia – and may form a fusiform aneurysm. This may produce symptoms in a number of ways. The brainstem may be directly compressed, resulting in hemiparesis and cranial nerve signs. Disruption of flow in the perforating arteries may occur due both to in situ thrombosis and to distortion of their origins, resulting in ischaemia and infarction in their territories. Luminal thrombosis may result in distal embolization, usually to the PCA territories.

PCA occlusion (Figure 4.13)

A homonymous hemianopia from infarction of the occipital cortex is the most common manifestation of PCA occlusion. This may spare the macula if the visual cortex is infarcted with sparing of the optic radiation. Partial syndromes may result in lesser visual loss – most commonly a quadrantanopia. If the PCA is occluded near its origin, this will result in ischaemia in the territory of its deep perforating branches and therefore infarction of the thalamus and upper brainstem. This most commonly results in a hemisensory deficit,

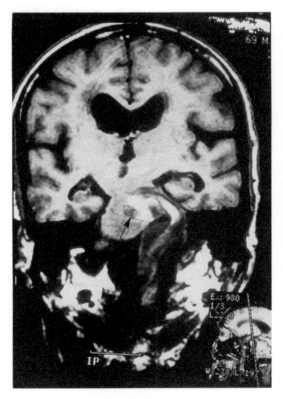

Figure 4.12   Fusiform aneurysm of the basilar artery seen on coronal MRI (arrow).

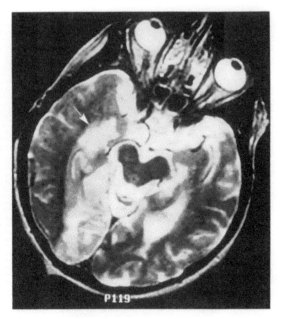

Figure 4.13 T_2-weighted MRI showing infarction after left PCA occlusion. Note the involvement of the medial temporal lobe (arrow).

but more extensive infarction and clinical consequences can occur. Bilateral cerebral artery occlusion may cause cortical blindness or rarely bilateral altitudinal field loss associated with loss of colour perception (achromatopsia) if the infarction is limited to the inferior or superior occipital cortex.

The thalamo-perforating or thalamic–subthalamic arteries arise from the proximal PCA. They supply the posteriomedial thalamus as well as the rostral midbrain, and unilateral infarction may result in a depression of conscious level, impaired upgaze, and neuropsychological disturbance with amnesia and mood disturbances. Bilateral thalamic infarction, which may occur acutely as a result of occlusion of a single trunk supplying both thalami, can cause subcortical dementia with impaired attention, apathy and poor motivation, in addition to amnesia. Memory loss can also occur from associated bilateral infarction

of the medial temporal lobes, which are often supplied by the PCAs (Figure 4.13).

The thalamo-geniculate perforating arteries arise from the more distal PCA and supply the ventrolateral thalamus in addition to the posterior limb of the internal capsule and the optic radiation. Ischaemia in the territory of the thalamo-geniculate arteries may result in the lacunar syndrome of a pure sensory stroke (see below). More extensive infarction may result in sensorimotor stroke. Involvement of the contralateral ventrolateral nucleus results in hemi-ataxia due to interruption of fibres in the dentatorubrothalamic pathway. Involvement of the optic radiation results in hemianopia or a quadrantanopia. Hemiballismus or hemi-chorea results from involvement of the upper brainstem. Although the sensory disturbance may frequently recover well, it may then be followed by development of Dejerine–Roussy syndrome, in which the initial sensory loss is replaced by paraesthesia and sometimes excruciatingly severe pain when the affected limb is touched, or even continuous pain (post-stroke pain or thalamic pain).

LACUNAR INFARCTS AND SYNDROMES

Occlusion of a single perforating artery results in a small focal area of infarction known as a *lacune*. This term was first coined to describe the pathological appearance of very small regions of infarction only a few millimetres across (Fisher, 1982). More recently, radiologists have defined lacunes on computed tomography (CT) or magnetic resonance imaging (MRI) as any small infarcts up to 1.5 cm in diameter. Some authorities prefer to use the term 'small deep infarct' to describe the radiological appearance, in order to include any small subcortical infarcts. The smallest lacunes are not detectable using current imaging techniques. The clinical consequences of a lacune depend upon its location, and if they occur at certain strategic locations (e.g. the internal capsule; Figure 4.10), a small region of lacunar infarction may result in a severe clinical deficit. Many lacunar infarcts are asymptomatic, but if they are symptomatic then the neurological deficit results from disruption of white matter tracts, most commonly involving hemiparesis or hemisensory loss without evidence of cortical dysfunction. The initial description of lacunar syndromes was prior to the advent of CT and relied on careful clinico-pathological correlation (Fisher, 1998). *In vivo* clinicoradiological correlation became possible with the advent of CT, but frequently lacunar infarcts are not visible on CT. The advent of MRI has greatly improved the detection of small lacunar infarcts and has allowed the identification of a large number of rarer lacunar syndromes. However, the majority of neurological defects caused by lacunar infarcts fall into one of four classical lacunar syndromes (Table 4.2). These are common and have characteristic clinical presentations that enable the diagnosis of lacunar syndrome to be made at the bedside. This has considerable utility in clinical practice because the underlying cause is usually lacunar infarction caused by small-vessel disease arising from hypertension or diabetes, and because lacunar stroke has a low mortality (Landi *et al.*, 1992). However, the diagnosis requires confirmation by imaging

Table 4.2 Common lacunar syndromes

- Pure motor stroke
- Pure sensory stroke
- Sensory motor stroke
- Ataxic hemiparesis/Dysarthria clumsy-hand syndrome

and investigation of other causes, because a small proportion of patients presenting with lacunar syndromes turn out to have large subcortical infarcts or localized cortical infarction of embolic or haemodynamic origin (Waterston *et al.*, 1990; Baumgartner *et al.*, 2003).

Pure motor stroke

This is the most common lacunar syndrome. In the classical syndrome, patients present with weakness of the face, arm and leg, without cortical signs, aphasia, hemianopia or disturbance of brainstem function. It is important to take a history of symptoms at the onset of the ischaemic event, as frequently patients will be seen some time following the event. If the event presents, for example, with an aphasia and right-sided hemiparesis, but by the time the patient is seen the deficit is merely a hemiparesis, the syndrome is not a lacunar syndrome and is likely to be caused by ischaemia in a larger region of the brain. The term 'pure motor stroke' has been extended to include patients who have weakness affecting only the face and arm, or the arm and leg. Such cases are best referred to as partial lacunar syndromes, but the majority are likely to be accounted for by ischaemia in the territory of the perforating arteries. In such cases, weakness should affect the whole of the face and arm or the whole of the arm and leg. Weakness affecting only one of these regions (e.g. just the arm) is more likely to be due to ischaemia in the cortex or to a peripheral nerve lesion. Particularly with the advent of MRI, cases of pure motor stroke have been reported with infarcts at multiple sites along the pyramidal tract, including the internal capsule, the coronal radiata, the cerebral peduncle, the pons and the medulla (Figure 4.14). However, the most common location appears to be the internal capsule. In cases of partial lacunar syndrome, infarcts occur more commonly in the corona radiata or the border between it and the internal capsule, where the corticospinal tract fibres are relatively more dispersed. Hemiparesis caused by lacunar infarction is more likely to progress over the first days after onset than other mechanisms of cerebral infarction, for reasons that are not clear (Steinke and Ley, 2002).

Pure sensory stroke

This presents with sensory loss affecting the face, arm and leg. It is much less common than pure motor stroke. It is believed to result most commonly from infarcts in the thalamus. Partial pure sensory strokes can occur in a similar fashion to partial pure motor syndromes.

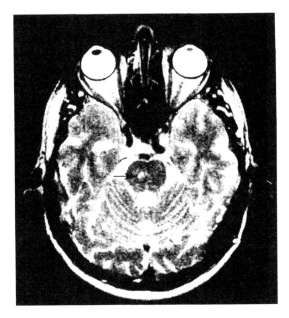

Figure 4.14 Lacunar infarct in the posterior circulation on the left side of the pons (arrow).

Sensorimotor stroke

This term describes hemiparesis and ipsilateral sensory loss without other features. In most studies, it is the second most common type of lacunar syndrome after pure motor stroke. The underlying lesion has been reported most commonly in the posterior limb of the internal capsule or in the corona radiata, and less commonly in the genu of the internal capsule or the anterior limb of the internal capsule and in the thalamus. In neuroimaging studies, infarcts in patients with sensorimotor stroke tend to be larger than those in patients with the other lacunar syndromes, although they still occur in a single perforating artery territory.

Ataxic hemiparesis and dysarthria clumsy-hand syndrome

These syndromes consists of hemiparesis and ipsilateral ataxia. The relevant lacunar infarct occurs most commonly in the basis pontis or the posterior limb of the internal capsule. Therefore limb ataxia in such patients does not necessarily imply a cerebellar or brainstem lesion. Dysarthria clumsy-hand syndrome is a variant in which the patient presents with dysarthria and clumsiness of one hand without severe weakness.

Other lacunar presentations

Lacunar infarcts in the basal ganglia may result in a unilateral movement disorder, including hemichorea and hemiballismus. Patients with multiple lacunar infarcts, who frequently also have more diffuse white matter changes, referred to as leukoaraiosis on neuroimaging, may present with dementia with a subcortical pattern of cognitive impairment, a small stepped gait apraxia, pseudobulbar palsy, or a parkinsonian syndrome with bradykinesia and rigidity (Chapter 6).

KEY REFERENCES

Anatomy of the cerebral circulation

Damasio H. A computed tomographic guide to the identification of cerebral vascular territories. *Arch Neurol* 1983;**40**:138–142

Middle cerebral artery territory infarction

Portera-Cailliau C, Doherty CP, Buonanno FS et al. Middle cerebral artery territory infarction sparing the precentral gyrus: report of three cases. *J Neurol Neurosurg Psychiatry* 2003;**74**:510–512

Striatocapsular infarction

Donnan GA, Bladin PF, Berkovic SF et al. The stroke syndrome of striatocapsular infarction. *Brain* 1991;**114**:51–70

Border-zone infarction

Del Sette M, Eliasziw M, Streifler JY et al. Internal borderzone infarction: a marker for severe stenosis in patients with symptomatic internal carotid artery disease. For the North American Symptomatic Carotid Endarterectomy (NASCET) Group. *Stroke* 2000;**31**:631–636

Gandolfo C, Del Sette M, Fincocchi C et al. Internal borderzone infarction in patients with ischemic stroke. *Cerebrovasc Dis* 1998;**8**:255–258

Mounier-Vehier F, Degaey I, Leclerc X et al. Cerebellar border zone infarcts are often associated with presumed cardiac sources of ischaemic stroke. *J Neurol Neurosurg Psychiatry* 1995;**59**:87–89

Vertebrobasilar artery infarction

Brandt T, Steinke W, Thie A et al. Posterior cerebral artery territory infarcts: clinical features, infarct topography, causes and outcome. Multicenter results: a review of the literature. *Cerebrovasc Dis* 2000;**10**:170–182

Caplan LR. Vertebrobasilar disease. *Adv Neurol* 2003; **92**:131–140

Chaves CJ, Caplan LR, Chung CS et al. Cerebellar infarcts in the New England Medical Center Posterior Circulation Registry. *Neurology* 1994; **44**:1385–1390

Glass TA, Hennessey PM, Pazdera L et al. Outcome at 30 days in the New England Medical Center Posterior Circulation Registry. *Arch Neurol* 2002; **59**:359–360

Voetsch B, DeWitt, LD, Pessin MS, Caplan LR. Basilar artery occlusive disease in the New England Medical Center Posterior Circulation Registry. *Arch Neurol* 2004;**61**:496–504

Wityk RJ, Chang HM, Rosengart A et al. Proximal extracranial vertebral artery disease in the New England Medical Center Posterior Circulation Registry. *Arch Neurol* 1998;**55**:470–8

Lacunar infarction

Baumgartner RW, Sidler C, Mosso M et al. Ischemic lacunar stroke in patients with and without potential mechanism other than small-artery disease. *Stroke* 2003;**34**:653–659

Fisher CM. Lacunar strokes and infarcts: a review. *Neurology* 1982;**32**:871–876

Fisher CM. Lacunes: small, deep cerebral infarcts. *Neurology* 1998;**50**:841–852

Landi G, Cella E, Boccardi E et al. Lacunar versus non-lacunar infarcts: pathogenetic and prognostic differences. *J Neurol Neurosurg Psychiatry* 1992;**55**:441–445

Steinke W, Ley SC. Lacunar stroke is the major cause of progressive motor deficits. *Stroke* 2002;**33**: 1510–1516

Waterston JA, Brown MM, Butler P et al. Small deep cerebral infarcts associated with occlusive internal carotid artery disease. A hemodynamic phenomenon? *Arch Neurol* 1990;**47**:953–957

CHAPTER 5

Epidemiology

About one in six people will have a stroke at some time in their life in industrialized countries. Of these, about a third die of their stroke and another third survive but remain disabled. Stroke is therefore responsible for a great burden of disability in the community (Wolfe, 2000). Small reductions in stroke incidence can have great population benefits. Epidemiological studies have allowed identification of a large number of risk factors of varying importance, many of which could be modified by lifestyle alterations or specific pharmacological treatment (Bonita, 1992).

DEFINITION OF STROKE

A uniform definition of stroke is vital for epidemiological studies. Most have used the World Health Organization (WHO) definition of stroke: 'rapidly developing clinical signs of focal (or global) disturbance of cerebral function, with symptoms lasting 24 hours or longer, or leading to death, with no apparent cause other than of vascular origin'. It should be noted that this definition includes ischaemic stroke, intracerebral haemorrhage and subarachnoid haemorrhage. However, it excludes transient ischaemic attacks (TIAs), subdural haematoma, and haemorrhage or infarction secondary to tumour or infection. It does not include differentiation of stroke into haemorrhage or infarction, let alone more detailed individual stroke subtypes – which is a serious deficiency of many studies using this definition.

STROKE INCIDENCE

Fatal stroke

Stroke accounts for 10–12% of all deaths in industrialized countries. About 88% of the deaths attributed to stroke are among people over 65 years of age. This age-related increase is seen in population studies (Figure 5.1). There is a marked variation in stroke mortality rates in both men and women in different parts of the world, with the highest-rate countries having a mortality about five times greater than the lowest-rate countries. Standardized mortality stroke rates per 100 000 population from WHO statistics are shown in Figure 5.2. Stroke is an increasing problem in the developing world, as much as in the more industrialized countries. The Global Burden of Disease Study showed that stroke is the third commonest global cause of death. In 1995, worldwide, there were 4.4 million deaths per year from cerebrovascular disease, which was third only to ischaemic heart disease (6.3 million) and malignant neoplasms (6.0 million) (Murray and Lopez, 1997).

Death rates from stroke and ischaemic heart disease have fallen markedly in most industrialized countries over the last few decades. This fall has not been uniform. As an example, the rate in Japan has fallen dramatically from a very high level to a level similar to that seen in other westernised countries (Figure 5.3). In contrast, stroke rates in some Eastern European countries have increased over the same period. In most populations, similar reductions or

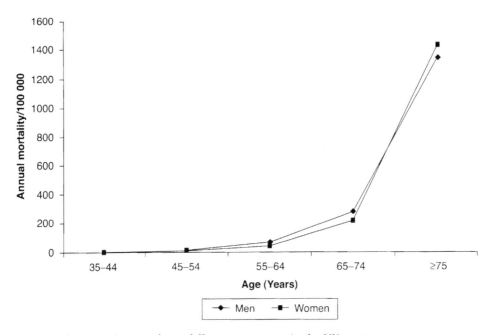

Figure 5.1   Mortality rates from stroke in different age groups in the UK, 1992.

increases have been seen in both men and women. Changes in age-standardized mortality rates from stroke in men and women between 1960–1964 and 1985–89 are shown in Figure 5.4. It is uncertain whether the reduction in stroke mortality seen in many populations is due to a decline in incidence or a lower case fatality. Variability in the accuracy of death certification may also play a part (Corwin et al., 1982). However, when community stroke registers have been specifically set up, as in the WHO MONICA Project, the evidence suggests that for the purposes of international comparisons, there is good agreement between mortality rates from official statistics and stroke incidence registers (Thorvaldson et al., 1995). In this study, case fatality rates (defined as the proportion of strokes that are fatal within 28 days of onset) averaged about 30%, although they ranged from the lowest rates of around 15% in the Nordic countries to the highest rates of 50% in Eastern European populations. However, although the standardized mortality rates (corrected for age) may be declining, the burden of stroke in the population as a whole is increasing because the proportion of elderly individuals is growing throughout the world.

Stroke incidence

Evaluation of the incidence of stroke in a given population requires the use of a standard WHO definition and prospective ascertainment of cases using comprehensive case-finding methods to identify non-fatal cases treated both in hospital and out of hospital, as well as patients who have died very shortly after the acute stroke event (Bamford et al., 1990). Few studies meet these criteria, but data from four studies which do are summarized in Figure 5.5. Such studies show that stroke incidence rises exponentially with age (Hollander et al., 2003). From these data, the cumulative incidence of stroke (i.e. the lifetime risk of having a stroke) can be calculated by means of life tables from age-specific incidence data. For example, in Table 5.1, the cumulative probability that a 45-year-old person will suffer a stroke by a certain age has been calculated from data based on New Zealand epidemiological studies. Although the risk of stroke is higher in men

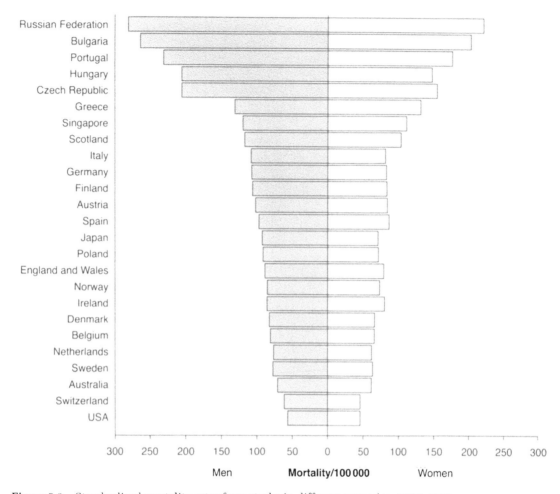

Figure 5.2 Standardized mortality rates from stroke in different countries, 1990–1992.

than in women, more women in total die as a result of stroke, because of their greater life-expectancy. Typically, first-ever strokes account for about 75% of all acute stroke.

Although a large number of studies have shown a reduction in stroke mortality over recent decades, this could be due to lower incidence or increased survival. Performing ideal epidemiological studies on stroke incidence is time-consuming, and very few 'ideal' stroke incidence studies have been repeated, or continued for long enough, to provide reliable information about changes in stroke incidence over time. Serial studies from Rochester, Minnesota, demonstrated that stroke incidence declined markedly during the 1950s and 1960s, but then increased. This later increase may represent increased case ascertainment as a result of computed tomography (CT) scanning and diagnosis of more minor strokes. In contrast, studies in Japan suggest that stroke incidence may be falling, while repeated studies using similar protocols and the same investigators in Auckland, New Zealand suggest they have not altered significantly. Further data from Soderhamn, Sweden and from Denmark suggest that stroke incidence may even be rising. In Oxfordshire, England, the age-specific incidence of major stroke has declined by over 40% in the last 20 years, while the incidence

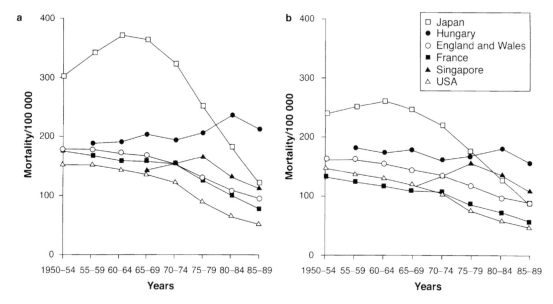

Figure 5.3   Change in age-standardized mortality rates from stroke in different countries over time from 1954 to 1989 in (a) men and (b) women.

of minor stroke has stayed much the same, without any change in case fatality (Rothwell *et al.*, 2004). It is therefore difficult to draw firm conclusions because of the paucity of data and potential inaccuracies of incidence data based on mortality or obtained from studies of non-fatal stroke. Even in large epidemiological studies, relatively few stroke events may result in wide confidence intervals for estimates of stroke incidence. It is also likely that changes in lifestyle or other factors will affect different causes of stroke in different ways, but it is only recently that epidemiological studies have taken stroke subtypes into account (Kolominsky-Rabas *et al.*, 2001). Some of the variability in mortality may reflect variations in stroke management (Wolfe *et al.*, 2000).

RISK FACTORS

Much of the information on stroke risk factors has been obtained from case–control studies. These may allow more detailed evaluation of individual stroke patients and differentiation between stroke subtypes, but are subject to potential bias in both patient and control case

selection. Such biases are less of a problem in prospective population studies. However, in the latter, the diagnosis of stroke is frequently based upon death certification or family doctor records, which may be less reliable and often fail to differentiate between ischaemic and haemorrhagic stroke. In addition, the number of strokes during the period of follow-up may be small, even in large prospective studies.

Strength of association and attributable risk

A risk factor for stroke is a characteristic of an individual indicating that he or she has an increased risk of stroke compared with an individual without that characteristic. Such an association does not necessarily imply causality. Determining causality depends upon a number of factors, including the strength of the association, its consistency over different studies and populations, its independence from confounding factors, a temporal sequence between risk factor and stroke, the presence of biological and epidemiological

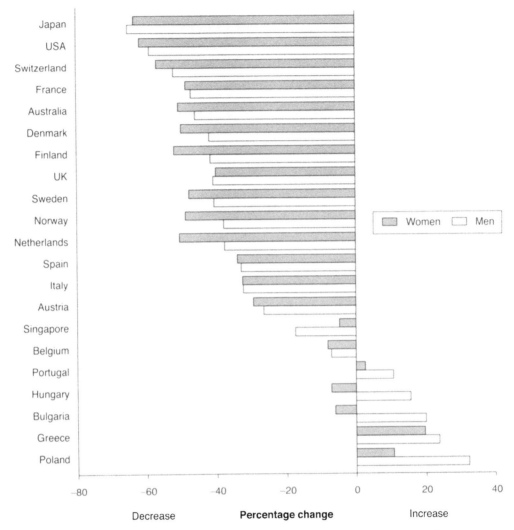

Figure 5.4 Changes in age-standardized mortality rates from stroke in different countries between 1960–1964 and 1985–1989.

plausibility, and the demonstration that removal or reduction of that risk factor reduces stroke risk.

The strength of an association between a risk factor and stroke can be expressed either as a relative risk or as an odds ratio. The relative risk describes the increase in the frequency of stroke in a population with that risk factor, compared with the frequency of stroke in a matched population without that same risk factor, in terms of multiplication of risk (Table 5.2). When the incidence of stroke in a given population is unknown, but information is available about the proportion of patients with and without the risk factor in patients with stroke, an odds ratio can be calculated as an expression of the strength of association (Table 5.3). Examples of the increase in risk associated with the commoner risk factors for stroke are given in Table 5.4.

The importance of any risk factor on a population basis will depend both upon its relative risk and upon the prevalence of that risk factor

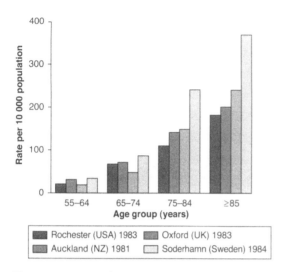

Figure 5.5   Annual incidence of stroke in different age groups in specific studies. Adapted from Bonita R. *Lancet* 1992;339:342.

Table 5.1   Cumulative probability (%) of a 45-year-old person having a stroke before the specified age in years

Age	Men	Women
65	3	3
75	10	6
85	24	18
90	33	28

in the population. Population risk can be indicated using the concept of attributable or absolute risk. The dependence of absolute or attributable risk upon the population prevalence of the risk factor can be illustrated with hypertension. For example, elevation of systolic blood pressure to greater than 180 mmHg confirms a greatly increased relative risk of stroke, which is much greater that the relative risk of stroke due to a blood pressure in the range 160–180 mmHg. However, such marked elevations of blood pressure are rare, while more modest elevations are much more common. Therefore the population-attributable risk associated with a blood pressure elevation in the range 160–180 mmHg is greater than that due to blood pressure elevation above 180 mmHg.

The most reliable identification of stroke risk factors comes from prospective cohort studies, (e.g. the Framingham Study). However, in most of these studies, there has been little or no division of stroke into cerebral haemorrhage and cerebral ischaemia, let alone any division of cerebral ischaemia into its different pathogenic subtypes. Most of these studies primarily tell us the risk factors for infarction rather than haemorrhage, because most strokes are due to infarction. Similarly,

because a large number of ischaemic strokes are related to the complications of atherosclerosis (e.g. carotid artery stenosis, embolism secondary to myocardial infarction, and atrial fibrillation secondary to coronary heart disease), these studies have similar risk factor profiles to those of coronary heart disease. However, there are some differences, particularly with regard to the importance of different risk factors for coronary heart disease and stroke.

Case–control studies allow much more detailed evaluation of each individual stroke in a standardized fashion. More recent studies have included imaging and can therefore allow differentiation between different stroke subtypes. Case–control studies are subject to potential bias, in both patient and control case selections. Nevertheless, they may provide useful information, particularly on relationships with particular stroke subtypes, for example suggesting that the risk factors for different types of stroke may vary. Imaging techniques (e.g. carotid duplex ultrasound) have allowed associations to be determined between individual components of the pathological process (e.g. carotid atherosclerosis) and risk factors on a population basis.

Well-recognized risk factors for stroke are listed in Table 5.5. It is convenient to divide these into risk factors that the individual is unable to influence (unmodifiable risk factors) and those that can be altered or treated to reduce risk (modifiable risk factors). Although risk factors may predict an increased incidence of first stroke for the population as a whole, they are not particularly useful at predicting stroke recurrence within the population of patients who have already had a stroke (Hillen

Table 5.2 Formula for calculating relative risk

Calculation of relative risk requires the risk of a particular risk factor (e.g. smoking) to be known. For example, in a cohort study, a group of subjects with and without the risk may be followed-up for a length of time and the number developing an outcome event (e.g. stroke) determined. If the numbers of patients developing a stroke during follow-up are as follows:

	Number with outcome during follow-up	*Number without outcome during follow-up*
Risk factor positive	a	b
Risk factor negative	c	d

- The risk of an outcome in those with the risk factor (A) is

$$\frac{a}{a+b}$$

- The risk of an outcome in those without the risk factor (C) is

$$\frac{c}{c+d}$$

- And the relative risk is

$$\frac{A}{C} = \frac{ac+ad}{ac+bc}$$

Table 5.3 Formula for calculating odds ratio

In a case–control study, the population risk is not known and hence the relative risk cannot be calculated. Instead, the proportion of patients with a particular risk factor (e.g. smoking) in a group of patients with an outcome event (e.g. stroke) is compared with the proportion of subjects in a matched control group with that risk factor using an odds ratio calculation. When the absolute risk of stroke is small, the odds ratio will be very similar to the relative risk. If the numbers of patients and controls with and without the risk factor are as follows:

	Patient group with stroke	*Control group without stroke*
Risk factor positive	a	b
Risk factor negative	c	d

- The odds of being exposed to the risk factor in cases (A) is

$$\frac{a}{c}$$

- The odds of being exposed to the risk factor in controls (C) is

$$\frac{b}{d}$$

- And the odds ratio is

$$\frac{A}{C} = \frac{ad}{bc}$$

et al., 2003). On the other hand, treatment of modifiable risk factors can be expected to reduce the risk of stroke both in the population as a whole and within individuals who have already had a stroke.

UNMODIFIABLE RISK FACTORS

Age

Increasing age is the strongest risk factor for cerebral infarction and primary intracerebral

Table 5.4   Relative risks associated with some of the major risk factors for stroke (the estimates of relative risk given are representative figures derived from different studies of each risk factor)

Risk factor	Relative increase in risk of stroke
Increasing age (55–64 versus >75 years)	5
Hypertension (160/95 versus 120/80)	7
Smoking (current status)	2
Diabetes mellitus	2
Social class (I versus V)	1.6
Ischaemic heart disease	3
Heart failure	5
Atrial fibrillation	5
Past transient ischaemic attack	5
Physical activity (little or none versus some)	2.5

Table 5.5   Risk factors for stroke

Unmodifiable risk factors
Age
Gender
Genetic factors
Ethnicity

Major modifiable risk factors
Alcohol
Aortic atherosclerosis
Atrial fibrillation
Carotid stenosis
Diabetes mellitus
Hyperlipidaemia
Hypertension
Ischaemic heart disease
Peripheral arterial disease
Physical activity
Prior stroke
Smoking
Socioeconomic conditions
Transient ischaemic attack

Minor modifiable risk factors
Diet
Fibrinogen
Homocysteine
Infection
Migraine
Obesity
Oral contraceptives
Snoring and sleep apnoea

haemorrhage. For example, the risk of stroke in people aged 75–84 years (14.3 per 1000 per annum) is 25 times the risk in people aged 45–54 (0.57 per 1000 per annum). This increase in risk is seen across different populations.

Gender

Male gender increases the risk of stroke at a given age, but, overall, more women will suffer stroke during their lifetime because of their greater life-expectancy and the greater importance of age as a risk factor (Di Carlo *et al.*, 2003). The excess risk seen in men is less than that seen in ischaemic heart disease and is much less marked in younger age groups. Women with stroke have different risk factor profiles and may be treated differently to men (Holroyd-Leduc *et al.*, 2000). This makes it uncertain whether differences between the genders in the incidence or outcome of stroke are genetic.

Genetic factors

Evidence from twin and family studies suggests that genetic factors contribute to the risk of stroke although the degree of risk is uncertain (Rastenyte *et al.*, 1998; Markus, 2004). Stroke and TIA were associated in the ongoing prospective Framingham Offspring Study with a parental history of coronary heart disease (relative risk 3.33), and a verified history of paternal (relative risk 2.4) or maternal (relative risk 1.4) stroke or TIA (Kiely *et al.*, 1993). In a prospective study from Finland, a parental history of stroke in either the father or mother predicted the risk of stroke independently from other risk factors (Jousilahti *et al.*, 1997). In the multivariate analysis, the risk associated with a positive parental history of stroke was 1.9 in men and 1.8 in women. In analysis by stroke subtype, the respective risk ratios for men and women were 1.5 and 1.8, respectively, for ischaemic stroke, 5.0 and 2.8 for subarachnoid haemorrhage, and 3.9 and 0.8 for intracerebral haemorrhage. The association between parental history of stroke and risk of stroke was stronger among subjects aged 25–49 years than among those aged 50–64 years. In addition, a number of case–control studies have found an increased frequency of family history of both stroke and ischaemic heart disease in the parents of individuals with stroke compared with control groups (Markus, 2004). The extent to which this association can be explained by inheritance of known cardiovascular risk factors varies in different studies. Many of the major cardiovascular risk factors (e.g. hypertension and diabetes) are themselves partly caused by genetic factors. Genetic predisposition to stroke may therefore occur directly through inheritance of such factors, independently by inheritance of currently unrecognized predisposing risk, or by inheritance of genetic factors that modulate the effect of known risk factors or increase susceptibility to known risk factors.

Twin studies in which the concordance rates between monozygotic and dizygotic twins are compared are a more robust method of estimating the heritability of a trait or disorder. One study found that the probandwise concordance rate of stroke for monozygotic twins was 17.7% while that for dizygotic twins was 3.6% (Brass *et al.*, 1992). However, there were few twin pairs with stroke in the study and therefore the confidence intervals were wide. Further studies are needed in this area.

Family history is a more important risk factor for subarachnoid haemorrhage than other types of stroke. One study found a relative risk of subarachnoid haemorrhage of 6.6 in first-degree relatives compared with second-degree relatives. The incidence in second-degree relatives was similar to that in the general population (Bromberg *et al.*, 1995). A number of studies have investigated the incidence of intracerebral aneurysms in the first-degree relatives of patients with subarachnoid haemorrhage. While in some families there are multiple members with aneurysms, in the majority of cases only one individual has had an aneurysm. The risk of aneurysm in a second sib is relatively small.

The marked differences in the rate of stroke between areas with a similar gene pool (e.g. Eastern and Western Europe) suggest that potentially modifiable environmental factors might be more important than genetic differences in determining stroke susceptibility. The results of migrant studies support this view. Japanese populations in the USA experience rates of stroke that are closer to those of American White populations than to those of Japanese populations in Japan. However, it is likely that there are complex interactions between genetic and environmental influences, and that many environmental influences will only increase the risk of stroke in those with pre-existing genetic susceptibility.

A number of relatively small studies have examined the relationship between polymorphisms or mutations in cardiovascular candidate genes and stroke. Associations have been suggested with a number of gene polymorphisms in the angiotensin-converting enzyme (ACE) gene, the factor V Leiden polymorphism, apolipoprotein E, and genes controlling homocysteine metabolism, including a polymorphism in the gene methylene tetrahydrofolate reductase (MTHFR). However, the results from different studies looking at these polymorphisms have been inconsistent. The disappointing results from candidate gene studies are likely to reflect small sample sizes and poor methodology. Guidelines for future stroke studies have been published (Dichgans and Markus, 2005) and large multicentre collaborations have been established to collect stroke DNA databases. Linkage analysis of Icelandic stroke patients identified a gene, encoding phosphodiesterase 4D, which appeared to be responsible in the Icelandic population for an approximately threefold increase in the relative risk of carotid and cardioembolic stroke (Gretarsdottir *et al.*, 2003). However, the same gene does not confer a major risk for stroke in two European populations studied (Bevan *et al.*, 2005). Further large population-based studies are required in this area before firm conclusions can be drawn (Hassan and Markus, 2005).

The above paragraphs have considered genetic influences that may affect the risk of stroke on a population basis. In addition, there are a number of rare genetic causes of familial stroke, which are inherited as either an autosomal dominant or autosomal recessive condition, or via mitochondrial DNA (Table 5.6). These are described in more detail in later chapters.

Ethnicity

There is an increased incidence of stroke in Afro-Caribbeans compared with Caucasians in both North American and Europe and this probably applies to both ischaemic stroke and intracranial haemorrhage (Wolf *et al.*, 2002). In the UK, Asian populations have a higher stroke mortality than Caucasians, which may be due partly to an increased incidence of central obesity, insulin resistance and diabetes mellitus. It has been suggested that the pattern of ischaemic stroke differs between the ethnic groups, with there being less extracranial, but more intracranial, atheroma in Afro-Caribbean and Asian compared with Caucasian populations. Intracerebral haemorrhage also appears to be more common in Asian populations. The extent to which these differences are genetic or the result of social and environmental differences are uncertain (Hajat *et al.*, 2001).

MAJOR MODIFIABLE RISK FACTORS

Alcohol

There is increasing evidence that mild and moderate alcohol consumption protects against both

Table 5.6 Genetic causes of familial stroke

Ischaemic stroke
- CADASIL syndrome
- MELAS syndrome
- Sickle cell disease
- Protein C deficiency
- Protein S deficiency
- Antithrombin III deficiency
- Familial hypercholesterolaemia
- Fabry's disease
- Homocystinuria

Intracerebral haemorrhage
- Cerebral amyloid angiopathy
- Hereditary arteriovenous malformations
- Hereditary haemorrhagic telangiectasia
- Haemophilia and other coagulation factor deficiencies

Subarachnoid haemorrhage
- Ehlers–Danlos syndrome
- Pseudoxanthoma elasticum
- Marfan's syndrome
- Polycystic kidney disease
- Other collagen deficiencies

ischaemic heart disease and ischaemic stroke (Djousse *et al.*, 2002; Reynolds *et al.*, 2003). However, heavy alcohol consumption is a risk factor for stroke, with a U-shaped curve best describing the relationship. The effect of alcohol may be mediated by effects on blood pressure. High alcohol levels may promote stroke by a number of other mechanisms, including induction of haemorrhage, atrial fibrillation or myocardial damage secondary to cardiomyopathy. The relationship between alcohol and stroke is described in more detail in Chapter 11.

Aortic atherosclerosis

Atherosclerosis in the arch of the aorta is increasingly recognized as an important source of thromboembolism to the brain (Amarenco *et al.*, 1994; Agmon *et al.*, 2002). It is not easily detected by routine examination or investigations, but can be seen on transoesophageal echocardiography. The proportion of stroke caused by aortic atherosclerosis is uncertain (Mendel *et al.*, 2002).

Atrial fibrillation

Non-rheumatic and rheumatic atrial fibrillation are both important risk factors for stroke (Mattle, 2003; Penado *et al.*, 2003). Atrial fibrillation accounts for about 12% of all stroke, and becomes increasingly common with advancing age. Above the age of 80, about a quarter of all strokes are attributable to atrial fibrillation. In some cases, the association may be coincidental because atrial fibrillation is also caused by ischaemic heart disease and hypertension, which themselves are both risk factors for stroke. However, the finding that there is an approximately 60% reduction in stroke risk following anticoagulation in patients with non-valvular atrial fibrillation suggests that the majority of strokes associated with atrial fibrillation are the result of cardiac embolism.

Carotid stenosis

Carotid bruit and asymptomatic carotid artery stenosis secondary to atherosclerosis demonstrated ultrasonically are both risk factors for stroke. The risk of ipsilateral stroke associated with asymptomatic carotid stenosis is not as high as might be expected, at about 2% per annum (Nadareishvili *et al.*, 2002; Halliday *et al.*, 2004). However, in the presence of recent ipsilateral symptoms, the risk of recurrent stroke associated with severe carotid stenosis rises to as high as 10–15% per annum (Rothwell *et al.*, 2003) (Chapter 15).

Diabetes mellitus

Diabetes is associated with an increase in the risk of stroke to approximately between 2 and 2.5 times that of a non-diabetic person (Jorgensen *et al.*, 1994). It has also been demonstrated to be a risk factor for carotid atherosclerosis. There is also an association between diabetes and hypertension that adds to the increase in risk. Some studies, based on stroke mortality, have led to an overestimation

of the strength of any association between diabetes and all stroke because stroke is more likely to be fatal in diabetic patients (Mergherbi *et al.*, 2003).

Hyperlipidaemia

Increased total cholesterol and low-density lipoprotein (LDL) cholesterol are strong risk factors for ischaemic heart disease, while high levels of high-density lipoprotein (HDL) cholesterol appear to be protective. The relationship to stroke in epidemiological studies following-up patients with different levels of cholesterol appears to be weaker. A meta-analysis involving 13 000 strokes in 450 000 people in 45 prospective cohorts found that, after standardization for age and the presence of ischaemic heart disease, there was no association between blood cholesterol and stroke except in those under 45 years of age at the time of screening (Prospective Studies Collaboration, 1995). However, because the subtypes of strokes were not available in most studies, the lack of any overall relationship might conceal a positive association with ischaemic stroke together with a negative association with haemorrhagic stroke. Supporting this view, a number of case–control studies have found an association between raised cholesterol and ischaemic stroke. More importantly, trials of various statins in patients with ischaemic heart disease have shown a significant reduction in stroke incidence in association with lowering cholesterol.

One of the largest trials of cholesterol-lowering therapy, the Heart Protection Study (HPS), included 1820 patients with cerebrovascular disease without prior coronary heart disease, among the total of 20 536 high-risk patients randomized with a history of ischaemic heart disease, other arterial occlusive disease or diabetes, between simvastatin and placebo (Heart Protection Study Collaborative Group, 2002). The patients were not required to have a high cholesterol, so long as it was above 3.5 mmol/l (135 mg/100 ml). Allocation to active treatment with simvastatin, 40 mg daily, was associated with an average reduction in cholesterol values over 5 years of treatment of 1.2 mmol/l (46 mg/100 ml) and a highly significant reduction in stroke incidence over 5 years of follow-up from 5.7% in controls down to 4.3% in those allocated treatment. The effect was primarily on ischaemic stroke, with little effect on the rate of cerebral haemorrhage. The results of several other trials of statin therapy recruiting only patients presenting with TIA or stroke are awaited. The role of plasma triglyceride as a predictive factor in ischaemic stroke is unclear.

Hypertension

Increasing blood pressure is a major risk factor for stroke (Collins and MacMahon, 1994). It is strongly and independently associated with both ischaemic and haemorrhagic stroke. The relationship between diastolic blood pressure and subsequent stroke is log–linear throughout the normal range, and there appears to be no threshold below which the stroke risk becomes stable – at least not over the normal range of blood pressures studied from 70 to 100 mmHg diastolic (MacMahon et al., 1990). The proportional increase in stroke risk associated with a given increase in blood pressure is similar in both sexes and almost doubles with each 7.5 mmHg increase in diastolic blood pressure (Figure 5.6). Recent evidence suggests that the relationship between stroke and systolic blood pressure is even stronger than that with diastolic blood pressure. In particular, 'isolated' systolic hypertension, with normal diastolic blood pressure, is associated with increased stroke risk, especially in the elderly (Vokonas et al., 1988). Approximately 40% of strokes can be attributed to a systolic blood pressure of more than 140 mmHg. The causal nature of the relationship is strongly supported by the results of randomized trials demonstrating that stroke can be prevented by lowering blood pressure with antihypertensive agents (Collins et al., 1990; Lawes et al., 2004). The reduction in stroke mirrors that predicted by epidemiological studies from the fall in blood pressure. However, few trials have

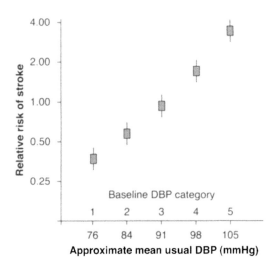

Figure 5.6 Relative risk of stroke related to usual diastolic blood pressure (DBP) in five categories estimated from remeasurements in the Framingham Study. From MacMahon S *et al.* Lancet 1990;**335**: 765–774.

shown a reduction in the risk of more than 40%, presumably because treatment rarely reduces blood pressure to normal values, there may be permanent damage to the blood vessels, and there are other non-hypertensive causes of stroke. In addition, treatment of hypertension appears to take some months to reduce the incidence of stroke and a few years for full benefit to be evident.

Hypertension appears to increase the risk of ischaemic stroke, by promoting both large-vessel atherogenesis and intracranial small-vessel disease. It has been shown to be strongly associated with carotid stenosis, carotid plaque and increased intima–media thickness demonstrated using carotid ultrasound.

Ischaemic heart disease

Atherosclerosis is a major cause of stroke and also causes ischaemic heart disease and peripheral arterial disease. These three symptomatic manifestations of atherosclerosis often coexist (Ness and Aronow, 1999). It is therefore not surprising that evidence of cardiovascular disease, particularly a history of myocardial infarction, is a risk factor for stroke (Wienbergen *et al.*, 2001; Lichtman *et al.*, 2002). Furthermore, some risk factors, particularly hypertension, are risk factors for cerebral infarction, cerebral haemorrhage and atheromatous disease, increasing the strength of such associations. An increased risk of stroke is therefore strongly associated with:

* symptoms of ischaemic heart disease
  – myocardial infarction
  – angina
* ECG abnormalities
* atrial fibrillation
* cardiac failure
* peripheral arterial disease
* aortic atherosclerosis

Peripheral arterial disease

Symptoms of peripheral arterial disease indicating significant atherosclerosis, such as claudication and/or evidence of a decrease in the ratio of blood pressure measured at the ankle compared with the arm (ankle–brachial index), are strong risk factors for stroke (Liu *et al.*, 2000; Tsai *et al.*, 2001).

Physical activity

A number of studies, both cohort and case–control, have demonstrated that lack of exercise is associated with an increased risk of stroke, while regular exercise is beneficial (Kiely *et al.*, 1994). Such an effect could act, at least in part, through reducing blood pressure.

Prior stroke

A history of previous stroke is one of the strongest predictors of further stroke (Jorgensen *et al.*, 1997; Hankey, 2003). The risk at other vascular events, particularly myocardial infarction and other symptoms associated with atherosclerosis (e.g. limb ischaemia), is also increased. For this reason,

trials of preventative treatment often choose the combination of recurrent stroke, myocardial infarction and vascular death as their primary outcome measure. The risk of recurrence is related to stroke subtype and is particularly high in the first few weeks after onset in patients with carotid artery stenosis (Lovett *et al.*, 2004).

Smoking

Cigarette smoking increases the risk of stroke to approximately double that of non-smokers (Wolf *et al.*, 1988). It appears to be important in both males and females and increases the risk at all ages. Studies have shown that it is a specific risk factor for ischaemic stroke and subarachnoid haemorrhage, as well as for all strokes. Epidemiological studies using non-invasive imaging of carotid atheroma and wall thickness by ultrasound have demonstrated that smoking is a strong independent risk factor for carotid atherosclerosis.

Socioeconomic conditions

There is a strong association between social class and other markers of socioeconomic status, and stroke risk (Hart *et al.*, 2000; Engstrom *et al.*, 2001). This is likely to act through a number of factors: smoking, poor diet and lack of exercise are all associated with low socioeconomic status and increased risk of stroke.

TIA

Not surprisingly, given that TIA has the same causes as stroke, a history of TIA is a major risk factor for stroke. It is important to recognize that the immediate risk after TIA is very high and TIAs are often followed by a completed stroke within hours or a day or two (Hill *et al.*, 2004). In a population-based study in Oxfordshire, England, the risks of recurrent stroke at 7 days, 1 month and 3 months after TIA were 8%, 12% and 17%, respectively (Coull *et al.*, 2003). The risks were almost identical in patients who had had a minor stroke. However, the long-term risk of stroke and other vascular events remains elevated indefinitely (Clark *et al.*, 2003). The risk of recurrence of stroke after TIA will depend on the presence of other risk factors. For example, when TIA is caused by carotid stenosis, the risk of recurrence is increased substantially.

MINOR MODIFIABLE RISK FACTORS

Diet

A large number of studies have demonstrated that increased salt intake is associated with increased blood pressure, although the strength of this association has been debated (Law, 1996). It has been estimated that a 100 mmol increase in sodium intake will increase blood pressure by 10 mmHg, leading to about a 34% increased risk of stroke.

It has been suggested that other dietary factors may increase or reduce stroke risk, but the evidence for this is less robust (Gariballa, 2000). A number of studies have suggested that higher vitamin C levels are associated with a lower risk of stroke. This may act through an antioxidant effect. The relationship with vitamin C may also explain the reports of a lower incidence of stroke associated with high fruit and vegetable intake. Folate may reduce stroke risk by reducing homocysteine concentration (see below).

Fibrinogen

There is a strong and consistent association between increased plasma fibrinogen and stroke (Bots *et al.*, 2002; Kofoed *et al.*, 2003). This relationship is partly confounded by smoking, which may partly increase stroke risk by raising fibrinogen levels. Fibrinogen levels are also affected by obesity, exercise, alcohol (negatively), diabetes, psychosocial factors, and inflammation and infection. It is not certain to what extent raised plasma fibrinogen is a causal factor for stroke or whether it is simply an indicator of other risk factors.

Homocysteine

Homocystinuria is an autosomal recessive condition in which very high levels of serum homocysteine are associated with an increased risk of stroke, particularly cerebral venous thrombosis, and arterial thrombosis at an early age. Increasing evidence suggests that moderately elevated levels of serum homocysteine within the normal range without homocystinuria are associated with stroke on a population basis (Kelly *et al.*, 2002). Such an association could act by promoting atherogenesis, promoting thrombosis or impairing endothelial function in small vessels (Sen *et al.*, 2002; Hassan *et al.*, 2004). Homocysteine levels are under both genetic and dietary control. A number of enzymes control homocysteine synthesis, including MTHFR. However, a number of recent studies have shown no association between a common polymorphism in the MTHFR gene and stroke risk, suggesting that poor diet may be responsible for the association between high homocysteine levels and stroke. Low vitamin B_{12} and, to a greater extent, low folate levels are associated with low homocysteine levels, and it has been demonstrated that folate supplementation reduces homocysteine levels. Trials are currently underway to determine whether folate supplementation will reduce stroke.

Infection

A number of case–control studies have shown an increased incidence of recent infection in cases of ischaemic stroke, as shown both by a history of recent respiratory tract or other infections and by serological testing (Bova *et al.*, 1996; Grau *et al.*, 1997). This association does not appear to be specific for any one type of organism or type of infection and may result from the effects of an inflammatory response leading to a prothrombotic state (Linsberg and Grau, 2003; Chamorro, 2004). This may partly account for the increased incidence of stroke seen in the winter months, although it is likely that lower ambient temperature also plays a part.

Migraine

See Chapter 11.

Obesity

The Whitehall Study showed that increased body mass index (BMI) was predictive of stroke in both smokers and non-smokers (Shinton *et al.*, 1991). Much of the association between BMI and stroke in studies is reduced when confounding variables (e.g. hypertension, diabetes, cigarette smoking and lack of exercise) are introduced into the analysis, suggesting that these contribute to the mechanisms through which obesity increases stroke risk. However, obesity remains an important predictor of stroke even after correction for other risk factors (Suk *et al.*, 2003; Tanne *et al.*, 2005).

Oral contraceptives

Case–control studies suggest that older high-dose oestrogen-containing oral contraceptives are associated with an increased risk of stroke, but the effect of current low-oestrogen-dose preparations is much less marked (Bousser and Kittner, 2000; Gillum *et al.*, 2000). This is discussed in more detail in Chapter 11.

Snoring and sleep apnoea

Both a history of snoring and evidence of sleep apnoea have been associated with an increased risk of stroke in control studies, but whether this relationship is cause-and-effect is uncertain (Yaggi and Mohsenin, 2004). The effect may be partly explained by an association of sleep apnoea with hypertension (Neau *et al.*, 2002). Whether treating sleep apnoea reduces stroke risk remains unknown.

OTHER RISK FACTORS

A large number of other risk factors have been associated with stroke, some of which are listed in Table 5.7.

Table 5.7 Additional possible risk factors for stroke

- Raised white blood cell count
- Large platelets
- Stress and type A behaviour
- Major life events
- Diagonal ear lobe crease
- Periodontal disease
- Blood group
- Serum uric acid
- Serum sialic acid
- Poor respiratory function
- Raised haematocrit
- High body iron stores

MULTIPLE RISK FACTORS

Epidemiological studies demonstrate that individual risk factors (e.g. the combination of smoking and hypertension) act independently to increase the risk of stroke (Wolf *et al.*, 1991). This means that the combined risk associated with more than one risk factor is calculated by multiplying each individual risk. Hence the combined effect is considerably greater than a simple additive effect. For example, if the individual relative increases in risk associated with smoking and hypertension are 2 and 7 times the normal population risk for a given age, an individual who has hypertension and also smokes will increase their risk of stroke by 14 times normal. If they also have diabetes, their risk will increase to 28 times normal. Obviously, such calculations are approximations, but can be helpful when advising patients about preventative measures.

PROGNOSIS OF STROKE

The outcome of a stroke depends on the underlying pathology and the size of the infarct or haemorrhage (Table 5.8). More patients with subarachnoid or intracerebral haemorrhage die within 30 days compared with patients with cerebral infarction, but patients who survive a haemorrhage have a slightly better outcome at 1 year (Bamford *et al.*, 1990). In all groups, 25–30%

Table 5.8   Prognosis of stroke[a]

	30-day fatality rate (%)	1-year fatality rate (%)	Survivors dependent on others at 1 year (%)
All strokes	19	31	35
All cerebral infarcts	10	23	35
Lacunar infarcts	1	10	34
Intracerebral haemorrhage	50	62	32
Subarachnoid haemorrhage	46	48	24

[a]Adapted from: Bamford J *et al. J Neurol Neurosurg Psychiatry* 1990;**53**:16–22 and Bamford J *et al. Stroke* 1987;**18**:545–551.

of patients remain significantly disabled and dependent on others. Patients with lacunar infarction have a better prognosis (Hankey, 2003). About 30% of patients with large cortical middle cerebral artery territory infarcts die within the first few days or weeks. Older age, coma at onset and persistent neglect predict a poor outcome.

KEY REFERENCES

General reviews

Bonita R. Epidemiology of stroke. *Lancet* 1992;**339**: 342–344

Wolfe CDA. The impact of stroke. *Br Med Bull* 2000; **56**:275–286

Incidence, prevalence and prognosis

Bamford J, Sandercock P, Dennis M et al. A prospective study of acute cerebrovascular disease in the community: the Oxfordshire community stroke project – 1981–1986. 2. Incidence, case fatality rates and overall outcome at one year of cerebral infarction, primary intracerebral and subarachnoid haemorrhage. *J Neurol Neurosurg Psychiatry* 1990;**53**:16–22

Corwin LT, Wolf PA, Kannal WP et al. Accuracy of death certification of stroke: the Framingham Study. *Stroke* 1982;**3**:8–18

Hillen T, Coshall C, Tilling K et al. Cause of stroke recurrence is multifactorial: patterns, risk factors, and outcomes of stroke recurrence in the South London Stroke Register. *Stroke* 2003;**34**: 1457–1463

Hollander M, Koudstaal PJ, Bots ML et al. Incidence, risk, and case fatality of first ever stroke in the elderly population. The Rotterdam Study. *J Neurol Neurosurg Psychiatry* 2003;**74**:317–321

Kolominsky-Rabas PL, Weber M, Gefeller O et al. Epidemiology of ischemic stroke subtypes according to TOAST criteria: incidence, recurrence, and long-term survival in ischemic stroke subtypes: a population-based study. *Stroke* 2001;**32**:2735–2740

Murray CJ, Lopez AD. Mortality by cause for eight regions of the world: Global Burden of Disease Study. *Lancet* 1997;**349**:1269–1276

Rothwell PM, Coull AJ, Giles MF et al. Change in stroke incidence, mortality, case-fatality, severity, and risk factors in Oxfordshire, UK from 1981 to 2004 (Oxford Vascular Study). *Lancet* 2004; **363**:1925–1933

Thorvaldson P, Asplund K, Kuulasmaa K et al. Stroke incidence, case fatality and mortality in the WHO MONICA Project. *Stroke* 1995;**26**:361–367

Wolfe CD, Giroud M, Kolominsky-Rabas P et al. Variations in stroke incidence and survival in 3 areas of Europe. European Registries of Stroke (EROS) Collaboration. *Stroke* 2000;**31**:2074–2079

Unmodifiable risk factors

Gender

Di Carlo A, Lamassa M, Baldereschi M et al. Sex differences in the clinical presentation, resource use, and 3-month outcome of acute stroke in Europe: data from a multicenter multinational hospital-based registry. *Stroke* 2003;**34**:1114–1119

Holroyd-Leduc JM, Kapral MK, Austine PC et al. Sex differences and similarities in the management and outcome of stroke patients. *Stroke* 2000;**31**: 1822–1827

Genetic factors

Bevan S, Porteous L, Sitzer M, Markus HS. Phosphodiesterase 4D gene, ischemic stroke, and asymptomatic carotid atherosclerosis. *Stroke* 2005;**36**:949–953

Brass LM, Isaacsohn JJ, Merikangas KR et al. A study of twins and stroke. *Stroke* 1992;**23**:221–223

Bromberg JG, Rinkel GJE, Algra A et al. Subarachnoid haemorrhage in first and second degree relatives of patients with subarachnoid haemorrhage. *BMJ* 1995;**311**:288–289

Dichgans M, Markus HS. Genetic association studies in stroke: methodological issues and proposed standard criteria. *Stroke* 2005;**36**:2027–2031

Gretarsdottir S, Thorleifsson G, Reynisdottir ST et al. The gene encoding phosphodiesterase 4D confers risk of ischemic stroke. *Nat Genet* 2003;**35**: 131–138

Hassan A, Markus HS. Practicalities of genetic studies in human stroke. *Meth Mol Med* 2005;**104**: 223–240

Jousilahti P, Rastenyte D, Tuomilento K et al. Parental history of cardiovascular disease and risk of stroke. A prospective follow-up of 14 371 middle-aged men and women in Finland. *Stroke* 1997;**28**:1361–1366

Kiely DK, Wolf PA, Cuppler LA et al. Familial aggregation of stroke. The Framingham Study. *Stroke* 1993;**24**:1366–1371

Markus H. Genes for stroke. *J Neurol Neurosurg Psychiatry* 2004;**75**:1229–1231

Rastenyte D, Tuomilento J, Sarti C. Genetics of stroke – a review. *J Neurol Sci* 1998;**153**:132–145

Ethnicity

Hajat C, Dundas R, Stewart JA et al. Cerebrovascular risk factors and stroke subtypes: difference between ethnic groups. *Stroke* 2001;**32**:37–42

Wolfe CD, Rudd AG, Howard R et al. Incidence and case fatality rates of stroke subtypes in a multiethnic population: the South London Stroke Register. *J Neurol Neurosurg Psychiatry* 2002;**72**:211–216

Modifiable risk factors

Alcohol

Djousse L, Ellison RC, Beiser A et al. Alcohol consumption and risk of ischemic stroke: the Framingham Study. *Stroke* 2002;**33**:907–912

Reynolds K, Lewis LB, Nolen JD et al. Alcohol consumption and risk of stroke: a meta-analysis. *JAMA* 2003;**289**:579–588

Aortic atherosclerosis

Agmon Y, Khandheria BK, Meissner I et al. Relation of coronary artery disease and cerebrovascular disease with atherosclerosis of the thoracic aorta in the general population. *Am J Cardiol* 2002; **89**:262–267

Amarenco P, Cohen A, Tzourio C et al. Atherosclerotic disease of the aortic arch and the risk of ischemic stroke. *N Engl J Med* 1994;**331**: 1474–1479

Mendel T, Popow J, Hier DB et al. Advanced atherosclerosis of the aortic arch is uncommon in ischemic stroke: an autopsy study. *Neurol Res* 2002;**24**:491–494

Atrial fibrillation

Mattle HP. Long-term outcome after stroke due to atrial fibrillation. *Cerebrovasc Dis* 2003;**16**:3–8

Penado S, Cano M, Acha O et al. Atrial fibrillation as a risk factor for stroke recurrence. *Am J Med* 2003;**114**:206–210

Carotid stenosis

Halliday A, Mansfield A, Marro J et al. Prevention of disabling and fatal strokes by successful carotid endarterectomy in patients without recent neurological symptoms: randomised controlled trial. *Lancet* 2004;**363**:1491–1502

Nadareishvili ZG, Rothwell PM, Beletsky V et al. Long-term risk of stroke and other vascular events in patients with asymptomatic carotid artery stenosis. *Arch Neurol* 2002;**59**:1162–1166

Rothwell MP, Eliasziw M, Gutnikov SA et al. Analysis of pooled data from the randomised trials of endarterectomy for symptomatic carotid stenosis. *Lancet* 2003;**361**:107–116

Diabetes mellitus

Jorgensen H, Nakayama H, Raaschou HO. Stroke in patients with diabetes. The Copenhagen Stroke Study. *Stroke* 1994;**25**:1977–1984

Mergherbi SE, Milan C, Minier D et al. Association between diabetes and stroke subtype on survival and functional outcome 3 months after stroke: date from the European BIOMED Stroke Project. *Stroke* 2003;**34**:688–694

Hyperlipidaemia

Heart Protection Study Collaborative Group. MRC/BHF Heart Protection Study of cholesterol lowering with simvastatin in 20 536 high-risk individuals: a randomised placebo-controlled trial. *Lancet* 2002;**360**:7–22

Prospective Studies Collaboration. Cholesterol, diastolic blood pressure and stroke: 13,000 strokes in 250,000 people in 45 prospective cohorts. *Lancet* 1995;**346**:1647–1653

Hypertension

Collins R, MacMahon S. Blood pressure, antihypertensive drug treatment and the risks of stroke and of coronary heart disease. *Br Med Bull* 1994;**50**: 272–298

Collins R, Peto R, MacMahon S et al. Blood pressure, stroke, and coronary heart disease. Part 2. Short-term reductions in blood pressure: overview of randomised drug trials in their epidemiological context. *Lancet* 1990;**335**:1534–1535

Lawes CMM, Bennett DA, Feigin VL, Rodgers A. Blood pressure and stroke: an overview of published reviews. *Stroke* 2004;**35**:1024–1033

MacMahon S, Peto R, Cutler J et al. Blood pressure, stroke, and coronary heart disease. Part 1, Prolonged differences in blood pressure: prospective observational studies corrected for the regression dilution bias. *Lancet* 1990;**335**:765–774

Vokonas PS, Kannel WB, Cupples LA. Epidemiology and risk of hypertension in the elderly: the Framingham Study. *J Hypertens* 1988;**6**:S3–9

Ischaemic heart disease

Lichtman JH, Krumholz HM, Wang Y et al. Risk and predictors of stroke after myocardial infarction among the elderly: results from the Cooperative Cardiovascular Program. *Circulation* 2002;**105**: 1082–1087

Ness J, Aronow WS. Prevalence of coexistence of coronary artery disease, ischemic stroke, and peripheral arterial disease in older persons, mean age 80 years, in an academic hospital-based geriatric practice. *J Am Geriatr Soc* 1999;**47**: 1255–1256

Wienbergen H, Schiele R, Gitt AK et al. Incidence, risk factors, and clinical outcome of stroke after acute myocardial infarction in clinical practice. MIR and MITRA Study Groups. Myocardial Infarction Registry. Maximal Individual Therapy in Acute Myocardial Infarction. *Am J Cardiol* 2001;**87**:782–785

Peripheral arterial disease

Liu XF, van Melle G, Bogousslavsky J. Heart and carotid artery disease in stroke patients with intermittent claudication. *Eur J Neurol* 2000; **7**:459–463

Tsai AW, Folsom AR, Rosamond WD, Jones DW. Ankle–brachial index and 7-year ischemic stroke incidence: the ARIC Study. *Stroke* 2001;**32**: 1721–1724

Physical activity

Kiely DK, Wolf PA, Cupples LA et al. Physical activity and stroke risk: the Framingham Study. *Am J Epidemiol* 1994;**140**:608–620

Prior stroke

Hankey GJ. Long-term outcome after ischaemic stroke/transient ischaemic attack. *Cerebrovasc Dis* 2003;**16**:14–19

Jorgensen HS, Nakayama H, Reith J et al. Stroke recurrence: predictors, severity, and prognosis. The Copenhagen Stroke Study. *Neurology* 1997; **48**:891–895

Lovett JK, Coull AJ, Rothwell PM. Early risk of recurrence by subtype of ischemic stroke in population-based incidence studies. *Neurology* 2004;**62**:569–573

Smoking

Wolf PA, D'Agostino RB, Kannel WB et al. Cigarette smoking as a risk factor for stroke. The Framingham Study. *JAMA* 1988;**259**:1025–1029

Socioeconomic conditions

Engstrom G, Jerntorp I, Pessah-Rasmussen H et al. Geographic distribution of stroke incidence within an urban population: relations to socioeconomic circumstances and prevalence of cardiovascular risk factors. *Stroke* 2001;**32**:1098–1103

Hart CL, Hole DJ, Smith GD. The contribution of risk factors to stroke differentials, by socioeconomic position in adulthood: the Renfrew/Paisley Study. *Am J Public Health* 2000;**90**:1788–1791

TIA

Clark TG, Murphy MF, Rothwell PM. Long term risks of stroke, myocardial infarction, and vascular death in 'low risk' patients with a non-recent transient ischaemic attack. *J Neurol Neurosurg Psychiatry* 2003;**74**:577–580

Coull AJ, Lovett JK, Rothwell PM. Population based study of early risk of stroke after transient ischaemic attack or minor stroke: implications for public education and organisation of services. *BMJ* 2004;**328**:326–330

Hill MD, Yiannakoulias N, Jeerakathil T et al. The high risk of stroke immediately after transient ischemic attack: a population-based study. *Neurology* 2004;**62**:2015–2020

Minor modifiable risk factors

Diet

Gariballa SE. Nutritional factors in stroke. *Br J Nutr* 2000;**84**:5–17

Law M. Commentary: evidence on salt is consistent. *BMJ* 1996;**312**:1284–1285

Fibrinogen

Bots ML, Elwood PC, Salonen JT et al. Level of fibrinogen and risk of fatal and non-fatal stroke. EUROSTROKE: a collaborative study among research centres in Europe. *J Epidemiol Community Health* 2002;**56**:14–18

Kofoed SC, Wittrup HH, Sillesen H et al. Fibrinogen predicts ischaemic stroke and advanced atherosclerosis but not echolucent, rupture-prone carotid plaques: the Copenhagen City Heart Study. *Eur Heart J* 2003;**24**:567–576

Homocysteine

Hassan A, Hunt BJ, O'Sullivan M et al. Homocysteine is a risk factor for cerebral small vessel disease, acting via endothelial dysfunction. *Brain* 2004; **127**:212–219

Kelly PJ, Rosand J, Kistler JP et al. Homocysteine, *MTHFR* 677→T polymorphism, and risk of ischemic stroke: results of a meta-analysis. *Neurology* 2002;**59**:529–536

Sen S, Oppenheimer SM, Lima J et al. Risk factors for progression of aortic atheroma in stroke and transient ischemic attacks patients. *Stroke* 2002; **33**:930–935

Infection

Bova IY, Bornstein NM, Korczyn AD. Acute infection as a risk factor for ischemic stroke. *Stroke* 1996;**27**:2204–2206

Chamorro A. Role of inflammation in stroke and atherothrombosis. *Cerebrovasc Dis* 2004; **17**(Suppl 3):1–5

Grau AJ, Buggle F, Ziegler C et al. Association between acute cerebrovascular ischemia and chronic and recurrent infection. *Stroke* 1997;**28**: 1724–1729

Lindsberg PJ, Grau AJ. Inflammation and infections as risk factors for ischemic stroke. *Stroke* 2003; **34**:2518–2532

Obesity

Shinton R, Shipley M, Rose G. Overweight and stroke in the Whitehall Study. *J Epidemiol Community Health* 1991;**45**:138–142

Suk SH, Sacco RL, Boden-Albala B et al. Abdominal obesity and risk of ischemic stroke. The Northern Manhattan Stroke Study. *Stroke* 2003;**34**:1586–1592

Tanne D, Medalie JH, Goldbourt U. Body fat distribution and long-term risk of stroke mortality. *Stroke* 2005;**36**:1021–1025

Oral contraceptives

Bousser MG, Kittner SJ. Oral contraceptives and stroke. *Cephalalgia* 2000;**20**:183–9

Gillum LA, Mamidipudi SK, Johnston SC. Ischemic stroke risk with oral contraceptives: a meta-analysis. *JAMA* 2000;**284**:72–78

Snoring and sleep apnoea

Neau JP, Paquereau J, Meurice JC et al. Stroke and sleep apnoea: cause or consequence? *Sleep Med Rev* 2002;**6**:457–469

Yaggi H, Mohsenin V. Obstructive sleep apnoea and stroke. *Lancet Neurol* 2004;**3**:333–342

Multiple risk factors

Wolf PA, D'Agostino RB, Belanger AJ et al. Probability of stroke: a risk profile from the Framingham Study. *Stroke* 1991;**22**:312–318

Prognosis

Bamford J, Sandercock P, Dennis M et al. A prospective study of acute cerebrovascular disease in the community: the Oxfordshire Community Stroke Project – 1981–86. Incidence, case fatality rates and overall outcome at one year of cerebral infarction, primary intracerebral and subaracnoid haemorrhage. *J Neurol Neurosurg Psychiatry* 1990;**53**:16–22

Bamford J, Sandercock P, Jones L, Warlow C. The natural history of lacunar infarction: the Oxfordshire Community Stroke Project. *Stroke* 1987;**18**:545–551

Hankey GJ. Long-term outcome after ischaemic stroke/transient ischaemic attack. *Cerebrovasc Dis* 2003;**16**(Suppl 1):14–19

CHAPTER 6

Vascular Dementia

DEFINITION

Various definitions of dementia exist, but all require a decline in intellectual function, involving several separate cognitive domains (Chui *et al.*, 1992; Roman *et al.*, 1993) (Table 6.1). Dementia resulting from vascular disease needs to be distinguished from confusion (an acute and quickly reversible disturbance of cognitive function) and focal single disturbances of cognitive function (e.g. isolated language disturbance or amnesia). Establishing the presence of dementia requires a cognitive examination including tests of attention, memory, language, frontal lobe functions and visuospatial skills. Unless these are carried out routinely, dementia is easily missed in the patient who has had a stroke, especially if attention is focused only on physical disability. In the presence of severe dysphasia, it may be difficult to test other aspects of cognitive function. Assessment by a skilled neuropsychologist can be very helpful.

A single infarct or haemorrhage is rarely sufficient to cause dementia, because of the discrete location of different domains of cognitive function within the different lobes of the hemispheres. Moreover, bilateral lesions are usually required to clinically disrupt memory or frontal lobe function. The term *multi-infarct dementia* is therefore sometimes used as a synonym for vascular dementia, but the latter term has the advantage of including dementia resulting from haemorrhage and ischaemic brain damage short of infarction. Vascular dementia is not necessarily progressive and indeed may improve when the onset of an episode of deterioration is associated with an acute stroke. In contrast to the degenerative dementias, vascular dementia is largely preventable.

INCIDENCE

The incidence of vascular dementia is difficult to establish, because of the lack of an agreed clinical or neuropathological definition, and the problem of selection bias. Overall, cerebrovascular disease is the only cause of dementia in about 20% of cases (Table 6.2). Both cerebrovascular disease and Alzheimer's disease become increasingly common with increasing age, and both pathologies contribute to intellectual decline in an additional 20% of cases (mixed dementia). Thus, in neuropathological series, vascular disease causes or contributes to dementia in nearly half the cases. As the population ages, vascular dementia will become increasingly important (Roman, 2002, 2003). In one epidemiological study carried out in Lundby, Sweden, the lifetime risk of developing vascular dementia was 30% in men and 25% in women, which was almost identical to the risk of developing Alzheimer's-type dementia (Hagnell *et al.*, 1992).

Dementia is surprisingly common in patients who have had stroke, with a prevalence of up to 30% in the first 3 years after stroke (Henon *et al.*, 2001). Risk factors for the development of dementia after stroke include advanced age, previous stroke, lacunar infarction, diabetes mellitus and left-hemisphere stroke. The

Table 6.1   Two examples of definitions of vascular dementia

	ADDTC criteria[a]	*NINDS–AIREN criteria[b]*
Dementia definition	Deterioration from a known level of intellectual function sufficient to interfere with the patient's customary affairs of life and not isolated to a single category of intellectual performance	Decline in memory as well as deficits in two other cognitive domains that impair function in daily living
Probable vascular dementia	Presence of all of the following: • Dementia • Evidence of two or more ischaemic strokes by history, neurological signs and/or neuroimaging; or a single stroke with a clear temporal relationship to the onset of dementia • At least one infarct outside the cerebellum on CT or MRI	Presence of all of the following: • Dementia • Focal neurological signs plus cerebrovascular disease on neuroimaging • Onset within 3 months of a stroke or abrupt onset of cognitive decline or fluctuating cognitive symptoms

Possible vascular dementia	May be diagnosed in the presence of dementia and:
	• History/evidence of a single stroke without clear temporal relationship or
	• All of the following:
	  – early-onset urinary incontinence and gait disturbance
	  – vascular risk factors
	  – extensive white matter change on neuroimaging
		May be diagnosed in the presence of dementia with focal neurological signs in:
		• The absence of neuroimaging
		• The absence of a clear temporal relationship between dementia and stroke
		• Patients with subtle onset and variable course of cognitive deficits and evidence of relevant cerebrovascular disease

[a]From Roman GC *et al. Neurology* 1993;**43**:250–260.
[b]From Chui HC *et al. Neurology* 1992;**42**:473–480.

Table 6.2   Frequency of common causes of dementia based on neuropathological series

Diagnosis	Frequency (%)
Alzheimer's disease	45
Pure vascular dementia	20
Mixed dementia	20
Other causes	15

incidence of new dementia developing in the first year after stroke is approximately 5%. It has not been established to what extent this is the result of coincidental Alzheimer's disease, but clinical features suggest that about two-thirds of cases are attributable to vascular dementia.

CAUSES OF VASCULAR DEMENTIA

Any cause of cerebrovascular disease may result in dementia if sufficient brain damage ensues. It is convenient to classify vascular dementia according to whether the predominant damage is cortical or subcortical (Table 6.3). Larger areas of damage are required for cortical infarcts or haemorrhage to result in dementia, and bilateral hemisphere infarcts are usually necessary. Recurrent cardiac embolism, for example in association with atrial fibrillation or valvular heart disease, is the most common cause. Recurrent cortical haemorrhage, usually resulting from cerebral amyloid angiopathy, is sometimes responsible. A combination of widespread small infarcts in both cortex and

Table 6.3   Causes of vascular dementia

Cortical
- Cardiac embolism
- Bilateral severe carotid stenosis
- Subarachnoid haemorrhage
- Recurrent intracerebral haemorrhage
- Cerebral amyloid angiopathy
- Vasculitis

Subcortical
- Bilateral paramedian thalamic infarction
- Binswanger's disease
- Lacunar state
- CADASIL
- Small vessel vasculitis

subcortical grey and white matter is sometimes seen in patients with dementia resulting from vasculitis, particularly granulomatous angiitis. Patients with cortical infarctions sufficient to cause dementia usually have clear cortical infarcts visible on computed tomography (CT) or magnetic resonance imaging (MRI). Pathologically, at least 50 ml of cortex need to be infarcted before dementia is likely.

SUBCORTICAL VASCULAR DEMENTIA

Subcortical vascular dementia results from ischaemia in the deep white matter and basal ganglia secondary to bilateral disease of the small blood vessels (Ward and Brown, 2002). This is usually hypertensive small vessel disease, but similar dementia can occur secondary to small vessel vasculitis (e.g. in systemic lupus erythematosus). Subcortical vascular dementia can result from small volumes of infarction, as low as 1–2ml. This is particularly striking in the syndrome of *bilateral paramedian thalamic infarction* (Guberman and Stuss, 1983; Reilly *et al.*, 1992). Patients with this syndrome usually present with sudden onset of a confusional state associated with disorders of ocular motility (Kumral *et al.*, 2001). The confusional state or coma evolves into a persistent pattern of subcortical dementia as the patient recovers consciousness.

When dementia results from multiple subcortical lacunar infarcts, the term '*lacunar state*' is sometimes used. *Binswanger's disease* (*subcortical arteriosclerotic encephalopathy*) is a variety of subcortical vascular dementia associated with diffuse atrophy of the subcortical white matter associated with severe arteriosclerosis of the perforating small blood vessels. Radiologically, Binswanger's disease is characterized by leukoaraiosis on CT (Figure 6.1) and often more obviously on MRI (Figure 6.2). Leukoaraiosis is recognized by the following features:

- Low attenuation on CT
- High signal on T_2-weighted MRI
- Patchy or diffuse changes with poorly demarcated edges
- Confined to subcortical white matter
- Maximum around the ventricular horns and in the centrum semiovale

Leukoaraiosis is distinguished from *white matter infarcts*, which:

- Are well demarcated
- Are circular, oval or wedge-shaped, and may include grey matter
- Follow vascular territories

The radiological features of leukoaraiosis can be caused by a number of other diseases, such as multiple sclerosis and metabolic disorders. However, in most patients with vascular risk factors, particularly hypertension, the cause is small vessel disease. The finding of leukoaraiosis on CT or MRI with suspected vascular dementia therefore supports the diagnosis of subcortical small vessel disease causing the dementia. However, leukoaraiosis can also be found in advanced Alzheimer's disease and is common in hypertensive patients and even in normal elderly subjects who are not demented. However, the radiological findings of leukoaraiosis in elderly patients have been shown to result from the same pathological changes to those seen in Binswanger's disease, and it is quite likely that leukoaraiosis is a risk factor for the subsequent development of vascular dementia.

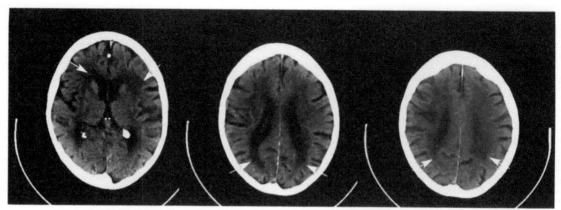

Figure 6.1   Axial CT at three levels showing typical features of leukoaraiosis with patchy low attenuation in the periventricular regions, most obvious adjacent to the horns of the lateral verticles (arrows).

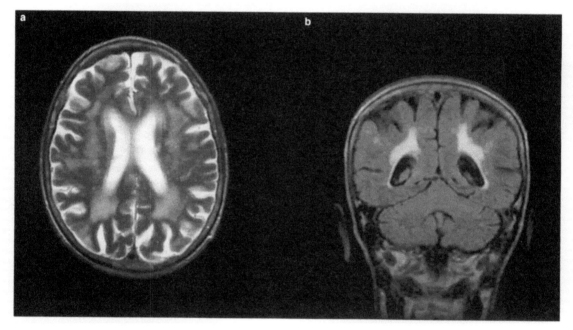

Figure 6.2   (a) Axial T_2-weighted and (b) coronal FLAIR MRI showing typical features of severe leukoaraiosis with extensive signal change in the deep white matter. (This is the same patient as in Figure 6.1.).

Pathologically, the microscopic changes of leukoaraiosis and in the white matter of patients dying of Binswanger's disease are those of ischaemic damage of the deep white matter without infarction (Ward and Brown, 2002). It is likely that the ischaemic damage results from hypoperfusion in the deep border-zone regions of the subcortical white matter, and in some cases subcortical vascular dementia follows episodes of hypotension or cardiac arrhythmia in patients who have thickening of the perforating small blood vessels.

The diffuse white matter changes seen in Binswanger's disease are almost invariably associated with the pathological finding of subcortical lacunar infarcts. The extent to which the dementia in patients with subcortical vascular disease is attributable to the lacunar infarcts as compared with the diffuse white matter changes remains uncertain, as do the exact degree and location of white matter damage required for the development of dementia.

Clinical features of subcortical vascular dementia

There is typically fluctuation in the clinical picture, with subacute accumulation of focal neurological symptoms and signs over weeks or months, in association with long plateau periods and the development of dementia of varying degrees. There may be a history of lacunar stroke. The fluctuating mental changes have features of subcortical involvement, with forgetfulness, abulia, emotional lability and impaired concentration. Bradyphrenia, a slowing of mental agility, may be very striking. In subcortical dementia, the patient may be very slow to remember a list of items but may eventually respond correctly, in contrast to the patient with cortical dementia, who tends to remember immediately or not at all. Confusional episodes may be a feature of subcortical vascular dementia, particularly in the later stages. Chronic hypertension is usual. However, in the later stages of Binswanger's disease, blood pressure measurements may decline markedly with rapid progression of the dementia.

The most useful clinical sign of subcortical vascular dementia is a small-stepped, wide-based gait (marche á petit pas). This is distinguished from the gait of idiopathic Parkinson's disease by the fact that the feet are held apart and the arms swing normally or even in an exaggerated fashion. Other clinical signs, particularly in advanced cases, include pseudobulbar palsy, extensor plantar responses and urinary incontinence. The combination of the small-stepped gait with cogwheel rigidity and impaired ocular movements may lead to the diagnosis of *vascular parkinsonism*.

CADASIL

Cerebral autosomal dominant arteriopathy with subcortical infarcts and leukoencephalopathy (CADASIL) is a rare, inherited cause of stroke and subcortical vascular dementia. It is described in detail in Chapter 11.

DIAGNOSIS OF VASCULAR DEMENTIA

The diagnosis of the cause of dementia without neuropathology is often difficult. The diagnosis of dementia resulting from large areas of cortical infarction is usually made fairly easily because of the clear history and findings of major stroke. However, the diagnosis of subcortical vascular dementia is more often missed. The main difficulty is distinguishing subcortical vascular dementia of insidious onset from Alzheimer's disease. A careful clinical history and examination, concentrating on the onset and time course of the history and the presence or absence of vascular risk factors, is essential. Vladimir Hachinski combined the common clinical features of multi-infarct dementia into an Ischaemic Score (Table 6.4), and it was suggested that a total Score of 4 or less indicated Alzheimer's disease and a Score of 7 or more multi-infarct dementia. Subsequent studies have shown that the Ischaemic Score has a rather poor correlation with neuropathological diagnosis and can be regarded as only a rough indicator of underlying pathology (Fischer *et al.*, 1991; Moroney *et al.*, 1997). The Ischaemic Score was developed before the general introduction of CT scanning, but even the addition of the CT to the Score does not greatly increase its sensitivity (Zekry *et al.*, 2002).

The most useful discriminator between vascular dementia and Alzheimer's disease is the finding of a wide-based, small-stepped gait suggesting subcortical ischaemia or corticospinal tract signs. Full investigation is important to exclude treatable vascular risk factors, and CT or MRI may show cerebral infarction or severe leukoaraiosis supporting the diagnosis. If available, positron emission

Table 6.4   The Ischaemic Score

Clinical feature	Score allocated
Abrupt onset	2
Stepwise deterioration	1
Fluctuating course	2
Nocturnal confusion	1
Relative preservation of personality	1
Depression	1
Somatic complaints	1
Emotional incontinence	1
History of hypertension	1
History of strokes	2
Evidence of associated atherosclerosis	1
Focal neurological symptoms	2
Focal neurological signs	2

Interpretation
• Score < 4 suggests a primary degenerative
  dementia (e.g. Alzheimer's disease)
• Score 4–7 suggests mixed dementia
• Score > 7 suggests vascular dementia

tomography (PET) or single-photon emission computed tomography (SPECT) may be helpful in the differential diagnosis by showing patchy focal reductions in cerebral blood flow and metabolism in patients with vascular dementia, compared with the focal temporoparietal reductions seen in Alzheimer's disease. Similarly, neuropsychological tests may show a patchy pattern of cognitive deficits in vascular dementia, compared with a more global deficit in Alzheimer's disease (McPherson and Cummings, 1996).

The distinction between vascular dementia and Alzheimer's disease is not made easy by the fact that the two conditions coexist in a substantial proportion of elderly patients (Roman, 2002). Moreover, even patients with apparently 'pure' Alzheimer's disease have an increased incidence of vascular risk factors and leukoaraiosis. It is not clear whether these findings indicate that vascular disease can promote the pathological changes of Alzheimer's disease or whether the association can be explained by mixed pathology.

The diagnosis of CADASIL is suggested by the combination of a young patient with a history of transient ischaemic attack (TIA) or stroke, the early onset of dementia and leukoaraiosis on imaging, together with the absence of hypertension and the positive family history of similar symptoms. The incidence of sporadic cases of CADASIL without a family history is currently uncertain. The diagnosis in some families may be confirmed by skin biopsy or DNA mutation analysis. The latter test may be time-consuming if a complete search for possible mutations in the *notch3* gene is made, because known mutations may occur in many sites in exons. However, about two-thirds occur in exons 4 and 3, which can be screened more rapidly.

MANAGEMENT

The prevention of vascular dementia by primary and secondary stroke prevention is of great public health importance. Treatment should include control of vascular risk factors, including stopping smoking, appropriate diet, and careful control of diabetes and hypertension. In patients with subcortical vascular dementia and leukoaraiosis, it is uncertain to what extent lowering blood pressure will reduce the perfusion of the deep white matter. It is therefore important to control hypertension as well as possible, without causing postural hypotension. There is some evidence that aspirin prevents further cognitive decline in patients with vascular dementia, and an antiplatelet agent should be prescribed unless contraindicated (Meyer *et al.*, 1989). There is no evidence that anticoagulation prevents vascular dementia, and it should be prescribed only if there is a clear indication (e.g. atrial fibrillation or recurrent cardiac embolism). The hazards of anticoagulation may be increased in patients with leukoaraiosis, and dementia itself may be a contraindication to anticoagulation, unless the patient's medication can be closely supervised. There is some indication from randomized trials that the cholinergic agents effective in Alzheimer's disease also benefit patients with vascular dementia, but further evidence is required to establish their place in the treatment of vascular dementia (Erkinjuntti et al., 2002; Black et al., 2003). There is no place for the use of cerebral vasodilators in dementia, except if they have a peripheral action in the treatment of hypertension.

KEY REFERENCES

Definition

Chui HC, Victoroff JI, Margolin D et al. Criteria for the diagnosis of ischemic vascular dementia proposed by the State of California Alzheimer's Disease Diagnostic and Treatment Centers. *Neurology* 1992;**42**:473–480

Roman GC, Tatemichi TK, Erkinjuntti T et al. Vascular dementia: diagnostic criteria for research studies. Report of the NINDS–AIREN International Workshop. *Neurology* 1993;**43**:250–260

Incidence

Hagnell O, Franck A, Grasbeck A et al. Vascular dementia in the Lundby study. 1. A prospective, epidemiological study of incidence and risk from 1957 to 1972. *Neuropsychobiology* 1992;**26**:43–49

Henon H, Durieu I, Guerouaou D et al. Poststroke dementia: incidence and relationship to prestroke cognitive decline. *Neurology* 2001;**57**:1216–1222.

Roman GC. Vascular dementia may be the most common form of dementia in the elderly. *J Neurol Sci* 2002;**203/204**:7–10

Roman GC. Stroke, cognitive decline and vascular dementia: the silent epidemic of the 21st century. *Neuroepidemiology* 2003;**22**:161–164

Subcortical vascular dementia

Ward N, Brown MM. Leukoaraiosis. In *Subcortical Stroke*. Donnan GA et al. (eds). Oxford University Press, Oxford, 2002

Bilateral paramedian thalamic infarction

Guberman A, Stuss D. The syndrome of bilateral paramedian thalamic infarction. *Neurology* 1983;**33**:540–546

Kumral E, Evyapan D, Balkir K et al. Bilateral thalamic infarction. Clinical, etiological and MRI correlates. *Acta Neurol Scand* 2001;**103**:35–42

Reilly M, Connolly S, Stack J et al. Bilateral paramedian thalamic infarction: a distinct but poorly recognized stroke syndrome. *Q J Med* 1992;**82**:63–70

Diagnosis of vascular dementia

Fischer P, Jellinger K, Gatterer G et al. Prospective neuropathological validation of Hachinski's Ischaemic Score in dementias. *J Neurol Neurosurg Psychiatry* 1991;**54**:580–583

McPherson SE, Cummings JL. Neuropsychological aspects of vascular dementia. *Brain Cogn* 1996;**31**:269–282

Moroney JT, Bagieela E, Desmond DW et al. Meta-analysis of the Hachinski Ischemic Score in pathologically verified dementias. *Neurology* 1997;**49**:1096–1105

Roman GC. Defining dementia: clinical criteria for the diagnosis of vascular dementia. *Acta Neurol Scand Suppl* 2002;**178**:6–9

Zekry D, Duyckaerts C, Belmin J et al. Alzheimer's disease and brain infarcts in the elderly. Agreement with neuropathology. *J Neurol* 2002;**249**:1529–1534

Management

Black S, Roman GC, Geldmacher DS et al. Efficacy and tolerability of donepezil in vascular dementia: positive results of a 24-week, multicenter, international, randomized, placebo-controlled clinical trial. *Stroke* 2003;**34**:2323–2330.

Erkinjuntti T, Kurz A, Gauthier S et al. Efficacy of galantamine in probably vascular dementia and Alzheimer's disearse combined with cerebrovascular disease: a randomised trial. *Lancet* 2002;**359**:1283–1290

Meyer JS, Rogers RL, McClintic K, Mortel KF. Randomized clinical trial of daily aspirin therapy in multi-infarct dementia. A pilot study. *J Am Geriatr Soc* 1989;**37**:549–55.

Causes

CHAPTER 7

Common Causes
of Ischaemic Stroke

This chapter will describe the common causes of stroke (Table 7.1). Rarer mechanisms are described in Chapter 11. The major mechanisms of ischaemic stroke are:

- Thromboembolism from atherosclerosis in the aorta or cervical blood vessels
- Cardiac embolism
- Local thrombosis superimposed on intracranial atherosclerosis
- Local occlusion of perforating vessels (small vessel disease or lacunar stroke)

At the end of the chapter, the mechanisms of platelet activation, thrombosis and thrombolysis are described.

ATHEROTHROMBOSIS

Atherosclerosis of the major vessels supplying the brain is an important source of cerebral embolism (Bogousslavsky *et al.*, 1988). The emboli are usually platelet aggregates or thrombus formed on atherosclerotic plaques, but occasionally consist of cholesterol and other atherosclerotic debris. Symptomatic atherosclerosis is most common at the bifurcation of the carotid artery into the external and internal carotid arteries, but emboli may also arise from the aorta, the carotid syphon, the common carotid artery, and the vertebral and basilar arteries (Figure 7.1). The causes of

Table 7.1 Common mechanisms of ischaemic stroke

Thromboembolism
- Atherosclerosis
  - Aorta
  - Carotid artery
  - Vertebral artery
- Cardiac disease
  - Atrial fibrillation
  - Valvular heart disease
  - Mural thrombus

Local intracranial thrombosis
- Intracranial atherosclerosis
- Small vessel disease (lacunar stroke)

atherosclerosis include ageing, hypertension, diabetes mellitus, smoking, abnormalities of lipid metabolism and genetic factors (Drouet, 2002). The mechanisms by which atherosclerosis leads to thrombosis are discussed below.

Atherosclerosis is the major cause of carotid and vertebral artery occlusion. In most cases, it is likely that the occlusion is caused by thrombosis superimposed on atherosclerosis, as described below. In young patients, thrombosis may occur as a result of other diseases of the arterial wall (e.g. dissection) (Chapter 11). This may cause transient ischaemic attack (TIA) or stroke as a result of embolism of thrombosis from the distal end of the clot to the

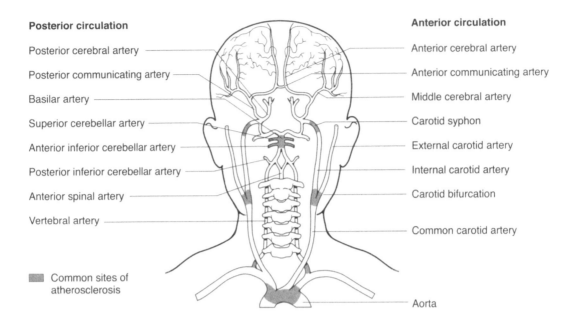

Figure 7.1   Common sites of atherosclerosis causing ischaemic stroke.

brain. Occlusion can also result in a stepwise progression of symptoms from propagation of thrombus. For example, vertebral artery occlusion may first cause only a TIA with transient vertigo and diplopia, but if the thrombus spreads to the basilar artery, the patient may develop a major life-threatening brainstem stroke a few hours or days later. Major vessel occlusion may also cause haemodynamic infarction because of the fall in distal perfusion pressure, but this is a much less common mechanism than thromboembolism. In many patients, carotid or vertebral artery occlusion occurs without symptoms because the circle of Willis, the external carotid artery and cortical pial anastomoses provide good collateral blood supply. If this is inadequate, border-zone infarction occurs (Chapter 4).

Cardiac embolism

Embolism from thrombus in the left atrium or ventricle accounts for 20–30% of ischaemic strokes (Bogousslavsky *et al.*, 1991; Ferro, 2003). The following strongly suggest cardiac embolism:

- Atrial fibrillation
- Valvular heart disease
- Recent myocardial infarction
- Intracardiac thrombus, atrial enlargement or ventricular aneurysm
- Prosthetic mitral or aortic valves
- Cardiac failure

It is likely that, in most cases, thrombus forms because of stasis in the left atrium or in areas of dyskinetic ventricular wall motion (see below). Atrial fibrillation is the most important cardiac cause and accounts for about 12% of ischaemic stroke and an even greater percentage in the elderly. In patients with calcific aortic or mitral valve disease, the embolic material may be degenerative portions of the valve itself. Congenital heart disease and patent foramen ovale (PFO) are potential routes for paradoxical embolism in patients with limb or pelvic vein thrombosis; however, in most cases, the relevance of a PFO in otherwise unexplained stroke or TIA remains uncertain (Chapter 11). Mitral valve prolapse is no longer considered an important cause of stroke.

Local intracranial thrombosis

Atherosclerosis of the medium-sized intracranial branches of the circle of Willis, and probably also the small branches up to the level of the origins of the perforating vessels, may lead to localized occlusion, usually as a result of superimposed thrombosis rather than progressive occlusion (Benesch and Chimowitz, 2000; Lutsep and Clark, 2000). Middle cerebral artery stenosis may cause distal embolism, although this mechanism has not been demonstrated *in vivo*. Intracranial atherosclerosis appears to be more common in the Asian and African-American population (Wong and Li, 2003). In Caucasians, middle cerebral artery occlusion is usually the result of cerebral embolism.

Small vessel disease

This causes lacunar stroke and accounts for about 30% of stroke (Fisher, 1998). Occlusion of small penetrating arterioles, usually secondary to hypertension or diabetes mellitus, leads to small infarcts (lacunes or lacunar infarcts) in the subcortical white matter, internal capsule, basal ganglia or brainstem (Besson *et al.*, 2000). The pathology of small vessel disease appears to be of two types (Lammie, 2000). Micro-atheroma may affect the origins of the perforating vessels, and then presumably stroke results from thrombosis secondary to superimposed thrombosis or occlusion. More commonly, the perforating vessels are affected by a degenerative disease of the wall, known as lipohyalinosis (Figure 7.2). This is a destructive lesion of small vessels between 40 and 200 μm in diameter, with loss of normal vessel architecture, mural foam cells and (in acute cases) fibrinoid necrosis. This may lead to progressive vessel occlusion, with or without superimposed thrombosis and ischaemia in the small zone of tissue supplied by the perforating vessels, which are end-arterioles with no collateral supply. Lacunar infarcts, being very small, are commonly asymptomatic and only cause stroke when vital pathways are close together and supplied by the perforating

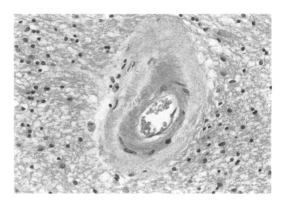

Figure 7.2   (See also Colour Plate VII, p. xii). Microscopic cross-section of a perforating vessel showing the characteristic changes of lipohyalinosis.

vessels for example in the brainstem, thalamus or posterior limb of the internal capsule. Lacunar infarction may be associated with progressive stroke, but the mechanism of the progression is unclear (Steinke and Ley, 2002). Small vessel disease with lipohyalinosis is also an important cause of cerebral haemorrhage (Chapter 8).

MECHANISMS OF THROMBOSIS

Thrombosis plays a fundamental role in occluding blood vessels in ischaemic stroke. An understanding of the mechanisms through which thrombosis occurs is therefore important in stroke for many reasons. In the first place, it may clarify the choice of agents for primary prevention of stroke (e.g. antiplatelet agents or warfarin) and also the mode of action of certain thrombolytic agents (e.g. urokinase and tissue plasminogen activator). Secondly, it is important in understanding the dynamic interplay between all aspects of the vascular system – endothelium, blood cells and plasma factors – and how they may contribute to thrombus formation. For example, the endothelium is not an inert pipe-like structure. Alterations of the expression of adhesion molecules on endothelial surfaces may occur in response to an adjacent underlying atheromatous plaque. These adhesion molecules enable leukocytes and platelets to stick to the endothelial wall with greater ease, encouraging thrombus formation. Factors secreted by these blood cells may in turn upregulate the expression of these adhesion factors. In turn, the adhesion and activation of neutrophils and platelets on the surface of the endothelium may encourage the release from these cells of agents such as platelet-derived growth factor (PDGF) and tumour necrosis factor α (TNF-α) that can cause structural damage to the endothelium and proliferation of fibroblasts and myointimal cells in the subendothelial layer. This will encourage plaque extension, denuding of the endothelium and enhanced local thrombus formation. This is described in more detail below.

Certain conditions are also known to generally enhance the coagulability of blood. These include infections, pyrexia and malignancy. Cytokines liberated by activated leukocytes at sites remote from a plaque may have an effect on the vascular endothelium in the region of atheroma. As mentioned, the effect may be upregulation of adhesion molecules. In addition, platelets and leukocytes become generally activated with an increased tendency to adhere to abnormal regions of the vascular endothelium. The association of stroke with recent infection (Chapter 5) may reflect these mechanisms.

Platelet activation

Atherosclerosis leads to thrombosis by a number of mechanisms. Severe vascular stenosis alters blood flow characteristics. Turbulence replaces laminar flow once the arterial lumen becomes narrowed by more than 70% or so (Figure 7.3). The resulting stresses on the blood vessel walls lead to loss of the endothelial lining and exposure of underlying collagen and glycoproteins, which have a procoagulant effect on the blood elements. Non-laminar flow also encourages margination of platelets and leukocytes where they can come into contact with the blood vessel wall. The high shear stress at sites of stenosis results in platelet

activation, and specific adhesion molecules are expressed on both circulating blood cells and platelets, as well as on the endothelial surface (Marquardt *et al.*, 2002). These latter may be upregulated in the vicinity of an atheromatous plaque. Platelet activation may also be promoted by ulceration or rupture of atheromatous plaque, exposing the lipid-rich core to the circulating blood. One of the platelet adhesion molecules, the integrin glycoprotein (GP) Ia/IIa, binds to collagen fibrils (Figure 7.4). Platelet adhesion to the vascular wall is also facilitated by the secretion of von Willebrand factor (vWF) by activated platelets and endothelial cells. This factor binds both to collagen in the vessel wall and to GPIb/IX expressed on the platelet surface, linking the two. Fibrinogen secreted by activated platelets binds to the GPIIb/IIIa receptor on adjacent platelets, forming cross-linkages and encouraging extension of the thrombus. Adenosine diphosphate (ADP), which is also released from activated platelets, binds to a specific platelet receptor. This increases the affinity with which the GPIIb/IIIa glycoprotein receptor binds fibrinogen and therefore strengthens platelet–platelet binding. In this way, the tendency for the expanding clot to be dissolved by fast-flowing blood is reduced by the increased strength of the interplatelet linkages.

PDGF is also secreted during the platelet release reaction. This enhances the growth, differentiation and proliferation of many cells, including subintimal myocytes and fibroblasts. These cells have receptors for cholesterol-rich lipoproteins, and their proliferation may increase the deposition of cholesterol within the atheromatous plaque. In this way, the process of thrombus formation may also enhance the progression of the atherosclerosis.

Thrombosis

The cascade of platelet factor secretion, glycoprotein binding and adhesion molecule upregulation results in amplification of the initiating signal and rapid enlargement and strengthening of the platelet plug. This is paralleled by a

a

Normal, laminar flow of blood,
with blood cells and platelets
generally occupying the centre
of the vessel

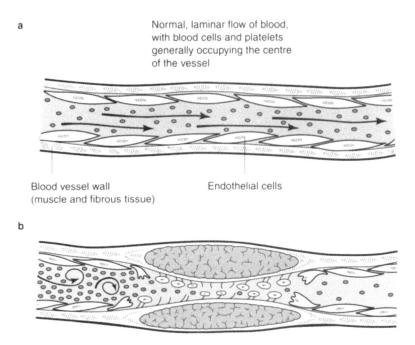

Blood vessel wall
(muscle and fibrous tissue)

Endothelial cells

b

Figure 7.3   (a) Normal laminar flow in a vessel without atherosclerotic stenosis. There is streamlined flow of blood throughout the blood vessel. The blood cells in general occupy a central position, with plasma occupying the outer regions adjacent to the vessel wall. The endothelial lining is intact. (b) A high-grade stenosis, with a subintimal atherosclerotic plaque causing turbulent flow (curved arrows) with sequestration and margination of platelets and white cells adjacent to the endothelial cells, which are denuded adjacent to the plaque.

dependent process that rapidly increases the conversion of fibrinogen to fibrin and provides a mesh-like network to support the expanding platelet plug. Exposure of the blood to collagen generates a complex with high-molecular-weight kininogen (HMWK) and prekallikrein (Figure 7.5). Factor XII becomes activated by this complex and in turn converts prekallikrein to active kallikrein and also activates factor XI. This sequence of events, termed reaction 1, continues in tandem with the initiation of reaction 2. Tissue factor, which is a lipoprotein present in cellular membranes of the cells in the subintimal layer, complexes with factor VII. In reaction 3, factor X is activated as a result of the previous two reactions. Activated factor X then converts prothrombin to thrombin in the presence of factor V, calcium and phospholipid. Thrombin then converts fibrinogen to fibrin and also enhances platelet adhesion and secretion (reaction 4).

Fibrinogen is split into fibrin and fibrinopeptides A and B. Fibrinogen is highly reactive and polymerizes rapidly into an insoluble complex composed of many chains of fibrin interlinked by activated factor VIII. This reaction is markedly accelerated when it occurs on the membrane surface of platelets. In this way, a fibrin–platelet thrombus may be formed over an area of abnormal or denuded endothelium, such as in the region of an atheromatous plaque.

It is most likely that this is a dynamic process. The thromboembolic potential of a plaque may well vary with time. This will be greatest around the time of plaque rupture or intraplaque haemorrhage and may be least when re-endothelialization occurs. It is this phenomenon that could account for the clinical observation that a completed stroke is most likely to occur within 1–3 months of a TIA or minor cerebral infarction.

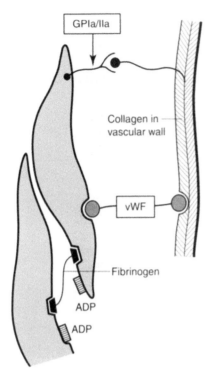

Figure 7.4 Simplified schematic of some of the interactions responsible for platelet thrombus formation. ADP, adenosine diphosphate; GPIa/IIa, glycoprotein Ia/IIa; vWF, von Willebrand factor.

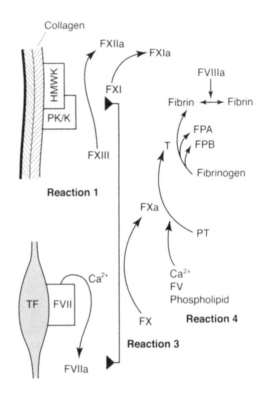

Figure 7.5 Simplified diagram of the clotting cascade. Ca^{2+}, calcium ion; FPA and FPB, fibrinopeptides A and B; FV, ... , factor V, ... (suffix 'a' indicates activated factor); HMWK, high-molecular-weight kininogen; K, kallikrein; PK, prekallikrein; PT, prothrombin; T, thrombin; TF, tissue factor.

Thrombolysis

The process of clot formation is balanced by that of clot lysis (Figure 7.6). It is believed that certain phases of the coagulation cascade are constantly activated; for example the reaction between tissue factor and factor VII may be continuously active. Thus thrombolysis is required in order to prevent in situ clotting of the blood. In the region of denuded or altered endothelium around an atheromatous plaque, the thrombotic cascade partially exceeds the ability of thrombolysis to contain it. However, a dynamic balance is eventually reached. Thrombolysis is triggered by (a) Hageman factor, (b) urokinase and (c) tissue plasminogen activator (tPA). As the clot is laid down, plasminogen is adsorbed onto its surface. tPA is released from endothelium in response to clot formation and by thrombin. This protease cleaves plasminogen, generating an active form, plasmin, which destroys polymerized fibrin, producing fibrin degradation products (FDPs), and these are subsequently sequestered by monocytes and macrophages. This reaction is markedly enhanced on the clot surface. Although tPA can degrade fibrinogen, its release into the general circulation is inhibited by binding to α_2 plasmin inhibitor. This prevents more widespread anticoagulation within the circulation from occurring and localizes the effect. In addition, plasminogen activator inhibitor is released in tandem from the

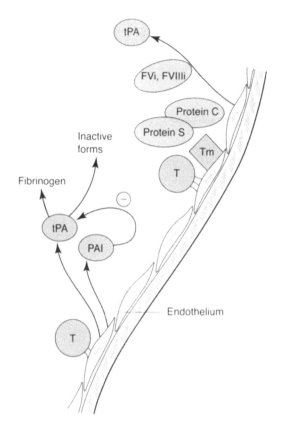

Figure 7.6 Schematic showing the pivotal role of thrombin (T) in the activation of the fibrinolytic pathway. FVi and FVIIIi, inactivated factors V and VIII; PAI, plasminogen activator inhibitor; Tm, thrombomodulin; tPA, tissue plasminogen activator.

endothelium, and this inhibits the actions of tPA. Pro-urokinase is also liberated from the endothelium and converted to urokinase within the clot. This furthers clot dissolution. Heparin-like molecules on the endothelial surfaces serve to activate antithrombin III and other antithrombin molecules. These complex with a number of the activated coagulation factors, limiting their function. Thrombin also complexes with thrombomodulin and protein C on the endothelial surface. The activated protein C thus formed has a number of functions: it can inactivate factors V and VIII and release tPA. This will shift the dynamic balance towards clot lysis and limitation of the

extent of clot formation. Activated protein C requires another liver-derived agent, protein S, for stabilization and optimization of activity.

The content of the clot is to some extent determined by haemorheological conditions. In veins, where slow flow prevails, the clot mostly comprises fibrin, with few platelets. The same may be true in a fibrillating left atrial appendage or in the region of a critical, extremely severe extracranial or intracranial stenosis. On the other hand, arterial thrombi mainly comprise platelets. This has some clinical significance (Feinberg *et al.*, 1999). It would therefore be predicted that prevention of clot extension or formation in the extracranial arterial vasculature would be best served by antiplatelet agents (e.g. aspirin or clopidogrel), in contrast to the venous side or atrial appendage, where warfarin might be a better choice. The finding that warfarin was superior to aspirin in trials of stroke prevention in patients with atrial fibrillation supports this prediction (Chapter 15).

KEY REFERENCES

Atherothrombosis

Bogousslavsky J, Van Melle G, Regli F. The Lausanne Stroke Registry: analysis of 1,000 consecutive patients with first stroke. *Stroke* 1988;**19**: 1083–1092

Drouet L. Atherothrombosis as a systemic disease. *Cerebrovasc Dis* 2002;**13**(Suppl):1–6

Cardiac embolism

Bogousslavsky J, Cachin C, Regli F et al. Cardiac sources of embolism and cerebral infarction – clinical consequences and vascular concomitants: the Lausanne Stroke Registry. *Neurology* 1991;**41**: 855–859

Ferro JM. Cardioembolic stroke: an update. *Lancet Neurol* 2003;**2**:177–188

Local intracranial thrombosis

Benesch CG, Chimowitz MI. Best treatment for intracranial arterial stenosis? 50 years of uncertainty.

The WASID Investigators. *Neurology* 2000;**55**: 465–466

Lutsep HL, Clark WM. Association of intracranial stenosis with cortical symptoms or signs. *Neurology* 2000;**55**:716–718

Wong KS, Li H. Long-term mortality and recurrent stroke risk among Chinese stroke patients with predominant intracranial atherosclerosis. *Stroke* 2003;**34**:2361–2366

Small vessel disease

Besson G, Hommel M, Perret J. Risk factors for lacunar infarcts. *Cerebrovasc Dis* 2000;**10**:387–390

Fisher CM. Lacunes: small, deep cerebral infarcts. *Neurology* 1998;**50**:841–852

Lammie GA. Pathology of small vessel stroke. *Br Med Bull* 2000;**56**:296–306

Steinke W, Ley SC. Lacunar stroke is the major cause of progressive motor deficits. *Stroke* 2002;**33**: 1510–1516

Mechanisms of thrombosis

Feinberg WM, Pearce LA, Hart RG et al. Markers of thrombin and platelet activity in patients with atrial fibrillation: correlation with stroke among 1531 participants in the Stroke Prevention in Atrial Fibrillation III Study. *Stroke* 1999;**30**:2547–2553

Marquardt L, Ruf A, Mansmann U et al. Course of platelet activation makers after ischaemic stroke. *Stroke* 2002;**33**:2570–2574

CHAPTER 8

Intracerebral Haemorrhage

About 10–15% of strokes are due to intracerebral haemorrhage, in which there is arterial bleeding directly into the brain substance, with the formation of a localized haematoma. This type of stroke is associated with a high mortality rate and survivors frequently have persistent disability. Subarachnoid haemorrhage can also be associated with intracerebral haemorrhage, if there is bleeding into the brain substance as well as into the cerebrospinal fluid spaces (Chapter 9).

CAUSES (TABLE 8.1)

Arteriovenous malformation (AVM)

This term is used to describe congenital malformations of blood vessels in the brain and spinal cord. There is usually a tangle of blood vessels with one or more feeding arteries and often a single large draining vein (Figure 8.1) without a capillary network between them, embedded in a stroma devoid of normal brain tissue. The abnormality is present at birth but may enlarge slowly during life. Bleeding may be precipitated by the increase in blood volume accompanying pregnancy. AVMs vary in size from quite small to enormous lesions that occupy almost the whole of one hemisphere. *Cryptogenic AVMs* are so small that they cannot be seen on angiography. Their existence is speculative, but it has been suggested that they are not seen at angiography because they are destroyed by the bleed and the associated inflammatory reaction. *Dural AVMs* or *fistulas* are tangles of dilated

Table 8.1 Causes of intracerebral haemorrhage

Abnormal blood vessels
- Vascular malformations:
  - Arteriovenous malformations
  - Saccular aneurysms
  - Cavernous angiomas
  - Septic and mycotic aneurysms
- Lipohyalinosis and microaneurysms
- Amyloid angiopathy
- Cerebral tumours
- Cerebral venous thrombosis
- Vasculitis
- Moyamoya syndrome
- Haemorrhagic transformation

Systemic bleeding tendency
- Haemophilia
- Leukaemia
- Thrombocytopenia
- Anticoagulants
- Antiplatelet agents
- Thrombolytic agents

Illicit drugs
- Amphetamines
- Cocaine

Hyperperfusion syndrome

Trauma

veins and small arteries derived from the dural and meningeal branches of the external carotid artery, associated with a site of rapid communication between the arterial and venous circulation. The majority are probably not congenital malformations, but acquired communications

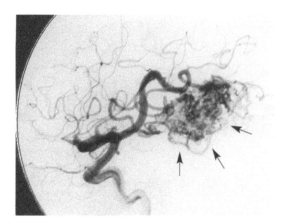

Figure 8.1 Cerebral angiogram showing a moderately sized arteriovenous malformation (arrows).

between dural arteries and veins. Such arteriovenous communications usually occur without an obvious precipitant, but may present after minor trauma or in association with a sudden rise in blood pressure (e.g. due to emotional upset) or after cerebral venous thrombosis. AVMs are an important cause of primary intracerebral haemorrhage, particularly in the young, although they account for no more than a third of all cases (Ruiz-Sandoval *et al.*, 1999). In the whole population over the age of 20, only about 1% of cases of intracranial haemorrhage are associated with an underlying AVM (Stapf *et al.*, 2002). The majority of such haemorrhages are lobar rather than located in the characteristic site of hypertensive intracerebral haemorrhage in the basal ganglia. AVMs are usually single and sporadic. In occasional cases, they can be multiple, particularly if there is an underlying systemic disorder (e.g. Osler–Rendu–Weber syndrome).

AVMs are clearly shown by angiography. Large feeding arteries are seen with rapid passage of blood to enlarged and tortuous veins, causing an early blush on the angiogram. In larger supratentorial AVMs, the arterial supply may be from a number of different systems; for example, both external and internal carotid arteries may feed the AVM. Thin-walled saccular aneurysms occur on feeding arteries in 10–20% of cases. These confer a particularly

high risk of recurrent haemorrhage of about 7%, against an annual recurrence rate of about 3% for AVMs without associated aneurysms.

Cavernous angiomas (cavernomas)

These are of unknown aetiology, but it has been suggested that at least part of the lesion forms as a localized reaction to small haemorrhages. They are mainly diagnosed from the characteristic magnetic resonance imaging (MRI) appearance of a central nidus of irregular bright signal intensity on T_2-weighted imaging, surrounded by a peripheral hypo-intense ring resulting from haemosiderin deposition due to previous episodes of bleeding (Requena *et al.*, 1991; Vogler and Castillo, 1995). No abnormalities are seen on angiography. Cavernous angiomas are predominantly supratentorial, most commonly affecting the temporal, frontal and parietal lobes. The most frequent infratentorial site is the pons. They are generally single lesions, but more than one can occur in an individual, particularly in families with hereditary cavernous angiomas. Cavernous angiomas may present with seizures, intracerebral haemorrhage or progressive neurological deficit. The last of these is more likely to occur in brainstem cavernous angioma. In the majority of cases, blood appears to leak slowly out of the lesion, rather than causing an acute haematoma, and this can result in a progressive neurological deficit. The majority of cavernous angiomas are asymptomatic and are frequently found on MRI performed for other reasons. The outlook in the vast majority of asymptomatic cases is benign.

Saccular aneurysms

These more usually cause subarachnoid haemorrhage (Chapter 9), but can cause an intracerebral haematoma with or without subarachnoid haemorrhage.

Lipohyalinosis and microaneurysms

In 1869, Charcot and Bouchard described multiple minute outpouchings of the small perforating blood vessels in the thalamus and corpus striatum and less often in the pons and cerebellum and cerebral white matter during postmortem examination of patients who had died from intracerebral haemorrhage. They called these miliary aneurysms. Their possible role in intracerebral haemorrhage was studied further in the 1960s by Ross Russell, who, in postmortem studies, found microaneurysms in a greater proportion of hypertensive patients than normotensive patients. These aneurysms measured 300–900 μm in diameter and were found on small arteries of 100–300 μm in diameter, commonly branches of the lateral lenticulostriate arteries in the region of the basal ganglion. These aneurysms were thin-walled and in some cases previous leakage as evidenced by haemosiderin-laden macrophages could be seen, while other aneurysms were thrombosed. Further studies confirmed the association with hypertension, and a hypothesis was developed that these structural abnormalities resulted from hypertension, and were the point at which cerebral haemorrhage occurred. More recently, this hypothesis has been questioned, and it has been suggested by some that the microaneurysms only account for a proportion of deep haemorrhages in hypertensive individuals (Takebayashi and Kaneko, 1983). Others have suggested that they may in fact represent artefacts caused by the injection technique, previous microhaemorrhages or misinterpretations of arteriole coils (Challa et al., 1992). On the basis of current evidence, it seems likely that they are important in at least a proportion of patients. However, the degenerative changes commonly found in the small perforating vessels of such individuals may be a more important site of haemorrhage (Lammie, 2002). This appearance, called lipohyalinosis, consists of a segmental process of fatty changes and fibrinoid necrosis and some areas of local thinning (see Colour Plate VII, p. xii). It is possible that haemorrhage may also occur at these points. Electron-microscopic studies of autopsy specimens have shown that the most common site of rupture appears to be at the distal bifurcations of the lenticulostriate arteries. In some cases, there appear to be multiple sites of rupture, and it is possible that the haemorrhage and local tissue distortion from one site of rupture may result in a cascade of rupture of neighbouring vessels. On balance, it seems likely that degenerative changes in the penetrating arteries lead to haemorrhage via direct rupture of thickened and weakened arterial walls and also in some instances from the walls of Charcot–Bouchard aneurysms. However, these aneurysms may largely be a marker of degenerative change and in many cases may not represent the focus from which haemorrhage occurs.

Cerebral amyloid angiopathy (CAA)

This is characterized pathologically by the deposition of amyloid in cerebral vessels, primarily small and medium-sized arteries of the cortex and leptomeninges (Yamada, 2000; Revesz et al., 2003). The classical birefringent amyloid material is seen on histological examination in the media and adventitia, which stains positive for Congo red. The incidence of these histological changes at postmortem increases steadily with age, occurring in as many as 60% of unselected autopsies of individuals older than 90 years. The incidence of haemorrhage secondary to amyloid angiopathy also increases with age and is rare before age 55. The mechanism of rupture of affected arteries is thought to be either a weakening of the vessel wall or the formation of microaneurysms at the sites of amyloid deposition. The amyloid seen in cerebral vessels is closely related to the amyloid comprising neuritic plaques in Alzheimer's disease, but it is entirely unrelated to the protein deposit seem in systemic amyloidosis. In early reports, CAA was primarily noted in patients with Alzheimer's disease, but it can occur without any clinical or histological evidence of this disease. It is strikingly restricted to vessels of the leptomeninges and grey matter, and usually stops abruptly when a penetrating vessel reaches a junction of cortex and subcortical white matter. Haemorrhages in CAA are almost exclusively lobar and often superficially close to the surface, with the site of rupture usually being at the grey–white matter junction.

Most cases of CAA are sporadic, but a number of hereditary forms exist. In Dutch familial amyloid, the amyloid is a β-protein similar to the amyloid plaque seen in Alzheimer's disease and to those in sporadic forms of CAA. In contrast, in the Icelandic form, the amyloid is antigenically different, being of the systatin C type. Haemorrhage tends to occur earlier in the Icelandic familial form, at a median age of about 30 years compared with 55 years in Dutch hereditary CAA.

Cerebral tumours

Bleeding into an underlying cerebral tumour is a relatively rare cause of intracranial haemorrhage, accounting for less than 10% of cases in most series. Haemorrhage can occur from either primary or metastatic tumours. Tumours with a particular tendency for intracranial bleeding include:

- Metastatic melanoma
- Choriocarcinoma
- Renal cell carcinoma

Cerebral breast and bronchogenic metastases rarely bleed, but, due to the greater frequency of these tumours, they should be considered in the differential diagnosis. Primary brain tumours that may bleed include glioblastoma multiforme and oligodendroglioma.

The underlying lesion may be obscured by a recent bleed. Neuroimaging features that suggest a tumour include:

- Spherical appearance of the haematoma
- Low-density area on computed tomography (CT) in the centre suggesting necrosis
- Multiple haemorrhages
- Enhancement after intravenous contrast

If there is any uncertainty, neuroimaging should be repeated after a few weeks to exclude an underlying lesion.

Cerebral venous thrombosis

Intracranial haemorrhage is an important feature of cerebral venous thrombosis caused by obstruction of sinus or cortical veins. It is often accompanied by ischaemic symptoms, including focal deficits and seizures. Bilateral haemorrhagic infarction in the parasagittal region should alert one to the diagnostic possibility of superior sagittal sinus thrombosis. This is covered in more detail in Chapter 12.

Vasculitis

Both systemic and primary central nervous system vasculitides can cause intracranial haemorrhage. In such cases, ischaemic infarction is often present as well.

Moyamoya disease

Haemorrhage is the most common presentation of Moyamoya disease in adults. This is covered in more detail in Chapter 11. Bleeding is most commonly caused by rupture of the collateral vessels formed in response to basal arterial occlusion.

Haemorrhagic transformation

This is a common complication of acute ischaemic infarction. Most commonly, scattered petechial haemorrhages occur within the necrotic tissue; these have little clinical consequence. Less commonly, a frank haematoma occurs, which only rarely results in mass effect and clinical deterioration. Haemorrhagic transformation is believed to arise following reperfusion of damaged vessels within a necrotic brain region. The major risk factor is a large volume of infarcted tissue. Haemorrhagic transformation is relatively common following stroke secondary to cerebral sinus thrombosis, presumably because the infarction is occurring at arterial pressure. The rate of haemorrhagic transformation is markedly increased in patients treated with thrombolysis for acute stroke.

Systemic bleeding tendency

Coagulation disorders are rare causes of intracranial haemorrhage. *Haemophilia*, which is due to factor VIII deficiency, results in intracranial haemorrhage in about 2–5% of patients, and approximately half of these will present with intracerebral haemorrhage and half with subdural haematomas. Haemophiliacs are also particularly susceptible to traumatic haematomas after head injury. The mortality rate of such haemorrhages, which are more common in younger individuals, is as high as 10% for subdural haematomas and 65% for intracerebral haemorrhages. Intracerebral haemorrhage is a well-recognized complication of *acute leukaemia*. Haemorrhage is most common in the lobar white matter, and its occurrence frequently coincides with systemic bleeding. Bleeding complications of *acute lymphocytic leukaemia* are often accompanied by a rapidly rising number of abnormal circulating leukocytes and a fall in platelet count – a condition referred to as 'blastic crisis'. *Thrombocytopenia* and *disseminated intravascular coagulation* can also result in intracerebral haemorrhage. Idiopathic thrombocytopenic purpura is associated with symptomatic intracerebral haemorrhage in about 1% of patients, and bleeding usually occurs when the platelet count drops below 10 000/mm^3.

Oral anticoagulants

Bleeding at various sites is the major hazard of the use of anticoagulants (Palareti *et al.*, 1996). Treatment with oral anticoagulants appears to increase the risk of intracerebral haemorrhage by approximately 8- to 10-fold in comparison with non-anticoagulated individuals with otherwise similar risk factors (Franke *et al.*, 1990; Sjalander *et al.*, 2003). Anticoagulant-related cases may account for as many as 10% of intracerebral haemorrhages. A number of factors have been reported to increase risk, including advanced age, hypertension, preceding cerebral infarction and head trauma. The risk of haemorrhage is related to the degree of anticoagulation (Hylek and Singer, 1994). In the SPIRIT Trial, in which warfarin was compared with aspirin for stroke prevention in patients with atherothrombotic stroke, the risk of intracerebral haemorrhage complicating warfarin therapy increased progressively with

an increasing international normalized ratio (INR), especially above an INR of 4 (SPIRIT, 1997). There is some evidence that the risk is specifically increased in individuals with radiological leukoaraiosis, presumably because this indicates degenerative small vessel disease due to lipohyalinosis (Smith *et al.*, 2002).

The management of anticoagulant-associated intracranial haemorrhage requires the reversal of any residual coagulation disorder with prothrombin complex concentrate or fresh frozen plasma in discussion with a haematologist. Warfarin should be discontinued and intravenous vitamin K given. Even in patients with a very strong indication for anticoagulation (e.g. prosthetic heart valves), the hazards of continuing anticoagulation are greater in the short term than the risks of stopping it. In patients with prosthetic heart valves, warfarin should be restarted after an interval of 4–6 weeks. In most other cases of warfarin-associated haemorrhage, further anticoagulation is contraindicated for life.

Antiplatelet agents

The Antithrombotic Trialists' Collaboration concluded that antiplatelet therapy, which was usually aspirin in patients with stroke or transient ischaemic attack (TIA), increased the risk of intracranial haemorrhage over a 2-year period by between 0.1% and 0.2% (Antithrombotic Trialists' Collaboration, 2002). The absolute risk was therefore extremely low, with one or two extra cerebral haemorrhages for every 1000 patients treated. When haemorrhage occurs in hypertensive individuals taking aspirin, the association is therefore usually not causal, but coincidental. However, in the primary prevention of vascular events in individuals without vascular risk factors, the risk of intracerebral haemorrhage from aspirin appears to largely outweigh any potential benefits of preventing cerebral thrombosis. In patients with vascular disease (secondary prevention), the benefits of antiplatelet therapy largely outweigh the risks. However, the combination of aspirin with clopidogrel is an exception to this rule, at least in the patients at high risk of recurrent stroke included in the MATCH study (mainly patients with recent stroke and diabetes). In this study, the addition of aspirin to clopidogrel increased the risk of cerebral haemorrhage and other major haemorrhages substantially, and this outweighed any benefit of combining the two agents (Diener *et al.*, 2004).

Thrombolytic agents

Intracerebral haemorrhage is an important complication of therapeutic thrombolysis. Intracerebral haemorrhage caused by thrombolysis for acute myocardial infarction generally occurs shortly after the onset of therapy, with about 40% of cases occurring during the drug infusion. The site of bleeding is most commonly the subcortical (lobar) white matter of the cerebral hemispheres. The prognosis of the condition is poor, with a mortality rate of between 44% and 88% in different series. In patients receiving thrombolysis using tissue plasminogen activator (tPA) for acute ischaemic stroke, haemorrhage occurs in about 6% of cases and is most common at the site of infarction, but can occur anywhere in the brain (NINDS, 1997; Berger *et al.*, 2001; Kase, 2001). Risk factors include a large stroke with major neurological deficit at the time of treatment, the appearance of mass effect and oedema on initial CT scan, and possibly a longer time interval between administration of thrombolysis and stroke onset (Larrue *et al.*, 2001). Thrombolysis also increases the proportion of patients who will progress to haemorrhagic transformation.

Drugs

Amphetamines can cause intracerebral haemorrhage after intravenous, oral or intranasal use. Haemorrhage usually occurs within minutes to a few hours after drug use and in the majority of cases is located in the subcortical white matter of the cerebral hemispheres. In about a half of the reported cases, transient hypertension has been documented and on angiography multifocal areas of spasm and dilation (referred to as 'beading') can sometimes be seen. It has been suggested that this

represents an amphetamine-related vasculitis, although it is possible that it is merely multifocal areas of spasm. Similar angiographic appearances have been reported following the use of other sympathomimetic agents, including ephedrine, pseudoephedrine and phenylpropanolamine. There are a large number of reports associating cocaine with both intracerebral and subarachnoid haemorrhage. They usually occur soon after (often within minutes of) the use of both the alkaloidal form of cocaine and its precipitate form known as 'crack'. Such haemorrhages are most common in the subcortical white matter but occasionally occur in the deeper portions of the hemispheres. On occasions, multiple haemorrhages can occur. Possible mechanisms include vasoconstriction and drug-induced vasculitis. Drug-induced stroke is discussed in more detail in Chapter 11.

There is a significant incidence of underlying cerebral aneurysm or AVM in patients presenting with subarachnoid haemorrhage associated with illicit drug use. Hence, patients with intracranial haemorrhage associated with drug use should still be fully investigated with angiography.

Hyperperfusion syndrome

This relatively rare syndrome is a well-recognized complication of carotid endarterectomy, with an incidence of 1% or less (Ascher *et al.*, 2003). The syndrome has also been described after carotid stenting (McCabe *et al.*, 1999). Patients usually present a few days following operation with a combination of headache, seizures and focal neurological signs. Neuroimaging may show haemorrhage and/or oedema in the carotid artery territory distal to the endarterectomy. Occasionally, patients present with massive intracerebral haemorrhage. The pathogenesis of the condition is poorly understood, but it appears to occur predominantly in individuals who have a haemodynamically compromised cerebral circulation prior to endarterectomy. The majority of such cases have contralateral carotid stenosis or occlusion, and transcranial Doppler or other haemodynamic tests show impaired perfusion reserve. It also appears to be more common in previously hypertensive patients in whom blood pressure is labile and elevated following operation. Rigorous postoperative blood pressure control is believed to reduce its frequency. Imaging studies, which have primarily been performed using transcranial Doppler, have shown increased flow velocities in the ipsilateral middle cerebral artery during the episode. Some studies have suggested that patients at risk can be identified by a rising middle cerebral artery flow velocity postoperatively.

RISK FACTORS (TABLE 8.2)

Hypertension

This is the major risk factor for intracranial haemorrhage. The hypertensive pathological histological changes that lead to haemorrhage are discussed above. *Ageing* may lead to similar changes. The most common locations for such hypertensive haemorrhages are in the basal ganglia, pons, and cerebellum. The risks of haemorrhage are related to the degree and duration of hypertension, rather than acute surges of blood pressure. Hypertension also increases the risk of haemorrhage from AVM and aneurysm.

Malignant hypertension This causes a vasculopathy, characterized physiologically by focal increases in cerebral blood flow secondary to impaired autoregulation and histologically by acute fibrinoid necrosis. Macroscopically, a combination of small petechial cerebral haemorrhages occurs in combination with oedema and focal ischaemic damage. Fibrinoid necrosis may be complicated by frank intracerebral haemorrhage. Neurologically, malignant hypertension may present with the symptoms of hypertensive encephalopathy (e.g. headache, confusion, visual disturbances, seizures, nausea and vomiting). TIAs or ischaemic or haemorrhagic stroke may complicate hypertensive encephalopathy or occur in malignant hypertension without other symptoms (Johnson *et al.*, 1988; Lip *et al.*, 1995). By definition, malignant hypertension is associated with papilloedema

Table 8.2 Risk factors for cerebral haemorrhage

- Hypertension
- Ageing
- Excess alcohol consumption

and there may also be renal involvement. Although the blood pressure is usually very high, malignant hypertension occasionally occurs with only a moderate increase in blood pressure. *Eclampsia* is a similar disorder and accounts for a significant proportion of cases of cerebral haemorrhage associated with pregnancy (Thomas, 1998).

Alcohol

Excessive alcohol intake (>21 units/week) is associated epidemiologically with an increased risk of intracranial haemorrhage. This association is likely to be mediated by a number of pathways, including induction of hypertension, coagulopathy from reduced liver synthesis of clotting factors and impaired platelet function.

CLINICAL PRESENTATION

Before the advent of CT scanning, considerable effort was spent devising scoring systems incorporating clinical features to differentiate between intracerebral haemorrhage and infarction. A degree of success was obtained, but such methods lacked specificity. Clinicians now rely on brain imaging as the only reliable method to distinguish between the two. Nevertheless, certain clinical features suggest intracerebral haemorrhage. If leakage of blood occurs into the subarachnoid space, a very severe headache, often with sudden onset, may occur with vomiting, neck stiffness and other signs of meningism. Even in the absence of subarachnoid blood, headache is more common in intracerebral haemorrhage than infarction. However, haemorrhages that are wholly contained within the brain parenchyma can present entirely without headache. A history of neurological symptoms that progress over minutes or hours, rather than reaching a maximum rapidly, favours a diagnosis of haemorrhage. However, the symptoms of infarction can also progress. Seizures are more frequent in intracerebral haemorrhage, occurring in as many as a quarter of individuals, although they are also seen in about 5% of patients with ischaemia, particularly early after onset. Occasionally, very small haematomas present with symptoms indistinguishable from TIAs. However, the majority of intracerebral haemorrhages cause longer-lasting stroke.

The focal signs and symptoms accompanying intracerebral haemorrhage reflect the location of the haemorrhage and are indistinguishable from ischaemia occurring in the same vascular territory (Kase, 2000). These are summarized in Table 8.3. Lobar haemorrhages frequently produce contralateral weakness or sensory loss, language disturbance, hemianopia or lesser field disorders, and parietal lobe signs. Their relationship to the cortex makes them more likely to be complicated by seizures. Putaminal haemorrhages typically cause contralateral hemiparesis with variable degrees of sensory loss, ataxia and (with larger haematomas) a homonymous hemianopia. Thalamic haemorrhages can result in contralateral sensory loss and weakness, while if they extend to or compress the superior midbrain, they may result in depressed consciousness and midbrain eye movement signs (e.g. loss of upgaze). Pontine haemorrhages often result in reduced consciousness, pinpoint pupils, bilateral weakness and pontine cranial nerve dysfunction, and may be severely disabling.

Cerebellar haemorrhages are particularly important to identify clinically as they may require surgical intervention, which can be life-saving. The onset can be deceptive, with initial non-specific brainstem symptoms (e.g. vertigo or double vision), followed a few hours or even days later by progressive clinical features, including gait, trunk or limb ataxia, nystagmus, headache, vomiting, and coma from brainstem compression. Hemiparesis

and hemiplegia are very rare in cerebellar haemorrhage. The clinical course of cerebellar haemorrhage can be difficult to predict at onset. On occasions, an abrupt deterioration may occur after a period of clinical stability. Obliteration of the ipsilateral quadrigeminal cistern on CT scanning is an early sign of mass effect. If this sign is absent, close clinical observation rather than immediate surgical evacuation may be warranted. Moderate degrees of cisternal compression predicted poor outcome unless the haematoma was evacuated early in the course. Severe mass effect on the quadrigeminal cistern carries a poor prognosis.

INVESTIGATION

CT scanning

This has transformed the diagnosis of acute intracerebral haemorrhage. Blood is easily seen and appears hyperdense on non-contrast-enhanced CT scans. The hyperdense appearance usually remains for 2 weeks or so, after which the haemorrhage becomes isodense. Later CT scans may not be able to distinguish between infarct and haemorrhage. Small haematomas may lose their hyperdense appearance after only a few days.

MRI

This is also very sensitive to intracerebral haemorrhage, providing the appropriate sequences are used. However, interpretation of haemorrhage on images is more complicated than with CT. Following haemorrhage, a series of events occurs that can be detected using MRI; these include initial deoxygenation of the blood within the haemorrhage, its subsequent chemical breakdown from haemoglobin into methaemoglobin, and finally the formation of iron-containing haemosiderin deposits. The time course of events is shown in Table 8.4. The hypointensity seen on T_2-weighted images, resulting from haemosiderin deposition during the chronic stage, can be accentuated by gradient echo MRI, also known as T_2^* imaging

Table 8.3 Clinical features of intracerebral haemorrhage according to anatomical location[a]

Type of intracerebral haemorrhage	Hemiplegia	Hemisensory syndrome	Aphasia	Homonymous visual field defects	Gaze palsy		Brainstem signs
					Horizontal	Vertical	
Putaminal	Generally dense	Frequent	Global > motor > conduction	In larger haematomas	Contralateral	No	No (only present with herniation)
Caudate	Absent or mild transient	Absent	No	No	Generally absent	No	No
Thalamic	Generally dense	Frequent, prominent	Occasional, thalamic variety	In larger haematomas	Contralateral, occasionally ipsilateral	Yes, upward	Skew deviation, Horner's syndrome, Parinaud's syndrome
Lobar	Prominent in fronto-parietal location	Prominent in frontoparietal location	In dominant temporoparietal location	In occipital haematomas	Contralateral in frontal haematomas	No	No (only present with herniation)
Cerebellar	Absent	Absent	No	No	Ipsilateral	No	Ipsilateral 5th- to 7th-nerve palsy, Horner's syndrome
Pontine	Variable, usually bilateral	Variable, usually bilateral	No	No	Bilateral	No	Pinpoint reactive pupils, ocular 'bobbing', decerebrate rigidity, respiratory rhythm abnormalities
Mesencephalic	Variable, usually present	Rare	No	No	No	Occasional, upward	Unilateral or bilateral third-nerve palsy

(Continued)

Table 8.3 (Continued)

Type of intracerebral haemorrhage	Hemiplegia	Hemisensory syndrome	Aphasia	Homonymous visual field defects	Gaze palsy		Brainstem signs
					Horizontal	Vertical	
Medullary	Generally absent	Occasional	No	No	No	No	Nystagmus, ataxia, hiccups, facial hypesthesia, dysarthria, dysphagia, 12th-nerve palsy, Horner's syndrome
Intraventricular	Generally absent	Rare	No	No	Occasional	Occasional	Rare (decerebrate rigidity)

[a]From Kase CS. Intracerebral haemorrhage. In *Neurology in Clinical Practice*, Vol 2. Bradley WG, Daroff RB, Fenichel GM, Marsden CD (eds). Butterworth-Heinemann, Boston, 2000: Table 58B.4.

Table 8.4 Radiographic appearance of intracranial haemorrhage

Duration after haemorrhage	Minutes–hour	Hours–days	Days–week	Weeks	Years
Source of radiographic signal	Extravascular blood	Deoxyhaemoglobin	Intracellular methaemoglobin	Extracellular methaemoglobin	Ferritin/ haemosiderin
Imaging technique:					
CT scan	↑↑	↑↑	↑↑	↑, ↔	↓, ↔
MRI: T_1-weighted	↓, ↔	↓, ↔	↑↑	↑↑	↓, ↔
MRI: T_2-weighted	↑	↑	↓↓	↑↑ + dark rim	↓
MRI: gradient echo	↓	↓↓	↓↓	↓↓	↓↓

CT, computed tomography; MRI, magnetic resonance imaging; ↑ or ↑↑, hyperintense signal; ↓ or ↓↓, hypointense signal; ↔, isointense signal.

(Figure 8.2). This is highly sensitive for detecting even small chronic intracerebral haemorrhages in individuals with diseases (e.g. amyloid angiopathy) (see below). MRI can therefore be used to distinguish between previous cerebral infarction and haemorrhage at a time when the appearances on CT are identical.

Certain radiological features characterize particular underlying causes of intracerebral haemorrhage. An AVM may be seen on MRI as a cluster of vascular channels with flow voids. Cavernous angiomas appear as small areas of high signal on T_2-weighted images surrounded by a ring of low intensity due to haemosiderin deposition. Haemorrhage secondary to tumours can contain complex mixtures of increased and decreased signal related to the presence of viable tumour, necrotic tissue, calcification and haemorrhage occurring at various time points. Cerebral vasculitis may be suggested by the concurrent appearance of both ischaemic and haemorrhagic lesions.

It is important to remember that the presence of recent haemorrhage can obscure underlying structural lesions (e.g. a saccular aneurysm, AVM or tumour). In some instances, particularly for suspected cases of saccular aneurysms, angiography in the acute or subacute phase is indicated. In other cases, particularly for lobar haemorrhage, repeat neuroimaging should be performed 2–3 months following the acute event.

Angiography

This is an important investigation in cerebral haemorrhage to exclude a treatable source of recurrence. The yield of conventional catheter angiography in patients with spontaneous intracerebral haemorrhage was examined in a prospective study of 206 cases in Hong Kong (Zhu et al., 1997). The frequencies of positive findings on angiography for haemorrhages occurring at different locations are shown in Table 8.5. The angiographic yield was highest for lobar intracerebral haemorrhages. Age and pre-existing hypertension were both found to be independent predictors of angiographic yield. In patients below 45 years of age the angiographic yield was 48% in putaminal, thalamic or posterior fossa intracerebral haemorrhage and 65% in lobar intracerebral haemorrhage. In older hypertensive patients, the yields were 0 and 10% respectively. However, in patients with isolated intraventricular haemorrhage, without widespread subarachnoid blood, the yield was high in both young individuals and old individuals (67% versus 63%) and most individuals were normotensive. In general, therefore, delayed angiography is indicated in all young patients with intracerebral haemorrhage and in selected older patients with lobar or intraventricular haemorrhage.

The presence of multiple haemorrhages on neuroimaging may give important diagnostic

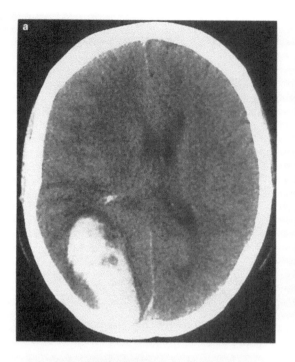

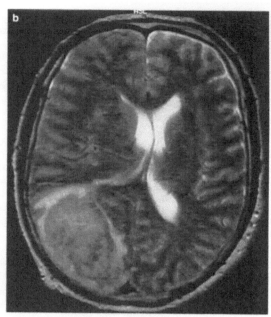

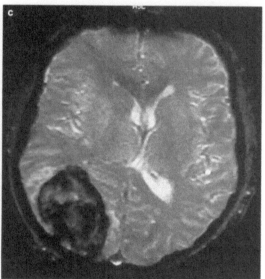

Figure 8.2   Appearances of an acute lobar intracerebral haemorrhage on (a) CT, (b) T_2-weighted MRI and (c) T_2^* gradient echo MRI.

clues (Table 8.6). Multiple haemorrhages of different sizes restricted to the lobar regions and grey–white matter junction should raise the possibility of amyloid angiopathy, particularly in elderly individuals without other known causes of intracerebral haemorrhage. Other important causes of multiple haemorrhage include metastatic tumours, coagulopathies from haematological disorders or therapy, vasculitis, and haemorrhage due to drug abuse. In the last two causes, regions of haemorrhage may accompany separate regions of infarction.

Table 8.5 Angiographic findings for various sites of intracerebral haemorrhage[a]

Site	No.	AVM	Aneurysm	Moyamoya disease	Sinus thrombosis	Angiographic yield
Lobar	90	30	7	2	5	44 (49%)
Putaminal	42	1	1			2 (5%)
Thalamic	33	4		2		6 (18%)
Caudate	4		1			1 (25%)
Intraventricular	17	10	1			11 (65%)
Cerebellar	15	5				5 (33%)
Brainstem	3	1				1 (33%)
Subdural[b]	2	1				1 (50%)
Total (206)	206	52	10	4	5	71 (35%)

[a]Modified from Zhu XL *et al. Stroke* 1997;**28**:1406–1409.
[b]Acute subdural haemorrhage.

Table 8.6 Causes of multiple intracerebral haemorrhages

- Amyloid angiopathy
- Metastases:
  - Melanoma
  - Bronchogenic carcinoma
  - Choriocarcinoma
  - Renal carcinoma
- Cerebral venous thrombosis
- Thrombolytic therapy
- Haematological disorders
- Haemostatic disorders and leukaemia
- Disseminated intravascular coagulation
- Head injury
- Cerebral vasculitis

TREATMENT

Neurological damage caused by intracerebral haemorrhage results both from local damage from the haematoma and from more generalized effects on intracranial pressure and cerebral perfusion. Neuroprotective agents might reduce direct tissue damage from the haematoma, but none has yet been shown to be effective. Acute treatment for intracerebral haemorrhage has therefore focused primarily on limiting the effects of increased intracranial pressure on brain tissue. Approaches that have been advocated include both aggressive medical interventions and surgery. There have been few controlled trials in this area and, perhaps because of this, clinical practice varies widely between different countries and different units.

MEDICAL MANAGEMENT

Initial management should be directed towards ensuring an adequate airway and ventilation as well as clinical evaluation. In particular, attention should be given to detecting signs of external trauma. General medical measures appropriate to any stroke patient (e.g. assessment of swallowing and early mobilization) are discussed in Chapter 16.

In 1995, over 500 randomized clinical trials were complete or ongoing for acute stroke and 78 for subarachnoid haemorrhage, but there had only been 4 small randomized surgical trials and 4 small medical trials in intracerebral haemorrhage. The four medical trials examined steroid versus placebo therapy, haemodilution versus medical therapy, and glycerol versus placebo. None of these four studies showed any significant benefit for the three therapies but all were likely to be under powered.

One area where management is unclear is in optimal blood pressure control. In general, recommendations for the treatment of elevated blood pressure in patients with intracerebral haemorrhage are more aggressive than for patients with ischaemic stroke. The theoretical rationale for this is that lowering blood pressure will decrease the risk of ongoing bleeding. However, overaggressive treatment of blood pressure may decrease the cerebral perfusion pressure and therefore theoretically worsen brain injury. It has been suggested that anti-hypertensive agents with a vasodilator action (e.g. glyceryl trinitrate) may themselves increase intracranial pressure. American guidelines suggest medical therapy if the systolic blood pressure is greater than 180 mmHg and the diastolic blood pressure is greater than 105 mmHg, or if the mean arterial pressure is greater than 130 mmHg on two readings separated by 20 minutes (Broderick *et al.*, 1999). However, these guidelines need to be tested in a randomized clinical trial.

Raised intracranial pressure is one of the major consequences of intracerebral haemorrhage and great efforts have been put into developing optimal regimens for its control. Again these have not been tested in clinical trials. Hyperventilation can be used to reduce intracranial pressure, but it will also reduce cerebral blood flow and therefore should be used only as an interim measure. Osmotic agents, including glycerol, mannitol and urea, extract water from the extracellular into the intravascular compartment of the brain and reduce intracranial pressure temporarily. There is no firm evidence that these drugs have benefit in intracerebral haemorrhage, but they are widely used in many centres. Mannitol 20% (0.25–0.5 g/kg every 4 hours) is one popular regimen. It has been suggested this should be given to patients with progressively increasing intracranial pressure values, or clinical deterioration associated with mass effect. To maintain an osmotic gradient, furosemide may be administered simultaneously. Serum osmolality should be measured twice daily in patients receiving osmotherapy and targeted to 310 mOsm/l. Intracranial pressure monitoring can guide treatment, but its use varies widely between centres – some

authorities recommend it for patients with suspected elevated intracranial pressure and reduced consciousness, while others base management on clinical and radiological measures alone.

A recent randomized trial has shown that treatment of intracerebral haemorrhage within 3 hours of onset with recombinant activated factor VII reduced early haematoma growth and improved outcome (Mayer *et al.*, 2005). There was a small increase in the rate of thromboembolic events and the treatment is therefore being tested in larger phase 3 trials.

SURGICAL TREATMENT

Theoretical potential benefits of surgical intervention include removal of clot, reduction in intracranial pressure, relief of hydrocephalus, and early treatment of underlying causes (e.g. arteriovenous malformations and saccular aneurysms). It is generally accepted that surgical removal of cerebellar haematoma can be life-saving. Patients often make a good recovery even from deep coma after evacuation of an acute cerebellar haematoma, because of relief of the associated brainstem compression. Approaches include operating only in patients with neurological decline, or trying to select out individuals who may be at high risk of neurological decline, in whom a prophylactic approach may be beneficial (Taneda *et al.*, 1987). For example, some neurosurgeons suggest operation in patients with haematomas greater than 3 cm in diameter, even if those patients are fully alert. Ventricular shunting may also be used to relieve hydrocephalus, but a shunt will not relieve the direct effect of the haematoma on the brainstem, and therefore additional clot evacuation is usually recommended. The benefits of evacuation of supratentorial haematoma are much less clear.

A number of surgical approaches have been used for haematoma evacuation for supratentorial haemorrhage. These include simple aspiration, open surgery, endoscopic evacuation and stereotactic aspiration. Simple aspiration was attempted in the 1950s, but only

Table 8.7   Recommendations for surgical treatment of intracerebral haemorrhage[a]

Non-surgical candidates
- Patients with small haemorrhages (<10 cm³) or minimal neurological deficits
- Patients with a Glasgow Coma Scale (GCS) score <4. However, patients with a GCS score <4 who have a cerebellar haemorrhage with brainstem compression may still be candidates for life-saving surgery in certain clinical situations

Surgical candidates
- Patients with cerebellar haemorrhage >3 cm who are neurologically deteriorating or who have brainstem compression and hydrocephalus from ventricular obstruction should have surgical removal of the haemorrhage as soon as possible
- Intracerebral haemorrhage associated with a structural lesion (e.g. an aneurysm, arteriovenous malformation or cavernous angioma) may be removed if the patient has a chance for a good outcome and the structural vascular lesion is surgically accessible
- Young patients with a moderate or large lobar haemorrhage who are clinically deteriorating

Best therapy unclear
- All other patients

[a]From Broderick JP *et al. Stroke* 1999;**30**:905–915.

allowed small amounts of clot to be removed and therefore was abandoned. The other approaches have been used by a number of centres, but there have only been five small completed randomized studies. The only firm conclusion that can be drawn from such studies is that the results from large multicentre trials are needed. One such trial, the International Surgical Trial in Intracerebral Haemorrhage (STICH), found that there was no benefit to neurosurgical evacuation of spontaneous cerebral haematoma in patients whom the randomizing surgeon was uncertain at the time whether surgery or medical treatment alone was the best option (Mendelow *et al.*, 2005). There is therefore little evidence for the benefit of neurosurgical evacuation in any group of patients, although there remains a strong view that some patients require surgical treatment. No firm conclusions about the efficacy of surgery in such patients can currently be drawn, and different centres have to develop their own clinical guidelines. The recommendations from an American committee drawn up before the results of STICH were available are shown in Table 8.7. Other authorities may suggest more conservative or more aggressive approaches.

The specific treatment of aneurysms and AVMs to prevent recurrent haemorrhage is discussed in Chapter 9.

PROGNOSIS

The overall prognosis of intracerebral haemorrhage is poor. In community-based studies, about 50% of patients are dead by 1 month after the onset, with half of these deaths occurring within the first 2 days. Only about 10% are able to live independently at 1 month and only 20% are independent at 6 months. At 1 year, only about 30% of patients are still alive, and of the survivors, a third remain dependent on others (Bamford *et al.*, 1990).

KEY REFERENCES

Arteriovenous malformations

Ruiz-Sandoval JL, Cantu C, Barinagarrementeria F. Intracerebral hemorrhage in young people: analysis of risk factors, location, causes, and prognosis. *Stroke* 1999;**30**:537–541

Stapf C, Labovitz DL, Sciacca RR et al. Incidence of adult brain arteriovenous malformation hemorrhage in a prospective population-based stroke survey. *Cerebrovasc Dis* 2002;**13**:43–46

Cavernous angiomas

Requena I, Arias M, Lopez-Ibor L et al. Cavenomas of the central nervous system: clinical and neuroimaging manifestations in 47 patients. *J Neurol Neurosurg Psychiatry* 1991;**54**:590–594

Vogler R, Castillo M. Dural cavernous angiomas: MR features. *AJNR Am J Neuroradiol* 1995;**16**:773–775

Lipohyalinosis and microaneurysms

Challa VR, Moody DM, Bell MA. The Charcôt–Bouchard aneurysm controversy: impact of a new histologic technique. *J Neuropathol Exp Neurol* 1992;**51**:264–271

Lammie GA. Hypertensive cerebral small vessel disease and stroke. *Brain Pathol* 2002;**12**:358–370

Takebayashi S, Kaneko M. Electron microscopic studies of ruptured arteries in hypertensive intracerebral haemorrhage. *Stroke* 1983;**14**:28–36

Cerebral amyloid angiopathy

Revesz T, Ghiso J, Lashley T et al. Cerebral amyloid angiopathies: a pathologic, biochemical, and genetic view. *J Neuropath Exp Neurol* 2003;**62**:885–898

Yamada M. Cerebral amyloid angiopathy: an overview. *Neuropathology* 2000;**20**:8–22

Oral anticoagulants

Franke CL, de Jonge J, van Swieten JC et al. Intracerebral hematomas during anticoagulant treatment. *Stroke* 1990;**21**:726–730

Hylek EM, Singer DE. Risk factors for intracranial haemorrhage in outpatients taking warfarin. *Ann Intern Med* 1994;**120**:897–902

Palareti G, Leali N, Coccheri S et al. Bleeding complications of oral anticoagulant treatment: an inception-cohort, prospective collaborative study (ISCOAT). *Lancet* 1996;**348**:423–428

Sjalander A, Engstrom G, Berntorp E, Svensson P. Risk of haemorrhagic stroke in patients with oral anticoagulation compared with the general population. *J Intern Med* 2003;**254**:434–438

Smith EE, Rosand J, Knudsen KA et al. Leukoaraiosis is associated with warfarin-related hemorrhage

following ischemic stroke. *Neurology* 2002;**59**:193–197

SPIRIT: Stroke Prevention in Reversible Ischaemia Trial Study Group. A randomized trial of anticoagulants versus aspirin after cerebral ischaemia of presumed arterial origin. *Ann Neurol* 1997;**42**:857–865

Antiplatelet agents

Antithrombotic Trialists' Collaboration. Collaborative meta-analysis of randomised trials of antiplatelet therapy for prevention of death, myocardial infarction, and stroke in high risk patients. *BMJ* 2002;**324**:71–86

Diener H-C, Bogousslavsky J, Brass LM et al. Aspirin and clopidogrel compared with clopidogrel alone after recent ischaemic stroke or transient ischaemic attack in high-risk patients (MATCH): randomised, double-blind, placebo-controlled trial. *Lancet* 2004;**364**:331–337

Thrombolytic agents

Berger C, Fiorelli M, Steiner T et al. Hemorrhagic transformation of ischemic brain tissue – asymptomatic or symptomatic? *Stroke* 2001;**32**:1330–1335

Kase CS. Cerebral hemorrhage after intra-arterial thrombolysis for ischemic stroke. The PROACT II Trial. *Neurology* 2001;**57**:1603–1610

Larrue V, von Kummer R, Muller A, Bluhmki E. Risk factors for severe hemorrhagic transformation in ischemic stroke patients treated with recombinant tissue plasminogen activator – a secondary analysis of the European–Australasian Acute Stroke Study (ECASS II). *Stroke* 2001;**32**:438–441

NINDS t-PA Stroke Study Group. Intracerebral hemorrhage after intravenous t-PA therapy for ischemic stroke. *Stroke* 1997;**28**:2109–2118

Hyperperfusion syndrome

Ascher E, Markevich N, Schutzer RW et al. Cerebral hyperperfusion syndrome after carotid endarterectomy: predictive factors and hemodynamic changes. *J Vasc Surg* 2003;**37**:769–777

McCabe DJ, Brown MM, Clifton A. Fatal cerebral reperfusion hemorrhage after carotid stenting. *Stroke* 1999;**30**:2483–2486

Malignant hypertension and eclampsia

Johnson K, Aitchison F, Beevers DG. Cerebellar infarction as a complication of malignant hypertension. *J Hum Hypertens* 1998;**12**:569–570

Lip GY, Beevers M, Beevers DG. Complications and survival of 315 patients with malignant-phase hypertension. *J Hum Hypertens* 1995;**13**:915–924

Thomas SV. Neurological aspects of eclampsia. *Neurol Sci* 1998;**18**:37–43

Clinical presentation

Kase CS. Intracerebral haemorrhage. In *Neurology in Clinical Practice*, Vol 2. Bradley WG, Daroff RB, Fenichel GM, Marsden CD (eds). Butterworth-Heinemann, Boston, 2000

Angiography

Zhu XL, Chan MSY, Poon WS. Spontaneous intracranial hemorrhage: Which patients need diagnostic cerebral angiography? A prospective study of 206 cases and review of the literature *Stroke* 1997;**28**:1406–1409

Medical management

Broderick JP, Adams Jr HP, Barsan W et al. Guidelines for the management of spontaneous intracerebral hemorrhage. A statement for healthcare professionals from a special writing group of the Stroke Council, American Heart Association. *Stroke* 1999;**30**:905–915

Mayer SA, Brun NC, Begtrup K et al. Recombinant activated factor VII for acute intracerebral hemorrhage. *N Engl J Med* 2005;**352**:777–785

Surgical treatment

Mendelow AD, Gregson BA, Fernandes HM et al. Early surgery versus initial conservative treatment in patients with spontaneous supratentorial intracerebral haematomas in the International Surgical Trial in Intracerebral Haemorrhage (STICH): a randomised trial. *Lancet* 2005;**365**: 387–397

Taneda M, Hayakawa T, Mogami H. Primary cerebellar haemorrhage: quadrigeminal cistern obliteration on CT scans as a predictor of outcome. *J Neurosurg* 1987;**67**:545–552

Prognosis

Bamford J, Sandercock P, Dennis M et al. A prospective study of acute cerebrovascular disease in the community: the Oxfordshire Community Stroke Project – 1981–86. 2. Incidence, case fatality rates and overall outcome at one year of cerebral infarction, primary intracerebral and subarachnoid haemorrhage. *J Neurol Neurosurg Psychiatry* 1990;**53**:16–22

CHAPTER 9

Subarachnoid Haemorrhage

Subarachnoid haemorrhage accounts for about 5% of stroke in all age groups combined, but is a more important cause in young patients, accounting for nearly 50% of stroke under the age of 45. The mortality of subarachnoid haemorrhage at 1 month is about 50%, which is much higher than in patients with cerebral infarction, but similar to the mortality of cerebral haemorrhage. Of the survivors, about a quarter have residual disability at 1 year and are dependant on others, but many of those that are independent have some intellectual impairment. Untreated, there is a very high risk of recurrent bleeding, but early neurosurgical treatment improves the prognosis considerably. Subarachnoid haemorrhage is also the only cause of stroke in which putative neuroprotective drug treatment with nimodipine has been shown to improve the outcome. Early diagnosis and treatment are therefore particularly important.

CAUSES

Subarachnoid haemorrhage is defined as bleeding beneath the arachnoid pia lining the surface of the brain. About 85% of subarachnoid haemorrhages are caused by ruptured saccular (berry) aneurysms, 10% are idiopathic, and the remainder result from arteriovenous malformations and rarer causes (Table 9.1). Risk factors include hypertension, smoking and heavy alcohol intake (Table 9.2) (Broderick *et al.*, 2003). Whether these risk factors cause cerebral aneurysm or simply increase the risk of an existing aneurysm rupturing is uncertain. The individual causes are discussed in more detail in the section on treatment later in this chapter.

Table 9.1 Causes of subarachnoid haemorrhage

Abnormal blood vessels
- Saccular aneurysm
- Arteriovenous malformation
- Dural arteriovenous fistula
- Mycotic aneurysm
- Intracranial dissection
- Vasculitis
- Spinal arteriovenous malformation
- Anterior spinal artery aneurysm
- Tumours
- Moyamoya disease
- Sickle cell disease

Bleeding diathesis
- Haemophilia
- Thrombocytopenia
- Warfarin therapy
- Thrombolytic therapy
- Antiplatelet therapy
- Drug abuse
- Trauma
- Idiopathic

CLINICAL PRESENTATION

Symptoms

In subarachnoid haemorrhage, the bleeding occurs into the cerebrospinal fluid (CSF) space

Table 9.2 Risk factors for subarachnoid haemorrhage

- Hypertension
- Smoking
- Alcohol

beneath the arachnoid pia and the blood therefore rapidly spreads throughout the CSF spaces. Many patients die suddenly, but in about half of the cases, the bleeding stops for long enough to allow the patient to get to medical attention. In survivors, the symptoms and signs of subarachnoid haemorrhage arise as a result of:

- Meningeal irritation
- Vascular spasm (leading to ischaemia)
- Raised intracranial pressure from the sudden increase in intracranial volume, or later from hydrocephalus
- Focal symptoms (headache, confusion, coma)

The clinical presentation of subarachnoid haemorrhage with severe generalized headache is characteristic. The headache is usually the most severe that the patient has ever had. The onset is so sudden that the patient may think they had been kicked or hit on the head from behind and can time the onset exactly. There is often vomiting and photophobia. The patient may also complain of neck stiffness, which may be delayed for several hours. Not infrequently, the bleed occurs during exertion, particularly sexual intercourse.

In severe cases, there is loss of consciousness at the onset of the bleed, followed by a rapid decline so that the patient succumbs soon after onset. If the bleed has been small, consciousness may recover within a few minutes, or the patient may remain drowsy or confused. About 50% of patients presenting to hospital have a history of loss of consciousness soon after onset.

The history of headache may not be obtained if the patient is drowsy or confused, and occasionally the headache is relatively mild. In addition, neck stiffness may not always develop.

The diagnosis can then be missed. It is therefore important to consider subarachnoid haemorrhage in the differential diagnosis of confusion and coma or any headache of sudden onset.

Sentinel headache A number of patients with established aneurysmal subarachnoid haemorrhage give a history of previous episodes of less severe headache (Linn *et al.*, 1994). These headaches usually last several days and in retrospect have the typical features of subarachnoid haemorrhage described above, suggesting that they are the result of small leaks from the aneurysm. Alternatively, in some cases, the headache may be caused by enlargement of the aneurysm. However, most patients with subarachnoid haemorrhage present without warning with severe symptoms of their first bleed.

Spinal subarachnoid haemorrhage Very rarely, subarachnoid haemorrhage occurs from a vessel in the spinal cord, usually from a spinal arteriovenous malformation (AVM) or less often from an aneurysm of the anterior spinal artery. In this case, headache may be absent or less prominent than usual and there may be additional back pain at the site of haemorrhage.

Differential diagnosis Differential diagnoses of severe sudden-onset headache mimicking subarachnoid haemorrhage may include:

- Meningitis
- Migraine
- Coital headache
- Exertional headache
- Benign thunderclap headache

Meningitis is the only other of these common conditions in which neck stiffness occurs, but the headache in meningitis is more gradual in onset and is accompanied by fever, which is usually absent in uncomplicated subarachnoid haemorrhage. Neck stiffness is usually absent in the other varieties of acute headache listed above, but the first attack of these conditions may be indistinguishable from subarachnoid haemorrhage. If there is any doubt the patient should be admitted for computed tomography (CT) and lumbar puncture (see below).

Clinical signs

The cardinal sign of subarachnoid haemorrhage is the presence of severe neck stiffness. This is usually such severe boardlike rigidity of the neck that the patient's head cannot be flexed more than a few centimetres off the bed. In contrast, rotation of the neck is relatively normal. Kernig's sign (limited straight leg raising) may also be present, but is a less reliable sign. In some bleeds, the neck stiffness may be less severe or never present at any time. Neck stiffness may also be absent if the patient is in deep coma. The accompanying raised intracranial pressure may lead to confusion, delirium, drowsiness or coma.

Focal neurological signs are usually absent at the presentation of subarachnoid haemorrhage, unless there has also been bleeding into the substance of the brain or compression of cranial nerves. In this case, the following focal deficits will help to diagnose the cause:

- Hemiparesis, dysphasia or parietal lobe deficits suggest that the bleed has occurred from a middle cerebral artery aneurysm associated with a haematoma within the middle cerebral artery territory.
- An ipsilateral third-nerve palsy suggests haemorrhage from an internal carotid aneurysm at the junction with the posterior communicating artery. The third-nerve palsy results from compression of the third nerve by the enlarging aneurysm (see below).
- Brainstem signs or bulbar cranial nerve palsies suggest a posterior fossa aneurysm or intracranial vertebral artery dissection (see below).
- Paraparesis with subarachnoid haemorrhage is very rare, but if present suggests a bleed from a spinal AVM or aneurysm. If there are no sensory signs, the paraparesis could also be the result of a bifrontal haematoma from an anterior communicating artery aneurysm.

Cranial bruit This sound, heard using a stethoscope over the skull or orbits, suggests a large AVM with increased flow within the malformation. There may also be audible bruits over the carotid arteries if there is considerable shunting of blood from the arterial to the venous side of the circulation. Most patients with AVM do not have audible bruits.

Subhyaloid haemorrhage This may be seen as a round haemorrhage in one or both optic fundi in patients with large subarachnoid haemorrhages.

Papilloedema This may develop within a day or two after onset because of persistent raised intracranial pressure or hydrocephalus.

Grading It is usual in neurosurgical practice to grade the severity of subarachnoid haemorrhage according to the conscious state of the patient and the presence or absence of focal motor deficit. One of the most widely used scales in the past was described by Hunt and Hess in 1968, but this has largely been replaced by the World Federation of Neurological Surgeons Scale (WFNS) (Table 9.3).

INVESTIGATION

Patients with suspected subarachnoid haemorrhage should be admitted and investigated in hospital as an emergency (Figure 9.1). CT should be carried out without delay and shows subarachnoid blood in 80–90% of cases scanned within 24 hours (Figure 9.2). If the bleed has occurred from an aneurysm, the location of the densest haemorrhage may provide a clue to the site of the haemorrhage:

- Blood situated predominantly in the frontal interhemispheric fissure suggests an anterior communicating artery aneurysm
- Blood predominantly in the Sylvian fissure suggests a middle cerebral artery aneurysm
- Blood predominantly in the suprasellar cistern on one side suggests an internal carotid

Table 9.3 World Federation of Neurological Surgeons Scale (WFNS) for grading the severity of subarachnoid haemorrhage

WFNS grade	Glasgow Coma Scale (GCS) Score	Focal deficit
I	15	Absent
II	13–14	Absent
III	13–14	Present
IV	7–12	Present or absent
V	3–6	Present or absent

aneurysm at the junction with the posterior communicating artery
• Blood predominantly in the basal cisterns suggests a basilar aneurysm

Occasionally, a large aneurysm may be visible on CT. An AVM may also be visible on the initial scan or may be suspected because of the presence of a large draining vein if contrast is given. AVMs are sometimes associated with some atrophy of the adjacent cortex, which may help to distinguish them from other mass lesions on CT. In most cases, the source of

bleeding will not be evident on CT. MRI is more sensitive, particularly if combined with magnetic resonance angiography (MRA).

A diagnostic CT saves the need for lumbar puncture, which may be hazardous if there is raised intracranial pressure. If the CT is normal or if CT is not available (and there is no evidence of raised intracranial pressure or mass lesion), a lumbar puncture should be carried out. In subarachnoid haemorrhage, the CSF is usually uniformly blood-stained, with a similar appearance in successive collection bottles. The white cell count will also be raised, but the ratio of white to red cells in the CSF should be identical to that of blood, i.e. approximately 1:1000, in contrast to meningitis, where the ratio will be increased. If the blood has been present for more than a few hours, it will have haemolysed, which helps to distinguish subarachnoid haemorrhage from a traumatic tap. Haemolysis leads to xanthochromia, which can be detected as a yellow tinge in the supernatant of the CSF if it is left to stand or by spectrophotometry in the laboratory. Xanthochromia may not be present for several hours after subarachnoid haemorrhage and, if appropriate, lumbar puncture

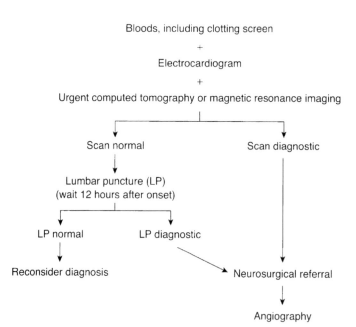

Figure 9.1 Investigation of suspected subarachnoid haemorrhage.

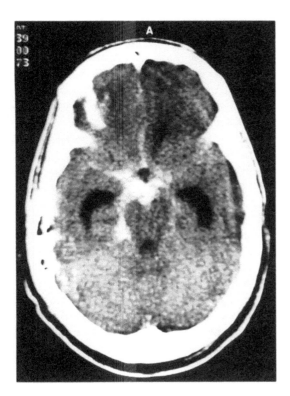

Figure 9.2 CT scan showing diffuse subarachnoid blood filling the basal cisterns.

that all patients with subarachnoid haemorrhage have a clotting screen to identify those with haemophilia and other bleeding disorders. The further investigation of confirmed subarachnoid haemorrhage requires referral to a specialist unit with neurosurgical facilities. Four-vessel cerebral angiography with views of the intracranial circulation of the carotid and vertebral arteries, including the external carotid circulation, is required to identify intracerebral aneurysm, AVM and dural arteriovenous fistula. Many of these are not seen on CT or MRI. Patients in whom an aneurysm in one arterial territory is discovered will require injections of the other arterial territories to exclude additional aneurysms, since they may be multiple. If there is more than one aneurysm, it can be difficult to tell which has bled, although the site of haemorrhage on CT and the presence of spasm adjacent to one aneurysm on angiography may be helpful. If an AVM is found, injections of all the cervical vessels, including the external carotid circulation, will be required to identify all the feeding vessels. Spasm in the acute stages may obscure an aneurysm, and normal angiography should be repeated 6 weeks after the onset of the subarachnoid haemorrhage to be certain that an aneurysm has not been missed.

should be postponed until 12 hours after the onset of symptoms. CT may only show subarachnoid blood for 1 or 2 days and lumbar puncture may only show blood for a few days after the ictus. However, xanthochromia detected by spectrophotometry is present for 2 weeks or longer. Some patients present, or are referred, with a history very suggestive of subarachnoid haemorrhage some weeks after onset. In these cases, if lumbar puncture with spectrophotometry and CT or MRI are normal, it may be necessary to carry out cerebral angiography to exclude an aneurysm or AVM. However, if CT and lumbar puncture are normal within 2 weeks of onset, the chances of the patient having had a subarachnoid haemorrhage are extremely small and there is no need to investigate further.

Apart from the routine blood tests to investigate stroke (see Table 2.6, p. 22), it is essential

COMPLICATIONS OF SUBARACHNOID HAEMORRHAGE (TABLE 9.4)

Rebleeding

The major hazard of subarachnoid haemorrhage is recurrent haemorrhage. This is much more likely if there is an underlying aneurysm or AVM than if no cause is found for the bleed. In aneurysm, the chances of a further haemorrhage are greatest in the first few weeks after onset. Studies before surgery was generally adopted suggested that about 50% of patients rebleed within a month (Winn *et al.*, 1977, 1978). Thereafter, the risk of rebleeding declines and tapers off to a rate of about 3% per annum in untreated patients (Figure 9.3). Seventy per cent of rebleeds are fatal.

Table 9.4 Complications of aneurysmal sub-arachnoid haemorrhage

Neurological
- Intracerebral haemorrhage
- Intraventricular haemorrhage
- Rebleeding
- Vasospasm
- Epilepsy
- Hydrocephalus
- Cerebral oedema

Cardiac
- Electrocardiogram changes
- Myocardial infarction
- Neurogenic pulmonary oedema

Endocrine
- Electrolyte disturbance
- Syndrome of inappropriate secretion of antidiuretic hormone (SIADH)
- Diabetes insipidus

Vasospasm

Subarachnoid blood irritates the arteries on the surface of the brain, causing vasospasm (i.e. excessive contraction of blood vessels). This may be localized to the artery that has bled or may be more generalized and seen on angiography as regions of focal constriction of one or more arteries. The exact component of blood that causes vasospasm is unknown. Vasospasm leads to a reduction in cerebral blood flow beyond the area of spasm, which may result in ischaemia and infarction. Angiographic vasospasm is found in as many as two-thirds of patients in the second week after the onset of subarachnoid haemorrhage, but only leads to cerebral symptoms in half this number. Diffuse ischaemia is responsible for persistence of confusion and coma after the initial bleed, whereas infarction causes the symptoms and signs of ischaemic stroke within the territory of the spasm. Although symptomatic spasm may be present from the onset of bleeding, it is uncommon within the first 2 days, reaches a maximum from 7–10 days after onset and then resolves after 2 weeks. Delayed ischaemia resulting from vasospasm is the major cause of disability in survivors of subarachnoid haemorrhage.

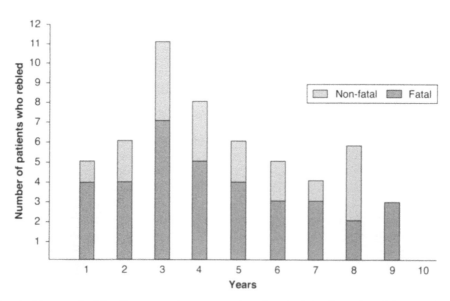

Figure 9.3 Incidence of rebleeding more than 6 months after initial subarachnoid haemorrhage in 213 patients with untreated cerebral aneurysms. Adapted from Winn *et al. Ann Neurol* 1977;**1**:358–370.

Transcranial Doppler measurement of flow velocity in the major intracerebral arteries can be useful to suggest the diagnosis of vasospasm in patients with aneurysmal subarachnoid haemorrhage (Sloan, 1995). Vasospasm leads to an increase in flow velocity across the area of vasoconstriction, and a middle cerebral artery velocity of over 200 cm/s is highly suggestive of vasospasm. Whether the identification of such stenoses by transcranial Doppler alters outcome has not been determined in a large controlled trial.

Neuropsychological damage

Subarachnoid haemorrhage from anterior communicating artery aneurysm is frequently followed by a syndrome of frontal neuropsychological damage because there is often ischaemia from spasm within both anterior cerebral arteries. Such patients have normal speech and limb function, but tend not to initiate activities or conversation. In severe cases of this syndrome, the patient suffers from a complete lack of initiative and drive (abulia) and may sit in a chair all day doing very little. These patients may be thought to have made a good recovery if they are not examined cognitively because they have no physical disability, but they often have difficulty returning to normal activities. Frequently, lesser disturbances in personality and mood are only detected on direct questioning of the patient's partner or relatives.

Epilepsy

This complicates about 10% of cases, usually as generalized seizures occurring on the first day. Less frequently, epilepsy occurs as a late complication.

Cardiac ischaemia

Subarachnoid haemorrhage is often associated with marked abnormalities on the electrocardiogram. The commonest is acute ST segment elevation, which may mimic acute myocardial infarction.

Neurogenic pulmonary oedema

This is a peculiar complication of subarachnoid haemorrhage, which is unexplained but can occur very rapidly in an otherwise stable patient.

Electrolyte disturbances

These disturbances, particularly a low sodium concentration and the syndrome of inappropriate secretion of antidiuretic hormone (SIADH), are common.

Intraventricular haemorrhage

This can occur at the time of aneurysm rupture and is associated with a poor prognosis.

Hydrocephalus

This can occur in the acute stages from clot obstructing the flow of CSF or as a late complication from obstruction to the absorption of CSF in the arachnoid villa. It should be suspected if the patient fails to improve after the acute stages or deteriorates after initial improvement. Occasionally, the syndrome of communicating or normal-pressure hydrocephalus develops many years after subarachnoid haemorrhage. The development of hydrocephalus may be an indication for therapeutic lumbar puncture or neurosurgical drainage.

Cerebral oedema

This may develop either as a result of ischaemia or in the postoperative patient from a failure of autoregulation.

Deterioration in conscious level

This may result from any of the above complications, and will require urgent re-investigation with scanning, blood gases, electrolyte measurement and chest X-ray.

TREATMENT

General measures

Careful attention to fluid balance, avoiding dehydration, is essential, together with routine care of the airway and pressure areas, and attention to swallowing assessment. Hypoxia should be avoided as it will compound any cerebral ischaemia. The patient may require admission to an intensive care unit and ventilation. Headache should be treated with analgesics (e.g. codeine) and vomiting prevented with an antiemetic (e.g. prochlorperazine). These drugs may adversely affect conscious level or alter neurological signs (e.g. mydriasis with codeine) and should be used with caution.

Neuroprotective therapy

The aim of treatment is to prevent rebleeding, cerebral ischaemia and other complications. Subarachnoid haemorrhage was the first cause of stroke in which treatment with a putative neuroprotective agent, the calcium antagonist nimodipine, was shown to be effective in reducing long-term disability. In the British Aneurysm Trial, oral nimodipine was given within 96 hours of onset of subarachnoid haemorrhage and was continued for 21 days (Pickard *et al.*, 1989). The relative incidence of cerebral infarction was significantly reduced by 34%, from 33% on placebo to 22% with nimodipine treatment. The number of patients with a poor outcome (death, vegetative state or severe disability) was reduced by a similar degree. Nimodipine does not have any benefit in established cerebral infarction, perhaps because of the adverse effect of a slight reduction in blood pressure. The mode of action of nimodipine is therefore uncertain, but it may work because the drug can be given in subarachnoid haemorrhage before the development of cerebral ischaemia, which is usually secondary to vasospasm. Alternatively, nimodipine may have a direct action on the mechanisms of vasospasm. In either case, nimodipine should be given as soon as the diagnosis has been confirmed.

Blood pressure

Subarachnoid haemorrhage is one of the few conditions in which bed rest is still recommended, because of concern that activity might precipitate rebleeding. Systemic blood pressure tends to rise in the acute stages, and hypertension is probably an adaptive response to vasospasm. Treatment with antihypertensive therapy should therefore be avoided because of concern that a reduction in blood pressure will increase the risk of ischaemia related to vasospasm, unless the blood pressure is very high (greater than 200/120 mmHg). Above this level, there will be more concern about the risk of rebleeding, and the blood pressure should be lowered cautiously.

Vasospasm

In patients who develop a focal deficit associated with vasospasm, allowing the blood pressure to rise spontaneously or treating with pressor agents (hyperdynamic treatment) may reverse the deficit and can be safely applied if an aneurysm has already been clipped. Hypervolaemic treatment using infusions of isotonic electrolyte solutions to expand the intravascular volume is also used to prevent and treat the ischaemic complications of vasospasm. Associated haemodilution may have additional rheological benefits. Admission to an intensive care unit may be necessary to monitor the effects of these treatments on the circulation. The combined use of hypervolaemic, hyperdynamic and haemodilution techniques is known as HHH therapy. Balloon angioplasty can be used to dilate focal areas of spasm in patients in whom other measures fail, but remains an experimental treatment.

Hydrocephalus

Acute hydrocephalus may require urgent ventricular shunting or repeated lumbar puncture.

Treatment after the patient has had the initial assessment and stabilization depends on the cause identified on investigation, as described in the following section.

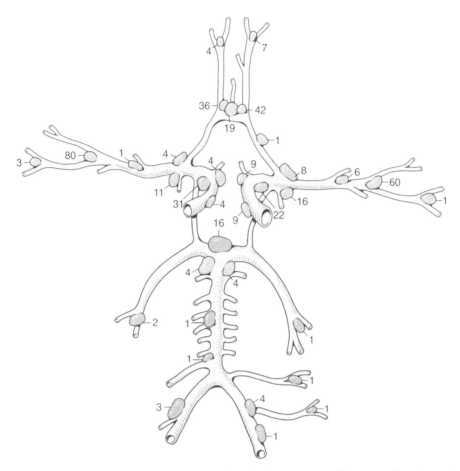

Figure 9.4 Diagram illustrating the common sites of cerebral aneurysms. The numerals indicate the number of aneurysms found at each site in 316 consecutive patients. From McCormick WF. In Rosenberg *et al.* (eds). *The Clinical Neurosciences*, Vol 3. New York: Churchill-Livingstone, 1983.

SPECIFIC CAUSES OF SUBARACHNOID HAEMORRHAGE

Cerebral aneurysms

These are saccular dilations of the medium- and large-sized arteries and are characteristically positioned in the fork of bifurcations of the main branches of the circle of Willis (Figure 9.4). The most common sites are listed in Table 9.5.

Aneurysms develop during adult life and were once thought to arise as the result of congenital weaknesses of the arterial muscular

Table 9.5 Sites of cerebral aneurysms

Site	Percentage
Anterior communicating artery	40
Internal carotid artery[a]	30
Middle cerebral artery	20
Posterior circulation[b]	10

[a]Includes the junction with the posterior communicating artery, the ophthalmic artery origin and the terminal internal carotid artery.
[b]Includes the basilar tip, the posterior inferior cerebellar artery origin and the posterior cerebral artery junction with the posterior communicating artery.

Table 9.6 Conditions associated with cerebral aneurysm

- Hypertension
- Smoking
- Genetic disorders:
  - Polycystic kidney disease
  - Neurofibromatosis type I
  - Marfan's syndrome
  - Pseudoxanthoma elasticum
  - Ehlers–Danlos syndrome
  - α_1-antitrypsin deficiency
  - Hereditary haemorrhagic telangiectasia
  - Coarctation of the aorta
  - Sickle cell disease
- Altered blood flow:
  - Arteriovenous malformation
  - Anomalies of the circle of Willis
  - Moyamoya syndrome

walls, although this theory is no longer widely held. In most cases, the factors that lead to the development of aneurysm are largely unknown. Hypertension and smoking are the main risk factors. A variety of other rare predisposing conditions are listed in Table 9.6. In the elderly, some aneurysms may arise secondary to atherosclerosis. Multiple aneurysms are found in a number of patients presenting with subarachnoid haemorrhage. However, a second subarachnoid haemorrhage resulting from a new aneurysm that develops after the initial angiogram is very unusual.

Treatment of cerebral aneurysms Urgent treatment is required in patients with subarachnoid haemorrhage in whom an operable aneurysm has been discovered, in order to obliterate the aneurysm and prevent rebleeding. Two methods of treatment are available: neurosurgical obliteration and endovascular treatment using detachable metal coils (coiling). Neurosurgical treatment of aneurysm usually involves the obliteration of the aneurysm by placing a titanium clip across its neck. Endovascular coiling requires an interventional neuroradiologist to navigate a small microcatheter through the arterial system to the aneurysm from a puncture site in the femoral artery. Detachable platinum coils are then inserted into the aneurysm to obliterate it (Figure 9.5). The coils stimulate thrombosis within the aneurysm. The technique may be the only effective way of treating patients who are not fit for surgery or in whom surgical access is difficult (e.g. in cases of aneurysms of the carotid siphon), and has the advantage of avoiding craniotomy. If the aneurysm is not completely

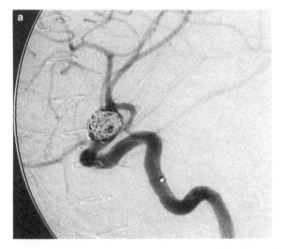
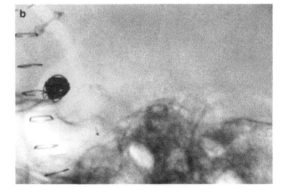

Figure 9.5 (a) Angiogram showing metal coils nearly obliterating a cerebral aneurysm after percutaneous insertion through a microcatheter. (b) Final view showing coils *in situ*.

obliterated, the coils may compact and the aneurysm recur. Patients treated by coiling may therefore require follow-up angiography.

The choice between these two techniques requires expert discussion and depends on the location and appearance of the aneurysm, the condition of the patient and the available experience. The randomized International Subarachnoid Aneurysm Trial (ISAT) has demonstrated that in patients with a ruptured aneurysm suitable for both techniques, the early outcome of coiling is superior to that of clipping, with less residual deficit during early follow-up (Molyneux *et al.*, 2005). At 1-year follow-up, 24% of patients allocated endovascular coiling were dependent or dead, compared with 31% of patients allocated neurosurgical treatment. The early advantage of coiling was maintained for up to 7 years.

The optimum time for treatment of recently ruptured aneurysms remains uncertain (Chyatte *et al.*, 1988; De Gans *et al.*, 2002). Early treatment as soon as possible after diagnosis will prevent early rebleeding, but may be more hazardous because of a higher risk of stroke due to vasospasm, which may be exacerbated by manipulation of the artery at surgery or endovascular treatment. Delaying treatment reduces the rate of perioperative stroke, but risks early rebleeding. The International Cooperative Study on the Timing of Aneurysm Surgery showed little difference in outcome between early and late surgery (Kassell *et al.*, 1990a, b). Different surgeons have different policies, but most favour early treatment for patients with good grades (Ross *et al.*, 2002). The decision when, and if, to treat patients in poor clinical condition will vary from centre to centre. In the past, surgery was restricted to younger patients, but nowadays the outcome in elderly patients is similar to that in younger age groups, and patients over the age of 65 contribute about 20% in most modern series. Rebleeding is extremely unusual after successful surgery, but may be slightly more common after coiling. In ISAT, the risk of rebleeding at 1 year after treatment was 2 per 1276 patient-years after allocation to endovascular treatment and zero per 1081 patient-years of follow-up after allocation to neurosurgery. The incidence of late rebleeding and the long-term outcome after coiling remain uncertain.

Idiopathic subarachnoid haemorrhage

No cause for subarachnoid haemorrhage is found in about 10% of fully investigated patients. In such cases, it is assumed that a small blood vessel on the surface of the brain has bled without underlying pathology. It is important that cerebral angiography be repeated after a delay of 6 weeks if the initial angiogram appears normal, because a small aneurysm may have been missed as a result of vasospasm reducing blood flow to the abnormal vessel. In one particular variant of idiopathic subarachnoid haemorrhage, known as *permesencephalic subarachnoid haemorrhage*, the bleeding is concentrated around the midbrain or is ventral to the pons, and the symptoms may be milder than those seen in aneurysmal subarachnoid haemorrhage. Most patients in whom no cause is identified make a full recovery and the prognosis for recurrence is very good. They can be therefore be reassured about the future, but should avoid risk factors for subarachnoid haemorrhage (e.g. smoking and aspirin therapy).

Arteriovenous malformation

AVM is an unusual cause of subarachnoid haemorrhage. It is far more common for AVMs to present with intracerebral haemorrhage (Chapter 8). Three options are available for the treatment of AVM to prevent recurrent haemorrhage: surgical resection, interventional neuroradiological techniques and stereotactic radiotherapy ('radiosurgery'). Interventional neuroradiological techniques include the injection of quick-setting 'super glue' (Figure 9.6) or insertion of detachable balloons into the nidus of the malformation using the approach described for aneurysm above. Interventional techniques may be used to reduce the size of large lesions prior to surgical resection. Deep lesions may be very difficult to resect without a high risk of causing major neurological deficit. Radiosurgery provides an

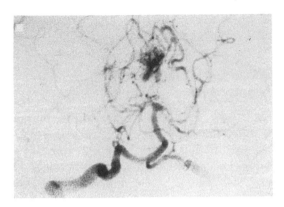

Figure 9.6   Angiogram illustrating a posterior circulation arteriovenous malformation. The lesion was subsequently obliterated by embolization with glue.

option for such lesions, but is only suitable for the smaller arteriovenous malformations. In some cases, it may be better to treat the AVM conservatively because of the risks of invasive treatment, particularly if the patient has presented with non-haemorrhagic symptoms (e.g. epilepsy).

Trauma

This is usually obvious from the circumstances of the accident. However, occasionally, a patient is found collapsed and no history is available. Signs of bruising to the head will suggest head trauma, and CT may show other abnormalities suggestive of trauma, such as skull fracture or intracerebral contusion. In these cases, it may be uncertain whether the patient has fallen because of the subarachnoid haemorrhage or whether the trauma of a fall has caused the haemorrhage. An acute subdural haematoma would usually suggest severe trauma, but can occasionally be associated with a ruptured aneurysm. Angiography should be performed if there is any doubt about the cause of the haemorrhage.

Bleeding diathesis

Subarachnoid haemorrhage is sometimes a presentation of a bleeding tendency, although intracranial haemorrhage is a far more common

manifestation. It should not be assumed that the haematological abnormality is the only cause of haemorrhage. Subarachnoid haemorrhage secondary to warfarin therapy or thrombolytic therapy is also rare. Patients who have had a subarachnoid haemorrhage associated with a bleeding tendency or anticoagulation therapy should still have cerebral angiography to exclude a source of bleeding.

Sickle cell disease

This is associated with both ischaemic stroke and subarachnoid haemorrhage. In children, the haemorrhage appears to occur from leptomeningeal collateral vessels formed as a result of distal branch occlusions and the moyamoya syndrome (Chapter 11). In adults there is an increased incidence of aneurysms.

Mycotic aneurysms

These are usually caused by embolism of infected material from endocarditis (Schold and Earnest, 1978; Salgado *et al.*, 1987). The patient is usually known to have endocarditis, but in some cases subarachnoid haemorrhage may be the presenting symptom. Mycotic aneurysms usually arise in distal branches of the middle cerebral artery and therefore present with intracerebral haemorrhage, but if the aneurysm is more proximal the presentation will mimic saccular aneurysm. Whether or not surgery is appropriate will depend on the size and location of the aneurysm, but antibiotic treatment is the mainstay of treatment. Anticoagulation should be avoided in the acute stages.

Intracranial dissection of intracranial vessels

This may cause bleeding into the subarachnoid space, if the dissection occurs in the intracranial portions of the artery. This is a rare cause of subarachnoid haemorrhage and usually involves the vertebral artery and occasionally the middle cerebral artery (Yamada *et al.*, 2004). The dissection may be caused by severe trauma, but more commonly it seems to arise spontaneously or after relatively minor trauma, particularly in the vertebral artery (Chapter 10). Most dissections involving the cerebral vessels arise in the carotid and vertebral arteries outside the dura, in which case subarachnoid haemorrhage cannot occur. In the intradural parts of the arteries, the adventitia and muscular layers of the arteries are thinner, so that subarachnoid haemorrhage and pseudoaneurysm formation may occur with the dissection (Chaves *et al.*, 2002). Clues to dissection as a possible cause of subarachnoid haemorrhage include:

- A history of trauma or forced neck movements
- Unilateral neck pain preceeding the onset of subarachnoid haemorrhage
- Early signs of ischaemia in the territory of the vertebral or middle cerebral artery
- Unilateral bulbar cranial nerve palsies

The management of intracranial dissection with subarachnoid haemorrhage is difficult. Unlike extracranial dissections, anticoagulation should be avoided. The sites of dissection are rarely easily amenable to surgery, but interventional techniques may be appropriate; for example, if there is an adequate collateral supply, it may be possible to occlude the artery with detachable balloons.

Cerebral venous thrombosis

This may rarely present with a history of sudden onset of headache, neck stiffness and blood in the CSF, typical of subarachnoid haemorrhage. Even without subarachnoid bleeding, cerebral venous thrombosis can be associated with neck pain and stiffness, which may be more marked on rotation of the neck – in contrast to subarachnoid haemorrhage, where neck stiffness is more marked in flexion. Usually, the headache in cerebral venous thrombosis is more gradual in onset and can be explained by raised intracranial pressure or distension of the venous sinuses. In some cases, the headache may be due to leakage of blood into the subarachnoid space, in which

case there may be a raised cell count or xanthochromia in the CSF without frank subarachnoid haemorrhage. The diagnosis is usually made by MRI or cerebral angiography, but it is important that the appropriate sequences should be imaged in a patient with unexplained subarachnoid haemorrhage to ensure that the diagnosis of cerebral venous thrombosis is not missed.

Cerebral vasculitis

This, from any cause, may be associated with subarachnoid haemorrhage, but more commonly the symptoms of cerebral vasculitis are the result of small vessel occlusion or intracerebral haemorrhage (Chapter 11).

Drug abuse

Abuse of drugs, particularly cocaine and amphetamine, is associated with subarachnoid haemorrhage, probably as a result of acute hypertension (Chapter 11).

Tumours

These may bleed into the cerebrospinal fluid if they are superficially located.

OTHER MANIFESTATIONS OF CEREBRAL ANEURYSM

Intracerebral haemorrhage from cerebral aneurysm

This can occur without subarachnoid haemorrhage. In this case, the presentation is indistinguishable from any other cause of intracerebral haemorrhage (Chapter 8). The site of the haematoma on CT may suggest the possibility of a bleed from an aneurysm.

Asymptomatic unruptured cerebral aneurysm

This may be found on CT, MRA or cerebral angiography by coincidence during the investigation of unrelated symptoms (Wardlaw and

Table 9.7 The 5-year cumulative rupture rates of cerebral aneurysms of various diameters in patients with no prior history of subarachnoid haemorrhage[a]

Site	Diameter of aneurysm			
	<7 mm	*7–12 mm*	*13–24 mm*	*>24 mm*
Cavernous carotid artery	0	0	3.0	6.4
Anterior circulation[b]	0	2.6	14.5	40
Posterior circulation[c]	2.5	14.5	18.4	50

[a]Adapted from Wiebers DO *et al. Lancet* 2003;**362**:103–110.
[b]Internal carotid (excluding cavernous portion), anterior communicating, anterior cerebral or middle cerebral artery.
[c]Vertebrobasilar, posterior cerebral or posterior communicating artery.

White, 2000). It is usual to clip an asymptomatic aneurysm in a patient who has already had one subarachnoid haemorrhage if the aneurysm is operable. However, the risk of haemorrhage associated with asymptomatic incidental aneurysms is much lower than the risk of recurrent haemorrhage in symptomatic aneurysms. The International Study of Unruptured Intracranial Aneurysms (ISUIA) assessed the natural history of unruptured intracranial aneurysms and reported that in patients with no history of subarachnoid hemorrhage from a different aneurysm, the cumulative 5-year rate of rupture of aneurysms depends on the location of the aneurysm and the size of the aneurysm at the time of detection (Table 9.7) (Wiebers *et al.*, 2003). In patients with aneurysms less than 7 mm in diameter, the 5-year risk of subarachnoid haemorrhage was zero if the aneurysm was in the anterior circulation and 2.5% if the aneurysm was in the posterior circulation. These figures do not justify the risks of surgery. The overall rate of surgery-related morbidity and mortality at 1 year in patients whose unruptured aneurysm was clipped was 12.6%, although the risk of surgery was less in younger patients with smaller aneurysms. In patients with larger aneurysms or a history of subarachnoid haemorrhage from another aneurysm, the risks of rupture of an asymptomatic aneurysm were higher, but were often exceeded or equalled by the risks of surgery or endovascular treatment of comparable lesions. The risks of endovascular coiling for unruptured aneurysm were less than those of surgery, but still exceeded the natural history in all but the larger aneurysms. Hence, most patients with small aneurysms should be treated conservatively and reassured that the risks of rupture are very low. In larger unruptured aneurysms, the long-term benefits of surgical or endovascular treatment may justify treatment in younger patients (Vindlacheruvu *et al.*, 2005). Decisions about surgical or endovascular repair of larger aneurysms require expert assessment of the individual patient's risks associated with their aneurysm and the various approaches to treatment. All patients should be advised about controlling risk factors (e.g. stopping smoking and treatment of hypertension).

Familial aneurysm

Close relatives of a patient with subarachnoid haemorrhage may be concerned about the risk of familial aneurysm. Saccular aneurysms are usually sporadic and not inherited. However, there are a few families in which aneurysm does seem to be inherited. In these families, in which two or more first-degree relatives have had a subarachnoid haemorrhage, the risk of an asymptomatic family member harbouring an aneurysm is about 10%. Even so, the benefits of screening individuals in a family in which aneurysm is known to be inherited are small because of the low chance of such an aneurysm rupturing and the risks of the cerebral angiography required to investigate the

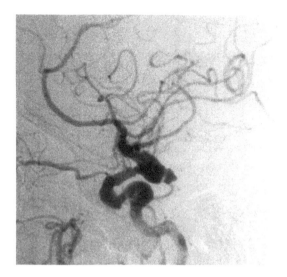

Figure 9.7 Digital subtraction angiogram showing a communicating artery aneurysm presenting with a painful third-nerve palsy.

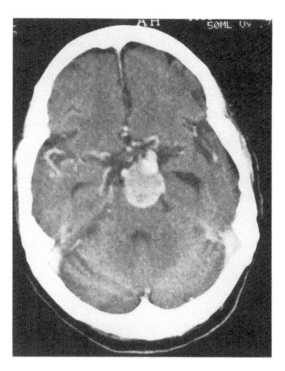

Figure 9.8 Contrast-enhanced CT showing a giant cerebral aneurysm.

patient. In families where only one member has had a subarachnoid haemorrhage, the chances of another member having an aneurysm that will subsequently bleed are very small and they should usually be reassured that investigation is not justified. Unfortunately, MRA is not yet sufficiently specific or sensitive to replace the need for catheter angiography in these patients. Policies of screening all family members of patients with subarachnoid haemorrhage are not cost-effective.

Third-nerve palsy

This is an important manifestation of an internal carotid artery aneurysm at the junction with the posterior communicating artery (often incorrectly called a posterior communicating artery aneurysm). The posterior communicating artery lies in close proximity to the trunk of the third cranial nerve as it passes from the brainstem to the orbit. An enlarging aneurysm on the artery can compress the third nerve and cause a third-nerve palsy. The palsy is almost invariably painful and the pupil is usually affected, as well as the levator palpebrae and the oculomotor nerve. The patient therefore presents with progressive

ptosis, double vision and pain, usually distributed around the eye. A painful third-nerve palsy should therefore always be investigated with cerebral angiography (Figure 9.7).

Internal carotid aneurysms

Aneurysms situated in the distal extradural intracranial segments of the carotid artery are less likely to present with subarachnoid haemorrhage and therefore usually present with symptoms of compression of adjacent structures once they are greater than 1 cm in diameter. Stretching of the carotid sympathetic chain may lead to retro-orbital pain or migrainous headaches. Petrous segment aneurysms are rare and present with abducens or trigeminal deficits. Intracavernous aneurysms are more common and cause compression of adjacent cranial nerves within the cavernous sinus (cranial nerves III, IV, V and VI) (Hahn *et al.*, 2000). Clinoid segment aneurysms present with facial pain or visual failure secondary to compression of the optic nerve. Ophthalmic segment aneurysms also present with unilateral optic nerve compression or sometimes bilateral visual loss or a bitemporal hemianopia from compression of the chiasm, which may mimic a pituitary tumour.

GIANT ANEURYSMS

These are 2.5 cm or more in diameter (Figure 9.8). They can be as large as 8 cm in diameter. These may be less likely to bleed than smaller aneurysms, but over one-third present with haemorrhage. The remainder present with symptoms suggesting a mass lesion, particularly epilepsy, or are found during the investigation of unrelated symptoms on CT or MRI. They may cause compression of adjacent structures. Giant aneurysms become filled with successive layers of thrombus, and may appear much smaller on cerebral angiography than they do on CT or MRI. Very rarely, they may present with transient ischaemic attack or stroke in the distribution of the artery beyond the aneurysm. This suggests the possibility of embolism of thrombus from the aneurysm, although it is usually not possible to prove that this has been the mechanism. Similar presentations may be caused by ectasia of one of the major cerebral arteries, particularly the basilar artery. In this condition there is dilation and often tortuosity of a segment of the artery. The aetiology of the ectasia is unknown, but it may be congenital in origin or secondary to atherosclerosis.

Giant basilar artery aneurysms

These tend to occur at the tip of the basilar artery projecting laterally and present with a third-nerve palsy or distortion of the brainstem causing dysarthria, ataxia or other brainstem symptoms (Figure 4.12, p. 54).

Giant vertebral artery aneurysms

These are very rare, but can compress the cranial nerves within the jugular foramen (IX, X and XI).

OTHER MANIFESTATIONS OF CEREBRAL ARTERIOVENOUS MALFORMATION

Intracerebral haemorrhage from cerebral AVM

This is more common than subarachnoid haemorrhage.

Epilepsy

This is one of the commonest manifestations of AVM. The epilepsy may occur at any age and can be focal or generalized.

Headache

This may be a presenting feature of an AVM, especially a larger malformation. It may mimic almost any variety of migraine. Prolonged migraine-like headache in a patient with a known AVM should raise the suspicion of haemorrhage.

Pulsatile tinnitus

This can be the presentation of an AVM, particularly a *dural arteriovenous fistula*. The patient complains of a pulsatile whooshing noise in the ears, which is often noticed to be in time with the pulse and to increase in volume with exercise or emotion. A cranial bruit may be audible to the examiner with a stethoscope placed over the skull, mastoid processes or orbits, but is not always present. If the AVM is very large, there may also be a flow murmur audible over the carotid arteries. Sometimes, pulsatile tinnitus is the result of high cervical carotid stenosis. Pulsatile tinnitus may be an indication for MRI and cerebral angiography, particularly if the patient finds the tinnitus very troublesome. However, quite often no abnormality is found.

Intracranial steal

This is a rare manifestation of very large AVMs. The massive increase in blood flow to the malformation diverts blood from the surrounding brain, leading to ischaemia and sometimes infarction, with focal signs or progressive dementia.

Cerebral venous thrombosis

There is an association between cerebral venous thrombosis and AVMs, particularly dural arteriovenous fistulas. Whether the association is cause and effect is uncertain, but the development of dural arteriovenous fistula after cerebral venous thrombosis, and conversely the occurrence of cerebral venous thrombosis in patients known to have AVMs, is well described.

KEY REFERENCES

Risk factors

Broderick JP, Viscoli CM, Brott T et al. Major risk factors for aneurysmal subarachnoid hemorrhage in the young are modifiable. *Stroke* 2003; **34**:1375–1381

Sentinel headache

Linn FH, Wijdicks EF, van der Graaf Y et al. Prospective study of sentinel headache in aneurysmal subarachnoid haemorrhage. *Lancet* 1994;**344**: 590–593

Rebleeding

Winn HR, Richardson AE, Jane JA. The long-term prognosis in untreated cerebral aneurysms: I. The incidence of late hemorrhage in cerebral aneurysm: a 10-year evaluation of 364 patients. *Ann Neurol* 1977;**1**:358–370

Winn HR, Richardson AE, O'Brien W, Jane JA. The long-term prognosis in untreated cerebral aneurysms: II. Late morbidity and mortality. *Ann Neurol* 1978;**4**:418–426

Vasospasm

Sloan MA. Transcranial Doppler monitoring of vasospasm after subarachnoid hemorrhage. In *Neurosonology*. Tegeler CH, Babikian VL, Gomez CR (eds). Mosby, St Louis, 1995:156–171

Neuroprotective therapy

Pickard JD, Murray GD, Illingworth R et al. Effect of oral nimodipine on cerebral infarction and outcome after subarachnoid haemorrhage: British aneurysm nimodipine trial. *BMJ* 1989;**298**: 636–642

Surgery and coiling of aneurysm

Chyatte D, Fode NC, Sundt TM Jr. Early versus late intracranial aneurysm surgery in subarachnoid hemorrhage. *J Neurosurg* 1988;**69**:326–331

De Gans, Nieuwkamp DJ, Rinkel GJ et al. Timing of aneurysm surgery in subarachnoid hemorrhage: a systemic review of the literature. *Neurosurgery* 2002;**50**:336–340

Kassell NF, Torner JC, Haley EC Jr et al. The International Cooperative Study on the Timing of Aneurysm Surgery. Part 1: Overall management results. *J Neurosurg* 1990a;**73**:18–36

Kassell NF, Torner JC, Jane JA et al. The International Cooperative Study on the Timing of Aneurysm Surgery. Part 2: Surgical results. *J Neurosurg* 1990b;**73**:37–47

Molyneux AJ, Kerr RSC, Ly-Mee Y et al. International Subarachnoid Aneurysm Trial (ISAT) of neurosurgical clipping versus endovascular coiling in 2143 patients with ruptured intracranial aneurysms: a randomized comparison of effects on survival, dependency, seizures, rebleeding, subgroups, and aneurysm occlusion. *Lancet* 2005;**366**:809–817

Ross N, Hutchinson PJ, Seeley H et al. Timing of surgery for supratentorial aneurysmal subarachnoid haemorrhage: report of a prospective study. *J Neurol Neurosurg Psychiatry* 2002;**72**: 480–484

Bleeding from mycotic aneurysm

Salgado AV, Furlan AJ, Keys TF. Mycotic aneurysm, subarachnoid hemorrhage, and indications for cerebral angiography in infective endocarditis. *Stroke* 1987;**18**:1057–1060

Schold C, Earnest MP. Cerebral hemorrhage from a mycotic aneurysm developing during appropriate antibiotic therapy. *Stroke* 1978;**9**:267–268

Intracranial dissection

Chaves C, Estol C, Esnaola MM et al. Spontaneous intracranial internal carotid artery dissection:

report of 10 patients. *Arch Neurol* 2002;**59**: 977–981

Yamada M, Kitahara T, Kurata A et al. Intracranial vertebral artery dissection with subarachnoid hemorrhage: clinical characteristics and outcomes in conservatively treated patients. *J Neurosurg* 2004;**101**:25–30

Wardlaw JM, White PM. The detection and management of unruptured intracranial aneurysms. *Brain* 2000;**123**:205–221

Wiebers DO, Whisnant JP, Huston J et al. Unruptured intracranial aneurysms: natural history, clinical outcome, and risks of surgical and endovascular treatment. *Lancet* 2003;**362**:103–110

Asymptomatic cerebral aneurysm

Vindlacheruvu RR, Mendelow AD, Mitchell P. Risk–benefit analysis of the treatment of unruptured intracranial aneurysms. *J Neurol Neurosurg Psychiatry* 2005;**76**:234–239

Cavernous sinus aneurysm

Hahn CD, Nicolle DA, Lownie SP, Drake CG. Giant cavernous carotid aneurysms: clinical presentation in fifty-seven cases. *J Neuroophthalmol* 2000;**20**:253–258

CHAPTER 10

Dissection

Carotid and vertebral artery dissection are increasingly recognized causes of stroke, particularly in the young. Dissection may also present with isolated headaches, Horner's syndrome, subarachnoid haemorrhage and even spinal cord pathology. Blood tracks along the split within the arterial wall and there may, or may not, be an intimal tear resulting in a false lumen.

EPIDEMIOLOGY

There are few epidemiological studies of the incidence of dissection, and those that have been carried out are likely to be under-estimates due to the incomplete case ascertainment. Studies in Dijon, France, and Rochester, USA, suggest an annual incidence of approximately 2–3 per 100 000. Approximately one-third of cases of dissection will present with stroke or transient ischaemic attack (TIA). Dissection appears to be rare above the age of 50, perhaps because atherosclerosis is protective. The incidence in young stroke (younger than 45 years) appears to be approximately 5–10%, while an incidence of up to 25% in individuals aged 16–29 years presenting with stroke has been reported.

CAUSES

The major causes of carotid and vertebral dissection are listed in Table 10.1. Direct trauma to the vessel wall may occur from the

Table 10.1   Causes of cerebral artery dissection

Major trauma
- Penetrating trauma
- Neuroradiological procedures
- Blunt trauma

Carotid dissection
- Stretching across the lateral processes of C2–3
- Basal skull fracture
- Peritonsillar trauma
- Strangulation
- Mandibular fracture

Vertebral dissection
- Atlanto-axial subluxation
- Cervical spine fracture
- Cervical spine hyper-rotation and hyperextension

Minor trauma
- Chiropractic manipulation
- Violent coughing
- Neck turning (e.g. during a parade)
- Sporting activities
- Fairground rides

Underlying arterial disease
- Fibromuscular dysplasia
- Marfan's syndrome
- Cystic medial degeneration
- Coiling or redundant loop
- Ehlers–Danlos syndrome
- Pseudoxanthoma elasticum

Idiopathic

guidewire or catheter during angiography and other interventional neuroradiological procedures, including angioplasty. The majority of dissections fall into the spontaneous category, but frequently there is a history of minor trauma. Chiropractic manipulation, a wide variety of sporting activities including tennis, skiing, volleyball and scuba diving, and trauma as mild as teeth brushing, nose blowing or violent coughing have been reported to be associated with spontaneous dissection. A number of diseases affecting the arterial wall appear to increase the predisposition to both vertebral and carotid dissection, including fibromuscular dysplasia (Chapter 11), Marfan's syndrome, Ehlers–Danlos syndrome, pseudoxanthoma elasticum and cystic medial degeneration.

In one study, more minor connective tissue abnormalities were reported on electron microscopy of skin biopsies from a large proportion of patients with atraumatic carotid dissection who had no clinical evidence of connective tissue disorders (Brandt *et al.*, 1998). In addition, coiling or redundancy in the internal carotid artery has been associated with an increased risk of dissection. Case reports have suggested that other diseases of the arterial wall (e.g. syphilis and polyarteritis) may be predisposing causes. It has been suggested that both hypertension and migraine may increase the risk of dissection. However, because both of these diseases are widely prevalent in the population and rigorous case–control studies are lacking, the association may be a coincidence. It should be remembered that fibromuscular dysplasia may cause both cervical artery dissection and renal artery stenosis with secondary hypertension.

PATHOGENESIS

Most carotid dissections occur just above the common carotid bifurcation at the origin of the internal carotid artery. Pathological investigations show haemorrhage into the subintima, the media and, less often, the subadventitia (Figure 10.1). The haematoma may involve the entire circumference or only a portion of the vessel. Subintimal haemorrhage tends to result in prominent narrowing of the lumen, while a haematoma in the outer media and subadventitia is more likely to cause arterial dilatation and pseudoaneurysm formation. In some cases, a primary intimal tear appears to be the initial event, and this allows tracking of blood along planes in the arterial wall. In some cases, the intimal tear may lead to intraluminal thrombus formation and vessel occlusion without the development of dissection or a haematoma in the vessel wall. In these latter cases, the cause of the thrombosis will not be evident on investigation and can only be confirmed at postmortem examination. On other occasions, a primary haematoma may form in the arterial wall, and this may or may not rupture inwards to create a false lumen. This type of dissection may occur as a result of haemorrhage from the vasa vasorum.

Dissection often tracks upwards as far as the skull base, resulting in a characteristic angiographic appearance (see below).

The dissection may have a number of consequences (Table 10.2):

- Thrombus formation at the site of an intimal tear with intraluminal clot formation. This can result in:
  - subsequent thromboembolism
  - vessel occlusion

- Reduction in luminal diameter secondary to the intramural haemorrhage. This can result in:
  - vessel occlusion
  - haemodynamic compromise

- Extension into the subadventitial layer and pseudoaneurysm formation. These pseudoaneurysms can occasionally expand and cause local pressure symptoms. Extracranial pseudoaneurysms very rarely rupture.

Intracranial dissections exhibit a predilection for the supraclinoid segment of the carotid artery, the middle cerebral artery, the fourth

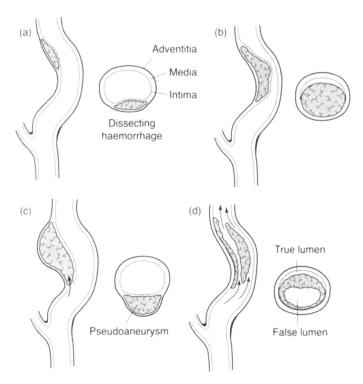

Figure 10.1   Lateral and cross-sectional views of the internal carotid artery to show the anatomy of dissections (a) initial phase of intramedial and subintimal dissecting aneurysm; (b) progression of intramedial haemorrhage; (c) intramedial haemorrhage, dissecting into subadventitial plane (rather than the subintimal plane as in a, b); (d) dissecting haemorrhage rupturing through the intima.

Table 10.2   Presenting features of cerebral artery dissection

Carotid artery dissection
- Headache
- Anterior neck pain
- Horner's syndrome
- Retinal ischaemia
- Carotid territory transient ischaemic attack (TIA) or stroke
- Pulsatile tinnitus

Vertebral artery dissection
- Headache
- Posterior neck pain
- Posterior circulation TIA or stroke
- Subarachnoid haemorrhage

segment of the vertebral artery, and the basilar trunk. Unlike extracranial dissections, intracranial dissections are commonly located between the internal elastic lamina and the media, leading to the assumption that most of these are the consequence of an intimal tear.

Most vertebral dissections occur in the extracranial portion of the artery and have similar pathological consequences to carotid dissection. Dissection of the intracranial vertebral artery is rare, but may present with subarachnoid haemorrhage, because of leakage of blood into the cerebrospinal fluid.

CLINICAL FEATURES

Extracranial carotid artery dissection

Carotid dissection may present with a variety of symptoms, depending on the pathological consequences of the dissection (Zetterling *et al.*, 2000).

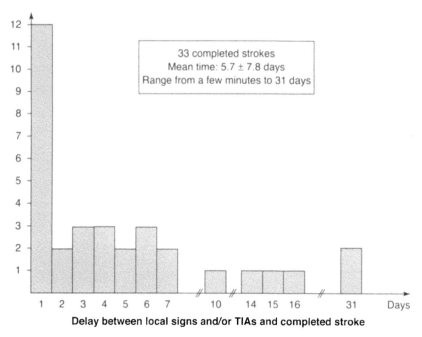

Figure 10.2   Histogram showing time from first presentation of extracranial carotid artery dissection to onset of stroke. Modified from Biousse V *et al. Stroke* 1995;**26**:235–239.

Headache   This is usually ipsilateral and localized to the side of the dissection in the face, orbit, temple, cheek or neck, and occasionally the pharyngeal regions, and may mimic migraine. It is sometimes associated with ipsilateral scalp tenderness. It may be of fairly sudden onset.

Horner's syndrome   This results from compression and interruption of sympathetic fibres running along the internal carotid artery adventitia and is usually incomplete, presenting with slight pupillary constriction and ptosis.

TIA and stroke   Carotid territory stroke, TIA, amaurosis fugax or retinal artery infarction is the presenting feature in approximately one-third of cases. Ischaemic symptoms may occur a number of days after the onset of other symptoms (e.g. headache) and are believed to be embolic in the majority of cases (Biousse *et al.*, 1995). Occasionally, stroke is delayed several

weeks after the presumed onset of dissection, for example when this can be timed to an episode of trauma (Figure 10.2).

Pulsatile tinnitus   This results from the patient's subjective perception of an ipsilateral bruit, which may also be heard on auscultation by the examiner. The bruit may be heard more distally than that usually heard over the carotid bifurcation in carotid artery stenosis secondary to atherosclerosis.

Cranial nerve palsies   The internal carotid artery lies close to the lower cranial nerves, and palsies affecting any of the cranial nerves IX–XII can occur as a presenting feature of carotid dissection (Sturzenegger and Huber, 1993). Hypoglossal palsy is the most common, occurring from compression of the hypoglossal nerve immediately below its exit through the anterior condylar canal. Dysgeusia may occur secondary to chorda tympani compression. Glossopharyngeal and vagal nerve palsies occur less commonly.

Extracranial vertebral artery dissection

This most commonly involves the third part of the vertebral artery between C1 and C2 (Hart and Easton, 1993). It may present with the following:

- *Pain* in the occipital region, the posterior neck, the mastoids, round the ears or occasionally around the shoulders.
- *TIA and stroke* affecting the vertebrobasilar territory, usually a lateral medullary syndrome or cerebellar infarct. If the thrombosis spreads to the basilar artery, the patient may present with devastating pontine or brainstem infarction.
- *Cervical spine symptoms:* the vertebral arteries lie close to the spinal nerve roots and the spinal artery arises from the vertebral artery. Cases have been reported in which vertebral dissection presents as a cervical spine problem, with symptoms and signs of root disturbance. Extremely rarely, vertebral artery dissection may cause ischaemia of the spinal cord.

Intracranial dissection

Intracranial carotid territory dissections usually affect the distal carotid artery in the siphon, or the first segment of the middle cerebral artery (Chaves *et al.*, 2002). The dissection may present with TIA or stroke, which is frequently severe. The dissection may only be diagnosed at postmortem. Subarachnoid haemorrhage has been reported, although it is more common with intracranial vertebrobasilar dissection.

Intracranial dissections affecting the vertebrobasilar circulation usually affect the intracranial vertebral artery, the basilar artery or the superior cerebellar artery (Naito *et al.*, 2002). They may present with pain affecting the occipital or posterior neck region, vertebrobasilar TIA, or brainstem and cerebellar infarction. These are often severe. Occasionally, they present with subarachnoid haemorrhage (Yamada *et al.*, 2004).

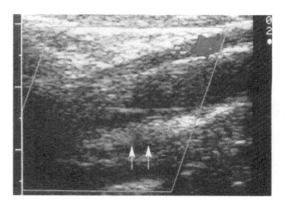

Figure 10.3 Carotid duplex showing carotid dissection with a free intimal flap (horizontal line 1 cm above small arrows).

INVESTIGATIONS

Extracranial carotid artery dissection

The different modalities for making the diagnosis are discussed below. Intra-arterial angiography is a gold standard in diagnosis, but increasingly non-invasive approaches, particularly ultrasonography and magnetic resonance imaging (MRI) are allowing diagnosis without angiography. Occasionally, angiography may be normal, particularly in subadventitial dissection, or may show complete occlusion without diagnostic features. In this case, MRI may be more helpful.

Ultrasonography In experienced hands, abnormal ultrasonographic findings can be found in the majority of extracranial carotid dissections (Steinke *et al.*, 1994) (Figure 10.3). However, studies using MRI have shown that ultrasound can miss more distal internal carotid artery dissections, particularly if there is no secondary stenotic lesion. The Doppler modality is most useful, and examination may need to include pulsed Doppler of the distal internal carotid artery via the submandibular approach if more distal stenoses resulting from dissection are to be detected. High-resolution B-mode imaging is of less use. A flap is only rarely visualized and frequently the abnormalities may occur distal to the extent of internal carotid artery imaged on B-mode. In combination with colour flow imaging, B-mode may allow a tapering to be visualized. A number of characteristic features of internal carotid artery dissection have been identified on ultrasound:

- High-resistance Doppler signal with bidirectional low-amplitude flow components and absent diastolic flow: typically the signal can be traced along the extracranial course of the internal carotid artery, thus allowing distinction from stump flow in atherosclerotic carotid occlusion. This pattern has been reported in two-thirds of cases in some series.
- Marked reduction of systolic and diastolic blood flow velocity may occur in cases in which the carotid obstruction is not severe enough to produce the characteristic high resistance Doppler pattern.
- A significantly increased Doppler shift frequency in turbulence in the upper cervical segment of the internal carotid artery may indicate distal stenosis and is best assessed by means of a 2 MHz pulsed-wave Doppler transducer.
- An appearance consistent with complete internal carotid artery occlusion: the absence of atherosclerotic plaque on B-mode imaging may suggest that the underlying process is dissection, as opposed to atherothrombosis.

Transcranial Doppler sonography of the intracranial vessels   This may demonstrate the effect of the carotid pathology on the post-stenotic intracranial circulation and allow identification of collateral blood flow. Since dissections narrow the carotid lumen rapidly, there is little time for intracranial collaterals to adapt to the altered haemodynamic pattern and therefore most patients have reduced middle cerebral artery blood flow velocity on the side of the dissection if examined early. Carotid–carotid collateral crossflow (i.e. reversed flow direction at the ipsilateral anterior cerebral artery and increased blood flow velocity of the contralateral anterior cerebral artery)

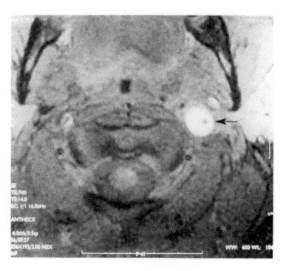

Figure 10.4   MRI, cross-sectional view, showing left carotid dissection (arrow). Note the enlarged diameter of the artery with an eccentric haematoma (white) and small lumen (dark).

may occur. Doppler embolic signals have been reported in the distal ipsilateral middle cerebral artery in individual cases, supporting the concept that embolization plays an important role in the pathogenesis of stroke associated with dissection.

Magnetic resonance imaging   Magnetic resonance angiography (MRA) may show a tapering occlusion (see 'Angiography' below) or string flow (pseudo-occlusion). However, MRA shows wall irregularities and lesser degrees of stenoses less well than conventional catheter angiography, and a tight tapering stenosis may appear as an occlusion due to signal dropout.

Structural MRI with cross-sectional views through the extracranial carotid artery is frequently diagnostic in cases imaged early, and, in combination with MRA, is now the investigation of choice. A diagnostic hyperintense signal, usually semilunar-shaped, in the wall of the carotid artery on both T_1- and T_2-weighted imaging is seen during the first week and indicates the presence of a mural haematoma (Figure 10.4). This cannot be

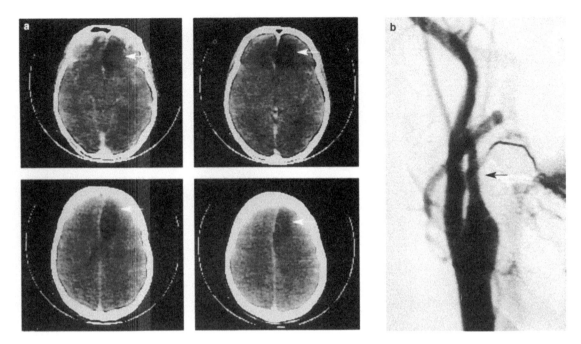

Figure 10.5   (a) CT scan showing anterior cerebral artery territory infarction (arrows). (b) Carotid angiogram from the same patient showing tapering occlusion of the internal carotid artery above the bifurcation (arrow), which is diagnostic of dissection.

detected in all cases. A reduction in arterial lumen and thickening of the arterial wall is also seen frequently.

Angiography   Conventional catheter angiography is usually diagnostic (Figure 10.5). The most characteristic finding is a tapering long stenosis ('rat's tail' appearance). If the stenosis is severe, the distal carotid may narrow into a 'string' sign. Dissection usually begins 2 cm or more distal to the origin of the internal carotid artery and then extends rostrally a variable distance, terminating before the entry of the artery into the petrous bone, where mechanical support limits further dissection. On angiography, a tapered narrowing can be identified, with normal luminal calibre being restored after entry of the vessel into the skull base. In some cases, an occlusion is seen, but tapering of the artery can frequently be seen proximal to the occlusion, allowing differentiation from occlusion secondary to atheromatous plaque or embolization. If a communication

exists between the cavity of the dissection and the true lumen, an extraluminal pouch of contrast is visualized as a dissecting pseudo-aneurysm. This is most commonly seen near the distal end of the dissection, close to the petrous bone. Small extraluminal pouches may be seen near the origin of the dissection. Some of the characteristic patterns are shown in Figure 10.6.

Other arteriographic findings may include occlusion of the intracerebral arteries from distal embolization, and fibromuscular dysplasia.

CT angiography (CTA) is being increasingly used and shows similar appearances, but with less resolution, to intra-arterial catheter angiography.

Extracranial vertebral dissection

Ultrasonography   Series examining the sensitivity of ultrasound in the diagnosis of vertebral dissection are small. In a significant proportion of cases, there may be no abnormalities detected on ultrasound. Abnormalities include

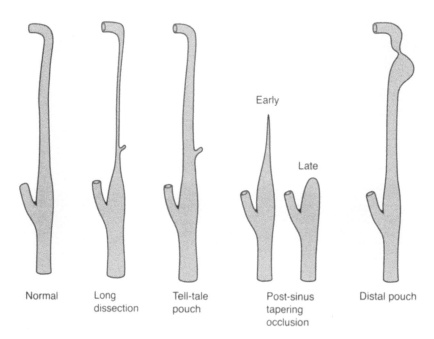

| Normal | Long dissection | Tell-tale pouch | Post-sinus tapering occlusion | Distal pouch |

Figure 10.6 Different patterns of angiographic abnormality seen in patients with carotid dissection. Adapted from Fisher CM *et al. Can J Neurol Sci* 1978;5:9–19.

a high-resistance signal in the vertebral artery, and no flow in a well-visualized vertebral artery. Occasionally, a dissecting membrane can be seen, or a localized increase in the diameter of the artery is visualized on B-mode imaging.

Magnetic resonance imaging Tapering or localized constriction of the vertebral artery may be seen on MRA, although less severe stenosis may be missed. Cross-sectional MRI may show wall thickening or an intramural haematoma, as seen in carotid artery dissection (see above), but there have been few controlled studies evaluating its sensitivity.

Angiography Similar findings to those seen in carotid dissection may occur, but tapering stenosis is a less consistent finding (Figure 10.7). Sometimes there may be just an area of localized narrowing. This may be difficult to differentiate from 'spasm', particularly if the dissection presents as a subarachnoid haemorrhage. MRI across the narrow segments may allow intramural haemorrhage of dissection to be distinguished from spasm. Aneurysmal

pouchings, double lumens or irregular zones of dilation and narrowing may be seen.

Intracranial dissections

These are usually diagnosed by angiography when a tapered narrowing or irregularity in the vessel wall is visualized or by structural MRI with cross-sectional views through the vessel wall.

TREATMENT

There are no large randomized trials on which to base treatment of either carotid or vertebral artery dissection. Most authors have advocated anticoagulation because the major risk appears to be from embolization and subsequent stroke. Commonly, intravenous heparin is given, followed by 3–6 months of anticoagulation with warfarin. Anticoagulation should be initiated as soon as possible because the risk of recurrent stroke appears to be greatest within the first 1–2 weeks (see 'Prognosis'

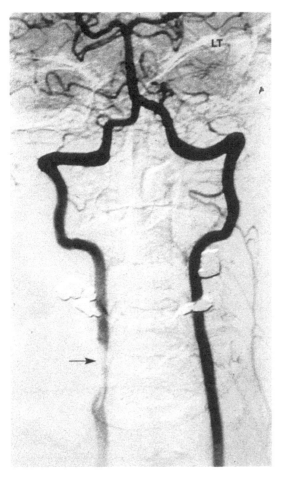

Figure 10.7 Angiogram showing right vertebral artery dissection (arrow).

below). Whether aspirin is as effective as warfarin is unknown. It is possible that some cases (e.g. those presenting with Horner's syndrome without significant vessel tapering on angiography) can be effectively treated with aspirin. In cases where there has already been a large cerebral infarct, it is sensible to delay anticoagulation because of the risk of haemorrhagic transformation, although the relative risks and benefits of this approach are uncertain. Anticoagulation should be avoided in patients with intracranial dissection because of the risk of subarachnoid haemorrhage (Kitanaka *et al.*, 1994). Prevention of stroke from dissection is discussed further in Chapter 15.

Surgical approaches to dissection are rarely necessary. If there is adequate collateral supply, carotid artery ligation has been proposed in the past to reduce the risk of embolization, but anticoagulation is now the preferred approach because recanalization frequently occurs spontaneously. Occasionally, surgery may be necessary for the treatment of large pseudoaneurysms. However, limited natural history data suggest that the risk of complications from extracranial pseudoaneurysms is very low. Surgery or interventional radiology may also be used in the treatment of intracranial vertebral artery dissections presenting with subarachnoid haemorrhage. Endovascular treatment with stenting has been successfully used to treat carotid dissection (Chapter 15) and may become more widely available in the future.

PROGNOSIS

The prognosis of dissection depends upon the presenting symptoms. Patients presenting with isolated headache or Horner's syndrome usually make a good recovery, although the anisocoria may be permanent. The prognosis of patients presenting with focal ischaemic events depends largely on the severity of the initial event. The major risk following presentation with minor symptoms is that of stroke or retinal ischaemia. A study of the time course of symptoms in patients with spontaneous carotid dissection suggests that the risk is greatest within the first 2 weeks (Biousse *et al.*, 1995). In this study, cerebral or retinal infarction occurred in 42 patients, and in 9 it was the first symptom. In the other 33, the interval between first symptoms (focal signs and or transient ischaemic attacks) and the onset of stroke ranged from a few minutes to 31 days, and it was less than 7 days in 82% of patients. This early risk of recurrence has been confirmed in a more recent Canadian study (Beletsky *et al.*, 2003).

The late recurrence of embolic symptoms is unusual after the first few weeks. Spontaneous recanalization frequently occurs over a period of weeks or months and can be serially monitored using ultrasound. The incidence of recurrent dissection is very low, except in patients with widespread fibromuscular dysplasia, where further episodes can occur.

KEY REFERENCES

Causes

Brandt T, Hausser I, Orberk E et al. Ultrastructural connective tissue abnormalities in patients with spontaneous cervicocerebral artery dissections. *Ann Neurol* 1998;**44**:281–285

Clinical features

Biousse V, D'Anglejan-Chatillon J, Touboul P-J et al. Time course of symptoms in extracranial carotid artery dissections: a series of 80 patients. *Stroke* 1995;**26**:235–239

Chaves C, Estol C, Esnaola MM et al. Spontaneous intracranial internal carotid artery dissection: report of 10 patients. *Arch Neurol* 2002;**59**:977–981

Hart RG, Easton JD. Dissections of cervical and cerebral arteries. In *Neurologic Clinics: Cerebrovascular Disease*, Volume 1. Barnett HJM (ed). WB Saunders, Philadelphia, 1983:155–182.

Naito I, Iwai T, Sasaki T. Management of intracranial vertebral artery dissections initially presenting without subarachnoid hemorrhage. *Neurosurgery* 2002;**51**:930–937

Sturzenegger M, Huber P. Cranial nerve palsies in spontaneous carotid artery dissection. *J Neurol Neurosurg Psychiatry* 1993;**56**:1191–1199

Yamada M, Kitahara T, Kurata A et al. Intracranial vertebral artery dissection with subarachnoid hemorrhage: clinical characteristics and outcomes in conservatively treated patients. *J Neurosurg* 2004;**101**:25–30

Zetterling M, Carlstrom C, Konrad P et al. Internal carotid artery dissection (review). *Acta Neurol Scand* 2000;**101**:1–7

Investigations

Steinke W, Rautenberg W, Schwartz A et al. Noninvasive monitoring of internal carotid artery dissection. *Stroke* 1994;**25**:998–1005

Treatment

Kitanaka C, Sasaki T, Eguchi T et al. Intracranial vertebral artery dissections: clinical, radiological features, and surgical considerations. *Neurosurgery* 1994;**34**:620–627

Prognosis

Beletsky V, Nadareishvili Z, Lynch J et al. Cervical artery dissection: time for a therapeutic trial? *Stroke* 2003;**34**:2856–2860

Biousse V et al. (See under clinical features above)

CHAPTER 11

Rare Causes

Rare causes of stroke (Table 11.1), although causing only a small proportion of cases of stroke and transient ischaemic attack (TIA) are important to recognize because they may require very different treatment. With some exceptions (e.g. temporal arteritis), rarer causes tend to be of greater importance in younger individuals, because atherosclerosis, hypertension and atrial fibrillation are less frequent. Many of these unusual causes are systemic diseases, in which stroke or TIA is only one possible presenting feature, and in which other neurological presentations (e.g. an encephalopathy or seizures) may also occur. In many cases, specialized investigations are required to make the diagnosis. Rare causes are discussed in this chapter in alphabetical order.

ATRIAL MYXOMA

Myxomas are the most common type of primary cardiac tumour. Atrial myxoma may occasionally present with stroke or TIA as a result of embolization of portions of the tumour to the cerebral circulation. The emboli may result in recurrent events and can cause peripherally sited neoplastic cerebral aneurysms. Signs of mitral valve disease may be present – either stenosis as a result of tumour prolapse into the mitral valve during diastole, or regurgitation as a consequence of injury to the valve by tumour-induced trauma. The findings on cardiac auscultation may vary from day to day. Myxomas

Table 11.1   Rare causes of stroke

- Atrial myxoma
- CADASIL
- Dissection
- Drug abuse
- Fabry's disease
- Fibromuscular dysplasia
- Haematological disorders (Table 11.2)
- Homocystinuria
- Infections
- Inflammatory vascular disorders
  - Behçet's disease
  - Giant-cell arteritis
  - Isolated angiitis of the central nervous system
  - Systemic lupus erythematosus
  - Systemic necrotizing vasculitis
  - Takayasu's arteritis
  - Other autoimmune/vasculitic disorders
- Migraine
- Mitochondrial disorders
- Moyamoya syndrome
- Oral contraceptives
- Paradoxical embolism
- Pregnancy
- Sneddon's syndrome
- Trauma

may also present with non-cardiac signs and symptoms, including fever, weight loss, malaise, arthralgia, clubbing, anaemia, and raised erythrocyte sedimentation rate (ESR). Diagnosis requires echocardiography (Figure 11.1) and cardiac catheterization. Surgical excision is usually the treatment of choice.

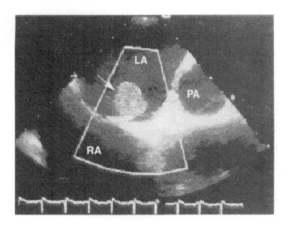

Figure 11.1 Echocardiogram showing an atrial myxoma (arrow). LA, left atrium; PA, pulmonary artery; RA, right atrium.

CADASIL (CEREBRAL AUTOSOMAL DOMINANT ARTERIOPATHY WITH SUBCORTICAL INFARCTS AND LEUKOENCEPHALOPATHY)

This is a hereditary cause of stroke and is transmitted in an autosomal dominant fashion (Hassan and Markus, 2000). Clinical features include multiple lacunar strokes and eventual progression to a subcortical dementia *(hereditary multi-infarct dementia)*. The age of onset is variable, but typically migraine starts in the third decade, and then TIAs, lacunar stroke and progressive cognitive impairment develop in the fourth and fifth decades (Desmond *et al.*, 1999). Sometimes, psychiatric disturbance or depression may occur early in the illness. Dementia occurs eventually in 90% of cases. In classical disease, death is usual in the sixth or seventh decade, but it is increasingly appreciated that some genetically affected individuals can survive to old age with only minimal symptoms.

The genetic defect results in a characteristic disorder of arterioles of between 100 and 400 µm in diameter, which show narrowing of the lumen, with hyaline degeneration of the media and reduplication of the internal elastic lamina at pathological examination. On electron microscopy, deposition of a unique granular electron-dense osmiophilic material (GOM)

is seen in the media, in close association with the vascular smooth muscle cells. Similar arterial changes have been reported in small arteries on skin and muscle biopsy. The exact nature of this substance is unknown, although it has been shown to be distinct from amyloid. The vasculopathy leads to multiple lacunar infarcts in the periventricular white matter, basal ganglia and pons, with diffuse loss of myelin in the cerebral white matter and ventricular dilation.

Computed tomography (CT) imaging shows lacunar infarction and marked leukoaraiosis. These changes are much better seen on magnetic resonance imaging (MRI), with characteristic extensive white matter abnormalities (Figure 11.2). The abnormalities are more extensive than is usually seen in leukoaraiosis from hypertension or ageing, and characteristically involve the temporal lobes and external capsule. MRI changes have been shown to precede the onset of clinical disease. Neuropathologically multiple small deep infarcts are seen, accompanied by diffuse myelin loss and a widespread vasculopathy of the small perforating arteries.

CADASIL is due to mutations in the *notch3* gene on chromosome 19 (Joutel *et al.*, 1996, 1997). The *notch3* gene encodes the Notch3 protein, which is a single-pass transmembrane protein with an extracellular portion containing 34 tandem repeats of an epidermal growth factor (EGF) motif, each of which contains 6 cysteine residues binding within the domain as 3 cysteine disulphide bonds. The mutations that have been demonstrated in CADASIL occur in these EGF repeats; all of these are missense mutations and occasionally small deletions resulting in the loss or gain of a cysteine residue. It is hypothesised that this leads to a disruption of the structure of the EGF domain and the formation of abnormal Notch3 dimers, or the binding of Notch3 protein to another protein as a result of the availability of an unpaired cysteine residue created by the mutation.

Diagnostic suspicion is aroused by the clinical picture, family history and MRI appearances. Skin biopsy may show the characteristic

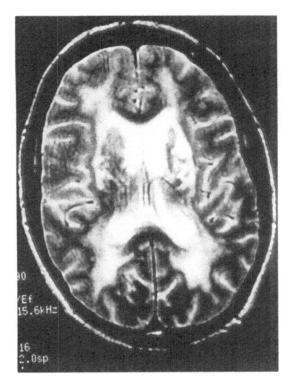

Figure 11.2 T$_2$-weighted MRI scan in CADASIL showing multiple lacunar infarctions and leuko-araiosis.

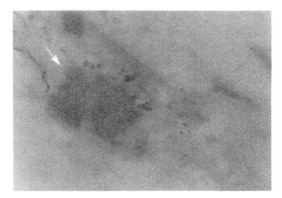

Figure 11.3 Electron microscopy of a skin biopsy in CADASIL showing typical granular osmiophilic material (courtesy of Dr L Bridges).

GOM on electron microscopy, which is diagnostic of the disease, but is only found in about 50% of biopsies (Figure 11.3). Definitive diagnosis is by genotyping. Mutations have been reported in a large number of exons of the *notch3* gene, but 60–70% cluster in exons 3 and 4.

There is no effective therapy for CADASIL. It is unknown whether treatment with antithrombotic agents or anticoagulants delays disease progression. However, smoking is associated with a lower age of onset of stroke in individuals with CADASIL and it is therefore logical to control modifiable vascular risk factors as vigorously as possible (Singhal *et al.*, 2004).

DISSECTION

This is an important cause of stroke, particularly in young individuals, and is covered in Chapter 10.

DRUG ABUSE

Abuse of illicit drugs is an important cause of stroke in some communities. The use of street drugs and alcohol may be associated with both haemorrhagic and ischaemic stroke. These complications are reviewed in this chapter. Stroke may also complicate the therapeutic use of prescription drugs (e.g. haemorrhagic stroke following streptokinase or anticoagulants) or overdose with similar prescription drugs. These associations are not covered in this chapter. The most important drug-related cause of stroke is smoking; this is covered in Chapter 5.

Alcohol

This was mentioned as a possible risk factor for stroke as early as 1725, but there has been disagreement over the strength and nature of the association. Much of this is due to difficulty in interpreting the available data for a number of reasons, including difficulty in accurately estimating alcohol intake and reliability of self-reported intakes; difficulty in disentangling the effects of different types of alcoholic drink; confounding with cigarette smoking, which is positively related, and exercise, which is negatively related to alcohol consumption; failure to differentiate between haemorrhagic and ischaemic strokes, which may have different relationships to alcohol, in a number of studies; and the small size and case–control design of many of the studies. Nevertheless, most evidence suggests that moderate or heavy alcohol consumption is associated with an increased risk of stroke, particularly haemorrhagic stroke, while low levels of alcohol consumption may exert a protective effect, particularly on ischaemic stroke (Ben-Shlomo *et al.*, 1992).

Haemorrhagic stroke and alcohol consumption
Overall, there is a positive direct linear association between alcohol consumption (>60 g ethanol daily) and the risk of both intracerebral and subarachnoid haemorrhage in diverse populations, including both urban and rural US populations and Japanese living in both Japan and Hawaii (Camargo, 1989). There is some evidence to suggest that following a reduction in alcohol consumption, the risk of haemorrhagic stroke falls rapidly. An association between binge drinking and subarachnoid haemorrhage secondary to pre-existing aneurysms has been reported. However, there is less evidence supporting this association. Moderate to heavy drinking may result in haemorrhagic stroke from a number of potential mechanisms, including the induction of hypertension, and disruption of coagulation by an effect on platelet function or a decrease in circulating levels of clotting factors produced by the liver.

Ischaemic stroke and alcohol consumption
Most data suggest there is a J-shaped relationship between coronary heart disease and alcohol consumption, with the lowest risk being associated with regular consumption of small amounts of alcohol of up to 21 units per week. A similar relationship appears to exist with ischaemic stroke, with there being a markedly higher risk at high levels of alcohol consumption and protective effects at moderate levels of consumption, with a slightly increased risk in abstainers. It has been argued that this association is less strong in Japanese and possibly Black populations. The increase in ischaemic

stroke risk associated with heavy drinking may be secondary to a number of mechanisms. These include the induction of hypertension, embolism from both atrial fibrillation and an alcoholic cardiomyopathy, and possibly other mechanisms including decreased cerebral blood flow and vasospasm, haemoconcentration and possibly changes in platelet aggregation.

Street drugs

There are a large number of reports of ischaemic and haemorrhagic stroke occurring during, or shortly after, the use of either illicit street drugs or over-the-counter (OTC) sympathomimetic drugs (Kelly *et al.*, 1992; Neiman *et al.*, 2000). The strongest association appears to be with cocaine, but there are also reports associating amphetamines and sympathomimetic agents, and occasional reports associating heroin, pentazocine, phencyclidine (PCP), lysergic acid diethylamide (LSD) and cannabis with stroke. There is little information about the proportion of strokes associated with the use or abuse of drugs in specific hospital populations. In one study, 167 of 178 stroke patients entered into the Maryland Stroke Data Bank between 1 September 1988 and 1 August 1989 were asked for a history of drug use or abuse (Sloan *et al.*, 1991). Information was incomplete in 51 of 167 (31%) of patients due to the neurological deficit preventing the patient from answering or failure to ask the relevant questions. Of the remaining 116 cases, 11 (9.5%) were associated with drug abuse. The age range was 25–56 years (mean 41 years). Stroke associated with drug abuse occurred in 4 of 62 (6%) cerebral infarcts, 2 of 28 (7%) intracerebral haemorrhages and 5 of 26 (19%) subarachnoid haemorrhages. Drugs included cocaine in 5 cases (45%), OTC sympathomimetics in 3 (27%), PCP in 2 (18%) and heroin in 1 (9%). Without a control group, it is difficult to assess the strength of these associations. However, one should have a high index of suspicion in all young cases of stroke for a possible association with drug abuse. In suspected cases, a urine sample should be taken on admission for drug screening.

Amphetamines and related drugs Both subarachnoid haemorrhage and intracerebral haemorrhage, as well as occasional cases of subdural haemorrhage, have been reported in association with amphetamine use (Petitti *et al.*, 1998; McGee *et al.*, 2004). In some cases, there is an underlying aneurysm or arteriovenous malformation (AVM). Ischaemic stroke is less common, but can occur with both amphetamine and amphetamine analogues. Vasculitis has been reported in a number of cases of both ischaemic and haemorrhagic stroke associated with amphetamine abuse. Experimentally, after repeated injections of methamphetamine, pathological examination shows small haemorrhages, infarctions, micro-aneurysms and perivascular cuffing by round cell infiltrates in small to medium-sized vessels. In patients, cerebral angiography has shown segmental narrowing and dilatations (or 'beading') of medium-sized intracerebral arteries. This appearance may recover following abstinence from amphetamines. Amphetamine also has a potent sympathomimetic action and induces a marked rise in blood pressure, which may contribute to the risk of haemorrhage, particularly in the presence of pre-existing vascular malformations. Vasoconstriction may also occur. Ecstasy (3,4-methylenedioxymethamphetamine, MDMA) has been associated with both cerebral infarction and intracranial haemorrhage.

Ingestion of phenylpropanolamine (PPA)-containing compounds has been associated with both subarachnoid and parenchymal haemorrhages (Kernan *et al.*, 2000). In most cases, haemorrhagic stroke occurs within hours of ingestion of the drug. The mechanism may be catecholamine-mediated vasospasm, coupled with an acute elevation of blood pressure, possibly a hypersensitivity reaction. Phentermine, which is used as an anorexiant, has been associated with ischaemic stroke. Ephedrine, a sympathomimetic agent that can be readily obtained without prescription, has been occasionally associated with stroke. Reports include both haemorrhagic and ischaemic stroke.

Cocaine This is the street drug most commonly associated with both ischaemic and haemorrhagic stroke. An underlying berry aneurysm or AVM is found in a significant proportion of patients with subarachnoid or intracerebral haemorrhage associated with cocaine use (McEvoy *et al.*, 2000). An important pathogenic mechanism may be the induction of hypertension, which may either cause bleeding from a pre-existing malformation or result in a spontaneous intracerebral haemorrhage. In ischaemic stroke, hemispheric stroke, often subcortical, is the most common site, but brainstem and cerebellar strokes and anterior spinal artery infarction have been reported. A number of mechanisms have been suggested for this association. These include vasospasm, vasculitis, cardiac arrhythmias, myocardial infarction and an increase in platelet aggregation. In a number of cases, there is a history of concomitant alcohol or other drug abuse, or hypertension and other cardiovascular risk factors. However, some cases lack any other definite stroke risk factors. Symptoms usually occur within a few hours of cocaine use, but this will partially depend upon the route of administration. Smoking results in a rapid increase in plasma concentration, with a short duration of action of about 20 minutes. Intranasal administration may result in raised plasma concentrations for longer than 1 hour. Absorption from mucous membranes is slow, resulting in a delayed onset of action.

One study in an inner city emergency trauma unit in the USA prospectively followed 31 081 admissions over a 3-year period (Peterson *et al.*, 1991). During this period, 33 patients were seen, with a total of 35 acute neurovascular events (infarction or haemorrhage) related to cocaine abuse. This represented 3% of the total 979 cocaine-related admissions. Fifty-four percent of the events were ischaemic and 46% haemorrhagic. Six patients died. The majority (63%) of ischaemic events were hemispheric and subcortical in distribution. Thirteen angiograms were performed in the 33 patients and 11 of these were abnormal, including the identification of 5 aneurysms and 2 arteriovenous malformations. No cases of 'angiographic vasculitis' were seen. Seventy percent of the patients exclusively abused crack cocaine and

94% of the neurovascular events were related to its use.

Heroin Stroke associated with heroin abuse is most commonly ischaemic, and intravenous injection is the usual route of administration (Brust and Richter, 1976). Cases have been reported both soon after heroin injection and following a delay of more than 24 hours. Rare cases of intracerebral haemorrhage have also been reported. A number of mechanisms may account for the association with heroin. Contamination of intravenous injections may result in infective endocarditis with septic embolism. Human immunodeficiency virus (HIV) infection from sharing needles may present with stroke. Some cases of cerebral angiography have shown changes consistent with an arteritis. Other possible stroke mechanisms that have been suggested include emboli from contaminants introduced during intravenous injection, hypotension, compression of the carotid artery while comatose, and a hypersensitivity reaction to either the heroin or an unknown adulterant.

Other street drugs Pentazocine, PCP and LSD have all been associated with rare reports of stroke. Marijuana has been associated with both TIA and stroke, although they seem to be rare and may not be caused by the drug.

FABRY'S DISEASE

Fabry's disease is a rare sex-linked recessive lysosomal storage disorder order in which there is a deficiency of α-galactosidase A (Brady and Schiffman, 2000). This results in an accumulation of glycosphingolipids in vascular endothelial smooth muscle cells and other cell types. These include renal glomerular epithelial cells, myocardial cells, dorsal root neurones and autonomic neurones. There is a wide spectrum of clinical findings. Ischaemic stroke, usually due to occlusion of small arteries, is a well-recognized complication. Other features include skin angiokeratosis, joint pain (which may resemble rheumatoid juvenile arthritis),

lancinating, burning limb pain, acroparaesthesia in the hands and feet from neuropathy, and the later development of corneal dystrophy, renal failure and myocardial involvement. Enzyme-replacement therapy is available.

FIBROMUSCULAR DYSPLASIA

Fibromuscular dysplasia (FMD) typically affects the medium-sized and large arteries of young and middle-aged women (Ortiz-Fandino *et al.*, 2004). It has a particular predilection for the extracranial distal cervical internal carotid artery and less commonly the vertebral artery. It also commonly affects the renal arteries, and can cause renal artery stenosis with secondary hypertension. Usually, FMD involves medial fibroplasia of the arterial wall, which results in a 'string of beads' appearance on angiography, with alternating areas of constriction and dilation (Figure 11.4). The intimal form of FMD is associated with smooth focal stenosis. Single or multiple cervical vessels can be involved. The disorder is of unknown aetiology, but seems to develop during adult life and is commonest in middle-aged women. It is often asymptomatic, and mild degrees of fibromuscular dysplasia have been reported in as many as 1% of angiograms performed for reasons other than cerebrovascular disease. The commonest presentation is with symptoms of dissection (Chapter 10), which may be recurrent. Occasionally, severe stenosis may cause TIA or stroke, or a cervical bruit without other signs. The diagnosis usually requires conventional catheter angiography, because the affected site is above the section of the artery visualized by ultrasound and is not well shown by magnetic resonance angiography (MRA).

HAEMATOLOGICAL DISORDERS (TABLE 11.2)

Haematological disorders account for 1–8% of ischaemic strokes in different series (Hart and Kanter, 1990; Markus and Hambley, 1998). Many primary haematological disorders have

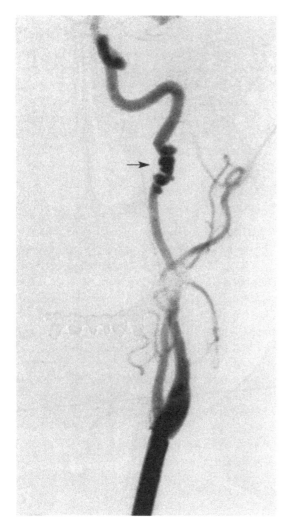

Figure 11.4 Carotid angiogram fibromuscular dysplasia of the distal internal cartoid artery (arrow).

Table 11.2 Haematological disorders associated with ischaemic stroke

Cellular disorders
- Essential thrombocythaemia
- Intravascular lymphoma
- Monoclonal gammopathies
- Paroxysmal nocturnal haemoglobinuria
- Polycythaemia rubra vera
- Sickle cell disease
- Thrombotic thrombocytopenic purpura

Thrombophilia
Congenital
- Natural anticoagulant disorders:
  - Protein C deficiency
  - Protein S deficiency
  - Factor V Leiden polymorphism (activated protein C resistance)
  - Antithrombin III deficiency
- Fibrinolytic system disorders
- Plasminogen deficiency
Acquired
- Antiphospholipid syndrome
- Anticardiolipin antibodies
- Lupus anticoagulant

been associated with ischaemic stroke and in many patients with stroke other aetiological factors are also present, making a cause-and-effect relation difficult to prove. Furthermore, some of these haematological factors, particularly deficiencies of the natural anticoagulants, are more potent causes of venous thrombosis, including cerebral venous thrombosis, than arterial thrombosis (Chapter 12). In patients with apparent arterial stroke associated with these haematological abnormalities, paradoxical embolism from the venous system should be considered as a possible cause of the arterial occlusion.

Essential thrombocythaemia

This is a myeloproliferative disorder in which the platelet count is above $600 \times 10^9/l$. In addition, the platelets are often functionally abnormal. Such abnormalities of platelet function occasionally result in a bleeding tendency, but thrombosis is more common. Stroke is a well-recognized complication (Arboix *et al.*, 1995). This condition needs to be distinguished from secondary thrombocythaemia arising in response to a wide variety of conditions, including inflammation, acute bleeding, iron deficiency, splenectomy and infection. Treatment of essential thrombocythaemia involves reducing the platelet count with cytotoxic agents (e.g. hydroxyurea). Aspirin is sometimes used to protect against thrombosis, but its benefit is uncertain as it can also increase the risk of haemorrhage.

Intravascular lymphoma

This is an uncommon malignancy, defined pathologically by neoplastic proliferation of lymphoid cells within lumens of capillaries, small veins and arteries with little or no adjacent parenchymal involvement. It used to be called malignant angioendotheliosis, but immunohistochemical studies have demonstrated that the cells are neoplastic lymphoid cells, more commonly of B-cell origin, and therefore it is now referred to as intravascular lymphoma or angiotrophic large-cell lymphoma. Most commonly, symptoms are confined to the skin or central nervous system (CNS) until later stages of the disease, when systemic features may develop. One neurological presentation is with recurrent stroke-like episodes, with haemorrhage and/or infarction on imaging (Baehring *et al.*, 2005). Intravascular lymphoma may progress to or present with a dementia, a spinal cord syndrome, and peripheral or cranial neuropathies. Clinically, it may produce an identical picture to primary angiitis of the CNS, including similar angiographic appearances, and distinction may only be possible on brain biopsy or postmortem.

Monoclonal gammopathies

These constitute a range of disorders that may occasionally be associated with cerebral infarction. They are due to monoclonal expansion of a single B stem cell in the bone marrow, or in a lymph node, with the excessive production of a monoclonal peak of either immunoglobulin G (IgG), IgA or IgM antibodies. The disorder comprises a variety of conditions, including benign monoclonal gammopathy of uncertain significance (MGUS), multiple myeloma, Waldenström's macroglobulinaemia, heavy-chain disease and light-chain disease. CNS manifestations include confusional states and blurred vision, thought to be caused by associated hyperviscosity and sludging. This may occasionally be associated with cortical venous thrombosis and rarely ischaemic stroke. In addition, renal amyloidosis may occur. Ophthalmological abnormalities and confusion are more common. Proteinuria with loss of both clotting factors and proteins involved in the fibrinolytic pathway may contribute to the increased thrombotic tendency. The disorders are diagnosed by serum and urine electrophoresis, skeletal survey, and bone marrow examination. Chemotherapy may be required in the more malignant cases; thrombosis in the context of hyperviscosity is best managed by hydration in the acute stages.

Paroxysmal nocturnal haemoglobinuria (PNH)

This condition occurs mainly between the ages of 20 and 40 years. The principal abnormality is a defect in the membrane of blood cells of all types preventing the permanent adhesion of a variety of membrane proteins and glycoproteins. Some of those missing proteins (decay accelerating factor and membrane inhibitor of reactive lysis) normally protect blood cells from the destructive effect of complexes of activated complement. Consequently, the integrity of the cell membrane is destroyed and patients usually present with a normochromic normocytic anaemia or pancytopenia. Despite the terminology, PNH rarely presents with haemoglobinuria. Platelet lifespan is normal, but complement activation results in excessive aggregation and hypercoagulability of these cells, with an increase in the incidence of thrombosis, primarily venous occlusion. This disorder is probably caused by the clonal expansion of a single abnormal stem cell and frequently progresses to aplastic anaemia and other myelodysplastic syndromes (MDS). The condition should be considered in patients with cerebral venous thrombosis or cryptogenic stroke associated with an anaemia or pancytopenia of unexplained origin (al-Hakim *et al.*, 1993). The condition is easily diagnosed by Ham's test, in which the patient's red blood cells are treated with acidified normal plasma. This activates complement, destroying only the abnormal cells.

Polycythaemia rubra vera (primary polycythaemia)

This is a myeloproliferative disorder resulting from clonal expansion of a transformed haematopoetic stem cell associated with pronounced overproduction of red blood cells and, to a lesser extent, expansion of granulocytic and megakaryocytic elements. The condition usually begins in late middle age. There is an absolute increase in red cell mass due to the abnormality of red cell production, with an increased haemoglobin concentration, red cell count and packed cell volume (haematocrit). There is usually an associated thrombocytosis and a variable neutrophilia. The plasma volume remains normal, while erythropoietin levels are reduced. Polycythaemic patients have approximately a 10–20% prevalence of stroke or TIA, with an annual incidence of 2–5% per annum (Gruppo Italiano Studio Policitemia, 1995). There is also an increased risk of cerebral venous thrombosis.

The increased haematocrit results in hyperviscosity and reduced cerebral blood flow. However, it is likely that most vascular symptoms result from superimposed thrombosis. It is likely that the associated platelet abnormality contributes to the increased risk of thrombosis in polycythaemia. Other neurological symptoms include headache, dizziness, visual blurring and confusion, possibly resulting from the reduction in cerebral blood flow. Treatment may involve phlebotomy, antiplatelet therapy, hydroxyurea and other cytotoxic drugs.

Secondary polycythaemia may occur in situations of chronic hypoxia (e.g. congenital cyanotic heart disease and smoking) and also with cerebellar haemangioblastomas and renal tumours. It has been suggested that secondary polycythaemia is a risk factor for stroke, but if this is the case then the association seems to be very weak and some studies have failed to report any association.

Sickle cell disease

Stroke is a frequent complication of homozygous sickle cell disease (HbSS), particularly in children. The disorder is due to the substitution of valine for glutamic acid at position 6 of the globin β chain. As a result, polymerization of the abnormal HbS haemoglobin can occur in regions of low oxygen saturation. These sheets of polymerized haemoglobin deform the red cell, reducing its resilience and impairing its ability to transit through capillaries without becoming impacted. If this occurs, the resultant tissue hypoxia accelerates sickling of red cells in adjacent vessels. This process is accentuated by the increased adhesion of affected cells to capillary endothelium. The polymerization of the abnormal haemoglobin is reversible. However, if repeated or prolonged hypoxia is experienced, sickling may become irreversible due to changes in membrane structure. The sickle forms then do not change shape during capillary transit and often cause irreversible obstruction of these vessels, local ischaemia and subsequent infarction.

Asymptomatic small vessel disease and cognitive impairment are common manifestations of cerebral sickling. In addition, stenosis of large extracranial or intracranial vessels, particularly the middle cerebral artery, may occur secondary to fibrous proliferation of the intima, and then lead to ischaemic stroke. Middle cerebral artery stenosis can be detected using transcranial Doppler by the finding of an increase in the blood flow velocity in the artery. Significant increases in the blood flow velocity have been shown to be a strong risk factor for subsequent stroke in children with sickle cell disease (Gebreyohanns and Adams, 2004). Occlusion of the distal internal carotid arteries may result in a moyamoya-like syndrome that can present in children and young adults with subarachnoid or intracerebral haemorrhage (see 'Moyamoya syndrome' below).

The mainstay of treatment of the cerebrovascular complications of sickle cell disease is exchange transfusion together with hydration and oxygen therapy (Kirkham and DeBaun, 2004). It has been suggested that prophylactic exchange transfusion in patients at particularly high risk could reduce the incidence of stroke and that transcranial Doppler ultrasonography to detect asymptomatic stenosis in the middle cerebral artery should be used to predict increased stroke risk. One study in the USA suggested that starting an exchange transfusion programme in neurologically asymptomatic children with raised blood flow velocity in the middle cerebral artery reduced the rate of subsequent stroke. Sleep apnoea in children with sickle cell disease may also be a risk factor for stroke.

Stroke may also complicate haemoglobin C sickle cell disease (HbSC). However, individuals heterozygous for HbS are not usually at an increased risk of cerebrovascular disease.

Thrombocytopenia

Idiopathic thrombocytopenic purpura (ITP) In adults, ITP tends to follow a more chronic course than the paediatric form of this disease. This condition is caused by an antibody to the platelet glycoprotein IIb/IIIa (GPIIb/IIIa) or GPIb/IX complex, which increases splenic sequestration of platelets as well as interfering with their function. The numbers of circulating platelets are reduced and their adhesion characteristics changed. The condition is more than three times more common in women. Intracranial haemorrhage is a common presentation of this condition (Cohen *et al.*, 2000). Patients usually respond to glucocorticoid treatment, but may also require plasmapheresis in the acute stage. Patients refractory to these regimens will require splenectomy. Other therapies include danazol and intravenous gammaglobulin infusion.

Thrombotic thrombocytopenic purpura (TTP) This is a rare but often fatal disorder characterized by thrombocytopenia, a micro-angiopathic haemolytic anaemia, renal failure, fever and neurological symptoms. The haemolytic anaemia occurs secondary to intravascular mechanical destruction of red cells. The peripheral blood smear is characteristic, showing deformed and unusual red cell fragments. The aetiology of this condition is unknown. Localized deposition of fibrin and platelet clots within arterioles occurs, leading to microvascular occlusion. The endothelium in the vicinity of this in situ thrombosis looks relatively intact. The clinical and pathological features are very similar to those of *disseminated intravascular coagulation (DIC)*, which can also present with stroke, but in TTP there is no measurable derangement of clotting. The condition may be associated with autoimmune states, including systemic lupus erythematosus (SLE), suggesting that there may be an immunological cause for the condition. Several abnormal proteins have been identified in this condition, including a platelet-aggregating protein, but their role in the pathogenesis is not clear. Many of the symptoms are due to the widespread small platelet microthrombi, which cause infarction in many organs including the brain. Neurological symptoms of TTP and DIC include a fluctuating encephalopathic picture with confusion and seizures, which may sometimes be accompanied by focal symptoms and signs. Both can occasionally present with isolated stroke or TIA. The thrombocytopenia on full blood count helps to suggest the diagnoses, but further studies of coagulation are required to distinguish between TTP and DIC. Both cerebral infarction and occasionally intracerebral haemorrhage may occur. Treatment involves infusion of fresh frozen plasma and platelet concentrates, coupled with exchange transfusion or extensive plasmapheresis in TTP. This has led to a considerable reduction in mortality. Antiplatelet agents or anticoagulants may increase the risk of haemorrhage. It should be remembered that treatment with heparin may also be complicated by thrombocytopenia.

Thrombophilia

The terms 'thrombophilia' and 'prothrombotic state' are used to describe an increased tendency to clinical thrombosis associated with laboratory evidence of abnormality in the coagulation pathway (Chapter 7). The main causes of thrombophilia are deficiencies of the natural anticoagulant factors (protein C, protein S and antithrombin III) and the factor V Leiden polymorphism. The natural anticoagulants (heparin cofactor II, antithrombin III, protein C and protein S) inhibit thrombosis in normal individuals. Proteins S and C are synthesized by the liver and released into the general circulation. Protein C is then activated by the thrombin/ thrombomodulin complex during thrombus formation and stabilized by protein S, which increases its potency. Activated factors V and VIII (which play key roles in the thrombotic cascade) are then degraded. Deficiencies of these may either occur congenitally or be acquired. Homozygotic inheritance of deficiencies of these factors usually causes fatal thrombosis in infancy. However, heterozygotes have much lesser degrees of deficiency, with levels approximately half normal, and are often asymptomatic. Protein C or S deficiency occurs in about 0.4% of the population. There have been a large number of studies linking deficiency of proteins C or S or, less often, antithrombin III with premature arterial disease, including stroke. However, many of these are case reports or small series with no control groups and it is difficult to be sure how important a cause of stroke these represent. Larger prospective series have shown no significant association between thrombophilia and stroke. For example, in a series of 219 patients from Western Australia with first ever ischaemic stroke, protein C or S deficiency or factor V Leiden polymorphism was found in 14.7% of patients and 11.7% of controls, which was not statistically different (Hankey *et al.*, 2001). The situation is complicated because in acute stroke, low concentrations of proteins C and S are fairly common and may reflect consumption. The degree of reduction in protein C concentration has been associated with the severity of stroke. Therefore if low levels of proteins C or S are found in the acute phase of stroke, the assays should be repeated after 3 months. In addition, a careful family history should be taken and family members tested. Low protein C and S concentrations may also occur in severe liver disease, the nephrotic syndrome and during pregnancy. Warfarin also lowers protein C and S levels.

Functional resistance to the anticoagulant effects of activated protein C seems to be the most common inherited prothrombotic state. This abnormality results from a point mutation in factor V at the exact site (Arg 506) where activated protein C normally cleaves and inactivates the Va procoagulant; this is referred to as the Leiden factor V mutation. A number of studies have suggested an association between activated protein C resistance, or the Leiden factor V mutation, and stroke, but larger case–control studies have failed to confirm the association. It should be remembered that the normal gene frequency of the heterozygote form may be as high as 5–10% and therefore finding the factor V mutation in a patient with stroke does not prove a causal association.

In contrast to arterial stroke, there is a strong and significant association between inherited heterozygous thrombophilia and venous thromboembolism, including cerebral venous thrombosis. Nevertheless, many patients with the haematological deficit never suffer a thrombotic event. Venous thrombosis is often precipitated by a prothrombotic event (e.g. bed rest) or occurs in association with other well-recognized risk factors (e.g. combined oral contraception or pregnancy).

In patients with arterial stroke and inherited thrombophilia, the association may be coincidence and the finding may not indicate an increased risk of recurrent thrombosis. Lifelong anticoagulation should therefore only be considered in patients in whom recurrent arterial thrombosis has been documented. Because of the stronger association of thrombophilia with venous thrombosis, the finding of inherited thrombophilia in a patient with apparent arterial ischaemia should always raise the possibility that an event that may appear arterial has in fact resulted from cortical venous thrombosis or paradoxical embolism from an asymptomatic deep vein thrombosis. Cerebral venous thrombosis associated with inherited thrombophilia is an indication for lifelong anticoagulation.

It is important that patients with known thrombophilia should not be started on warfarin without additional heparin cover for at least the first week of anticoagulation, because warfarin lowers protein C and S concentrations before other vitamin K-dependent coagulation factors. An association has been reported between warfarin-induced skin necrosis and protein C deficiency, which, although rare, can be serious. It usually presents with localized pain followed by petechial rash and ecchymoses. This can progress to widespread full-thickness necrosis. Decision about the management of thrombophilia should be made in consultation with an experienced coagulation specialist. Aspirin is an appropriate treatment for patients with thrombophilia if the decision is made not to anticoagulate.

Antithrombin III deficiency   Antithrombin III complexes with a variety of serine–protease clotting factors. The deficiency state is an autosomal dominant condition. Deficiencies may be due to decreased absolute levels of antithrombin III or to the production of a deficient molecule in adequate concentration. Occasionally, the deficiency may be acquired, in which case it will be associated with hepatic or renal diseases, use of oral contraceptives or ʟ-asparaginase therapy. Arterial and venous cerebral infarcts have occasionally been reported in relation to deficiency of this protein.

Plasminogen deficiency   Families have been described with recurrent venous thrombosis and embolism due to defects in fibrinogen or plasminogen or with decreased synthesis or release of tissue plasminogen activator (tPA). There have been a few case reports associating such abnormalities with stroke, particularly cerebral venous thrombosis, although it appears to be rare.

Antiphospholipid antibodies   The *lupus anticoagulant* and *anticardiolipin antibodies* are closely related autoantibodies, belonging to a group of antibodies that react with proteins associated with phospholipids, including the phospholipid moieties of DNA or RNA (Keswani and Chauhan, 2002). They are most commonly found in patients with SLE, but may also occur in patients without the disease, and are associated with both arterial and venous thrombosis. In the absence of SLE, they may form one part of the *antiphospholipid antibody syndrome*, which can present with recurrent miscarriages, arterial and venous thrombosis, and pulmonary embolism. Livedo reticularis, cardiac valve vegetations and thrombocytopenia have also been described in association with the syndrome. However, anticardiolipin antibodies are not specific to the antiphospholipid

syndrome and may occur in normal subjects, patients with other autoimmune disorders, and patients with malignancy, HIV infection or taking a variety of drugs.

Lupus anticoagulant is detected in blood samples in the laboratory by a prolongation of clotting time, probably as a result of interfering with the procoagulant effects of membrane phospholipids in their interactions with platelets and the clotting system. However, it is unclear how antiphospholipid antibodies produce increased coagulability. They may bind to specific endothelial cell regions; in addition, they might decrease the amount of prostacyclin production at that site. The result would be heightened platelet aggregability and the initiation of coagulation. Also, activated protein C activity is supported by membrane-bound phosphatidylethanolamine. It is possible that the lupus anticoagulant and the anticardiolipin antibody react with this moiety, resulting in reduced local thrombolysis.

By definition, anticardiolipin antibodies interact with the ubiquitous phospholipid, cardiolipin. Their presence can consequently be associated with a false-positive VDRL test for syphilis (the reagent being cardiolipin). In this case the fluorescent treponemal antibody (FTA) test for syphilis is unreactive. Generally, the presence of the lupus anticoagulant is best assessed by prolongation of the kaolin cephalin time (KCT) and Russell viper venom test. The addition of normal plasma to the blood sample fails to correct the prolongation. Prothrombin time (PTT) is somewhat less accurate in detecting the presence of this antibody. As the antibodies also interact with the phospholipids on platelet membranes, they can cause platelet sequestration and thrombocytopenia. An enzyme-linked immunosorbent assay (ELISA) test is used for the detection of IgG, IgA or IgM anticardiolipin antibodies.

The association between antiphospholipid antibodies and stroke has been controversial. A number of large case–control studies have failed to show an association between anticardiolipin antibodies and stroke, suggesting that it is not an important cause on a population basis – at least when present in low titres. In a minority of patients, antiphospholipid antibodies, particularly when present in high titres and when associated with the lupus anticoagulant, appear to be associated with premature stroke. Such patients may present with thrombosis of a large or medium-sized intracerebral artery resulting in stroke, or with TIA. The symptoms of cerebral ischaemia may be atypical (e.g. amaurosis fugax in the absence of carotid artery stenosis).

The finding of anticardiolipin antibodies in association with stroke or TIA is not a routine indication for anticoagulation, because of the uncertainty about whether the finding indicates an increased risk of recurrence. However, anticoagulation with warfarin should be considered when stroke occurs as part of the full-blown antiphospholipid antibody syndrome, if there are very high titres of anticardiolipin antibodies and other evidence of connective tissue disorder, if there is a persistently positive lupus anticoagulant, or in the presence of recurrent symptoms.

One unusual neurological manifestation of the antibody seen in patients with SLE is as an acute ischaemic anterior optic neuropathy presenting as a dense central scotoma with little recovery, probably caused by in situ thrombosis of the posterior ciliary artery. This may be associated with an ischaemic myelopathy and may consequently mimic multiple sclerosis. Often, patients with SLE in whom such neurological manifestations occur have disease activity in other organs (joints, skin, blood, heart, liver or muscle). However, this is not always the case. Another manifestation of SLE, pseudotumour cerebri, may be due to occlusion of small veins draining into the dural sinuses caused by the localized prothrombotic effect of these antibodies.

HOMOCYSTINURIA

Raised plasma homocysteine levels are a risk factor for stroke (Chapter 5). In homocystinuria, a recessively inherited defect in cystathionine synthase leads to the accumulation of homocysteine behind the metabolic block, with the excretion of its disulphide form, homocystine, in the urine. Features include a 'marfanoid appearance', mental retardation, light hair, downward dislocation of the lenses and premature vascular disease (Yap, 2003). Stroke is a well-recognized complication of hereditary homocystinuria. Cerebral venous thrombosis is more common than ischaemic stroke.

INFECTIONS

A number of infections (e.g. bacterial endocarditis) may result in stroke. In addition, there is an epidemiological association between recent infection and stroke. These issues are covered in Chapter 5.

INFLAMMATORY VASCULAR DISORDERS

Stroke is a feature of most of the vasculitic connective tissue disorders, including SLE, polyarteritis nodosa (PAN), rheumatoid arthritis and Behçet's disease (Berlit et al., 1993). Neurological involvement is usually seen in patients in whom the systemic disorder has already been diagnosed. Stroke and, less often, TIA are often accompanied by other neurological features suggesting vasculitis (e.g. headache and encephalopathy). In some of these conditions, aseptic meningitis and cerebral venous thrombosis (Chapter 12) can also occur, widening the differential diagnosis. Occasionally, stroke can be the presenting feature of these diseases, although often, on close enquiry or investigation, there is usually some evidence of systemic involvement. Stroke is often a presenting feature in giant cell arteritis and Takayasu's arteritis, in contrast to the other systemic vasculitides. Cerebral vasculitis usually presents with symptoms of cerebral infarction, but can also cause subarachnoid and intracerebral haemorrhage, particularly in PAN.

Behçet's disease

This is most common in individuals from Turkey and the Mediterranean regions and usually presents with an arthritis and urogenital ulceration. Uveitis and recurrent phlebitis are other features. Neurological involvement may also occur, sometimes as a presenting feature. A chronic aseptic meningitis is one of the commoner neurological symptoms, and even in patients without symptomatic meningitis but with other neurological involvement, a lymphocytosis is often found on cerebrospinal fluid (CSF) examination. Stroke may occur from an associated vasculopathy affecting the medium-sized and small vessels, which more commonly involves the brainstem. Areas of focal ischaemia are most easily seen on MRI and enhancement with gadolinium may show blood–brain barrier breakdown. The cerebral veins may also be involved, resulting in cerebral venous thrombosis. The disease is treated with steroids and other immunosuppressive agents.

Giant-cell arteritis (temporal arteritis)

This is a vasculitis that may affect any medium-sized or large artery, but by far most commonly affects the ophthalmic artery and branches of the external carotid artery (Caselli et al., 1988). It derives its name from the characteristic giant cells, which are seen on biopsy of an affected artery accompanied by other pathological changes of a vasculitis. Giant-cell arteritis occurs in elderly individuals, usually over the age of 60, and most commonly presents with headache, which is described as a boring or throbbing pain predominantly temporal in location. It may present with uniocular visual loss, which is usually permanent but may occasionally be initially temporary (i.e. amaurosis fugax). Other frequent features include facial pain and scalp tenderness from external carotid artery involvement, and occasionally jaw claudication. On examination, tenderness, nodularity or lack of pulsation may be found on palpation of one or both temporal arteries. There is an overlap between this condition and polymyalgia rheumatica, in which patients present with malaise and myalgia, particularly in the shoulder and hip girdle. In both conditions, the ESR and C-reactive protein (CRP) are both markedly raised on first presentation. Involvement of the extracranial vertebral artery and the internal carotid artery occurs less frequently. Patients may then present with TIA or stroke. Pathological studies show that the vasculitis involves only extracranial vessels up to the level of the dura, suggesting that intracranial vascular symptoms result from artery-to-artery embolism. Giant-cell arteritis is a self-limiting disease which usually runs its course over 1–2 years, although this is variable.

In patients with classical disease presenting with headache or facial pain, visual loss and a raised ESR, the diagnosis of giant-cell arteritis is usually easy to make. Sometimes, there is also disturbance of liver function, particularly raised alkaline phosphatase, and a chronic normocytic anaemia. Urgent confirmation of the diagnosis and treatment should be instituted to avoid the risk of permanent blindness occurring secondary to irreversible ischaemic damage to the optic nerve. Even in patients who have had complete visual loss in one eye, there is a significant risk of involvement of the contralateral eye and, to a lesser extent, involvement of other intracranial arteries. Definitive diagnosis can only be made on biopsy, which is usually taken from the superficial temporal artery. A reasonable length of artery needs to be biopsied, because the disease can result in skip lesions. In some cases, biopsy of both temporal arteries may be needed to make the diagnosis. Occasionally, disease can still be present even if a good biopsy is negative. Initial treatment is with high-dose corticosteroids (prednisolone 40–80 mg/day). If biopsy has to be delayed, steroid treatment should be initiated and biopsy performed within the next few days. Steroids usually result in a rapid resolution of headache, facial pain and the symptoms of polymyalgia, if these are present. The dose of prednisolone should be tailed off over the next few months, but usually steroids need to be maintained at a low dose for a variable duration, sometimes for a number of years. The ESR can be used to monitor the effectiveness of treatment, although occasionally relapses can occur with a normal ESR. If prolonged steroid therapy is required, other immunosuppressive agents (e.g. azathioprine) are sometimes added.

Isolated angiitis of the CNS

By definition, this disease is an angiitis or vasculitis only involving the CNS (Hankey, 1991). Histology may show granuloma formation in the arteriolar walls (hence the older name for the disease: *granulomatous angiitis*). Most commonly, small intracranial vessels are involved and the patient may present with an encephalopathy, a progressive dementia or multiple stroke-like episodes. By definition, systemic disease does not occur, although frequently in such patients it can be difficult to determine unequivocally whether there is any systemic involvement, particularly in some patients who present with a raised ESR. Multiple areas of tissue ischaemia and infarction, often confined to deep white matter, are seen on CT or MRI scanning and there may be enhancement with gadolinium. Angiography is only occasionally abnormal (Figure 11.5). The concentration of protein is usually slightly raised in the CSF and a moderate increase in the CSF lymphocyte count is often present. Establishing the diagnosis can be extremely difficult and it can often only be made on meningeal or brain biopsy. There are a number of case reports in which patients in whom a definite diagnosis has been made in this manner have responded extremely well to immunosuppressive agents, particularly cyclophosphamide. Untreated cases are usually fatal within 6 months of presentation. However, the disease is too rare for there to have been any large series or controlled trials of treatment.

Systemic lupus erythematosus

SLE frequently involves the nervous system, the features including headache, psychiatric presentations, encephalopathy, stroke and TIA as well as peripheral nervous system

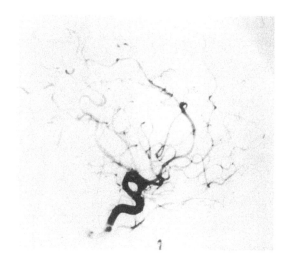

Figure 11.5 Carotid angiogram in a patient with cerebral vasculitis showing irregularity and beading of the distal arterial tree.

involvement (Brown and Swash, 1989). Stroke and TIA can occur as a result of a number of pathogenic processes. Involvement of small intracranial vessels may present with ischaemic, or sometimes haemorrhagic, symptoms. In those few cases in which pathological material has been obtained, appearances are not usually consistent with a florid vasculitis but rather a bland intimal proliferation involving the small vessels. Such brain involvement can be best imaged by MRI scanning, and frequently meningeal enhancement can be demonstrated by the use of gadolinium contrast (Figure 11.6). In such patients, the optimal treatment is immunosuppression with steroids and other agents (e.g. cyclophosphamide). Thrombosis may occur in large and medium-sized vessels, often in patients who have the lupus anticoagulant (see above) (Figure 11.7). In such patients, the optimal treatment is anticoagulation with or without immunosuppression. Patients with SLE may also develop an aseptic endocarditis (Libman–Sachs endocarditis), resulting in cerebral embolism and stroke. Renal disease in SLE may lead to stroke from renal hypertension or cerebral venous thrombosis from protein C deficiency secondary to proteinuria.

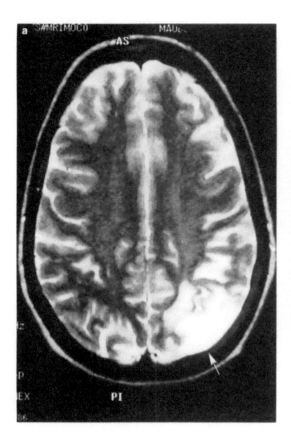

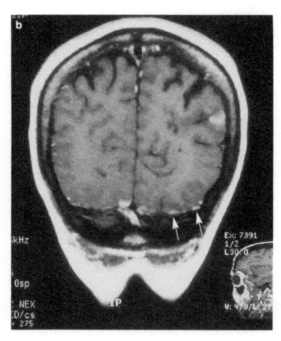

Figure 11.6 (a) SLE presenting with posterior parieto-occipital infarction shown on T_2-weighted MRI (arrow). (b) T_1-weighted MRI showed enhancement of the meninges (arrows) after gadolinium injection.

Systemic necrotizing vasculitis

The systemic necrotizing vasculitides include the related disorders Wegener's granulomatosis, PAN, and Churg–Strauss syndrome (Shannon and Goetz, 1989). Vasculitis most commonly affecting the medium-sized intracerebral vessels may occur and present with stroke, TIA or more diffuse CNS involvement, including vascular dementia. Occasionally, the disease can present with CNS involvement. An eosinophilia is often found on full blood count, and the anti-neutrophil cytoplasmic antibody is frequently elevated. Remission can be obtained with steroid and immunosuppressive therapy.

Takayasu's arteritis

This is also known as 'pulseless disease' and is an arteritis of the large vessels that predominantly affects the aorta and its branches at their origin (Lupi-Herrera *et al.*, 1977). This results in regions of vessel irregularity, focal stenosis or occlusion (Figure 11.8). Takayasu's arteritis usually affects young women, most commonly from the Far East, and is often accompanied by a systemic illness with fever, weight loss, malaise, arthralgias, night sweats and a raised ESR. It may present with ischaemia in the brain, in the arms (arm claudication), or sometimes in the kidneys and the lower limbs. Aortic regurgitation and coronary artery involvement may also occur. Clinical pointers to the disease on examination include a diminished or absent radial pulse or blood pressure, a blood pressure discrepancy of more than 30 mmHg between the left and right arms, cardiac murmurs and bruits. The nature of the neurological involvement will depend upon which arterial territories are affected.

The diagnosis is usually made on angiography with visualization of the entire aortic

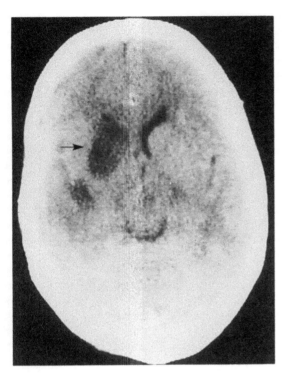

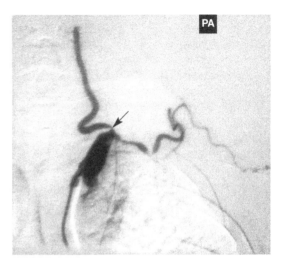

Figure 11.8   Left subclavian angiogram of a patient with Takayasu's aortitis showing severe left vertebral artery origin stenosis (arrow) and distal left subclavian artery occlusion. The axillary artery fills by collaterals.

Figure 11.7   CT scan showing acute striatocapsular infarction (arrow) associated with the lupus anticoagulant secondary to SLE.

arch and the renal and visceral arteries. The diagnosis may also be evident on contrast-enhanced MRA of the arch and proximal vessels. During the acute phase of the disease, thickening of the aortic arch has been reported, while in the chronic phase, arterial wall thinning has been seen. Treatment is with corticosteroids and is usually required for at least 2 years. The prognosis is usually good, with a 5-year survival rate of about 80%.

Other vasculitic/ autoimmune diseases

There are rare reports of *rheumatoid arthritis* and *Sjögren's syndrome* complicated by TIA or stroke. Rheumatoid arthritis may also cause vertebrobasilar ischaemia due to mechanical compression of the vertebral artery secondary to atlanto-occipital dislocation.

MIGRAINE

Ischaemic stroke is a very rare direct complication of migraine with aura. In these cases, patients with a history of migraine develop a typical visual aura that does not recover in the usual way and then persists as a permanent neurological deficit. Such deficits are almost always visual field defects (homonymous scotomata or hemianopia). The pathogenic mechanism of stroke in such cases is uncertain.

In addition to stroke complicating a typical migraine attack, a history of migraine appears to be a risk factor for stroke, particularly in young women. A number of studies have investigated whether a history of migraine is a risk factor for subsequent stroke (i.e. not necessarily occurring during a migraine attack). These studies have tended to show a positive association, with an odds ratio for ischaemic stroke associated with migraine history in the range of 2–3 (Tietjen, 2000). Some studies have suggested that this association is found largely, if not exclusively, in young individuals, particularly women on the combined oral contraceptive (Chang *et al.*, 1993). However, it is possible that some, if not all, of the relationship is related to recall and

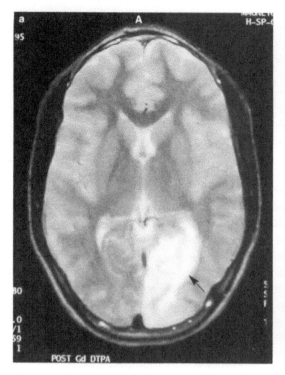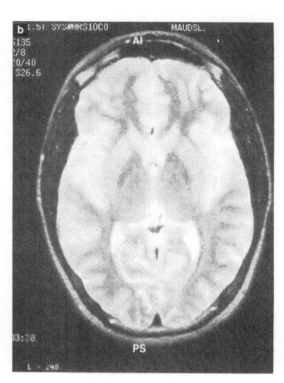

Figure 11.9   (a) MRI scan showing occipital lobe infarction in MELAS (arrow). (b) Two months later, a repeat MRI showed a marked improvement.

case ascertainment bias. Case–control studies have established that treatment of migraine with ergotamine or triptans is not associated with stroke (Hall *et al.*, 2004). It is important to recognize that migraine, like headache, can occur secondary to stroke rather than the migraine being the cause of the stroke. Moreover, the migraine is a frequent feature, sometimes with typical visual aura, in patients with carotid dissection, when it may precede the stroke (Olesen *et al.*, 1993). Thus, it is important to fully investigate patients with apparent migraine and stroke for other causes, particularly dissection, before attributing the stroke to migraine.

MITOCHONDRIAL DISORDERS

Mutations in mitochondrial DNA can result in a variety of syndromes that may involve the neurological system (Jackson et al., 1995). The phenotype that is most often associated with stroke is MELAS (mitochondrial encephalopathy with lactic acidosis and stroke-like episodes) (Ciafaloni et al., 1992). Individuals with MELAS usually present as children or young adults with recurrent stroke-like episodes. Infarction characteristically affects the occipital lobes, with a distribution that does not necessarily correspond to the distribution of the main cerebral arteries. Frequently, such ischaemic episodes are accompanied by epilepsy with both partial and secondary generalized seizures. Individuals may make a good recovery from initial episodes, but with recurrent episodes irreversible neurological damage and dementia usually occur. Other features that may occur include migraine, sensorineural deafness and episodic vomiting. There may also be other features characteristic of mitochondrial disorders (e.g. proximal muscle weakness, pigmentary retinopathy, myoclonus, ataxia, cardiomyopathy and external ophthalmoplegia) and there can be an overlap between the phenotypes of MELAS and other mitochondrial disorders. The mechanism of stroke is uncertain, but may involve local endothelial dysfunction with swelling of the intima and secondary occlusion of the smaller arteries.

The characteristic posterior involvement of the brain on neuroimaging, accompanied by epilepsy, often points to the diagnosis (Figure 11.9). During the early stages, the neuroimaging abnormalities may markedly improve or even disappear, often corresponding to clinical improvement. In patients in whom the diagnosis is suspected, lumbar puncture should be performed, and the CSF lactate is often raised. Magnetic resonance spectroscopy (MRS) may also demonstrate abnormal lactate production within the brain (Chapter 3). Muscle biopsy may show characteristic ragged red fibres. The diagnosis can be confirmed on mitochondrial DNA analysis. This can usually be demonstrated in white blood cells but sometimes can only be shown on muscle biopsy. The most common mutation is a 3243 mutation, but other mutations have also been associated with MELAS. Furthermore, in some individuals with a characteristic clinical picture, none of the previously reported characteristic mutations has been found.

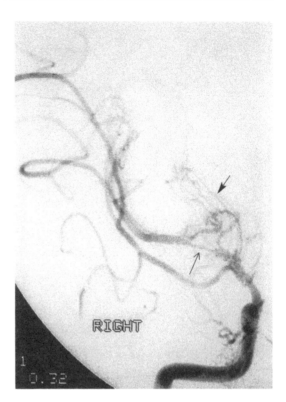

Figure 11.10 Angiogram of patient with moyamoya disease showing severe intracranial stenosis (open arrow head) and new vessel formation (closed arrow head).

MOYAMOYA DISEASE

Moyamoya disease is a rare condition, which is diagnosed from the appearances of the intracranial blood vessels on radiological imaging (moyamoya arteriopathy). The abnormalities of the blood vessels associated with moyamoya disease develop during early or mid childhood, but then may progress until late childhood or early adult life. Specifically, the appearances of the arteriopathy are those of bilateral occlusion or severe stenosis of the terminal portions of the internal carotid arteries and the proximal portions of the anterior cerebral and middle cerebral arteries. The disease rarely involves the posterior circulation. As a result of these occlusions, many small collateral lenticulostriate vessels develop beyond the occlusion and this pattern looks like a puff of smoke on an angiogram – hence its name (*moyamoya*: puff of smoke in

Japanese) (Figure 11.10). The diagnosis may also be suggested by the MRI appearance of multiple flow voids secondary to the enlarged lenticulostriate vessels in the basal ganglia. The abnormalities of the blood vessels are usually bilateral. Unilateral cases are encountered, but then the disease may spread subsequently to both hemispheres. The disease appears to be more frequent in the Orient and was first described in Japan, where the incidence is about 1 case per million of the population. It appears to be even rarer in other ethnic groups, but is occasionally found in Caucasians in the Western hemisphere (Chiu *et al.*, 1998).

Moyamoya disease is of unknown cause. Occasionally, identical angiographic appearances are encountered secondary to a known disease of the intracranial cerebral blood vessels, when the terms moyamoya syndrome,

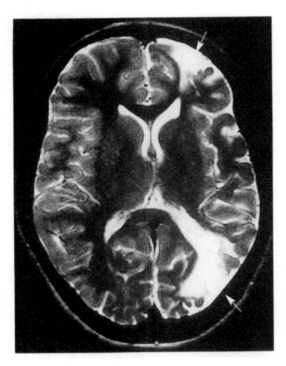

Figure 11.11 T_2-weighted MRI scan from a patient with moyamoya disease showing infarction in the anterior and posterior cortical border zones (arrows).

atypical moyamoya or secondary moyamoya disease may be used. These predisposing diseases include sickle cell disease, prothrombotic disorders, vasculitis and basal meningeal infections.

The condition usually presents in childhood with focal neurological deficits secondary to stroke caused by the vessel occlusion. Children may also present with mental retardation or cognitive problems. Silent infarction may occur, especially in the watershed areas (Figure 11.11). In adulthood, presentation with subarachnoid or intracerebral haemorrhage due to bleeding from the collateral vessels is more common. Often the diagnosis is not made until after the patient presents with a stroke from cerebral haemorrhage in young or middle-aged adult life. Headaches, presumably secondary to dilation of collateral vessels, may also occur.

The optimal treatment of moyamoya disease is uncertain. Extracranial-to-intracranial bypass, with anastomosis of the temporal branch of the external carotid artery to a superficial branch of the middle cerebral artery, is often recommended, particularly in children and young adults (Golby *et al.*, 1999). This may appear to improve outcome. Other revascularization procedures have been used, including omental transplantation. It is postulated that chronic hypoxia results in the new vessel formation, and this can be reduced by a revascularization procedure. However, there have been no controlled trials evaluating these surgical approaches. In patients who present late in the disease after formation of the collateral vessels, surgery has a limited role and management is uncertain. Children are often treated with aspirin or anticoagulation with warfarin, but in adults there is a risk that although these drugs might reduce the risk of further vessel occlusion, it is likely that they will increase the risk of haemorrhage. Hence, in adults, anticoagulation and antiplatelet agents should probably be stopped and pharmacological therapy should concentrate on treatment of any associated vascular risk factors and therapeutic lowering of blood pressure.

ORAL CONTRACEPTIVES

Recent evidence concerning the association between combined oral contraceptive medication and stroke is conflicting. Early studies suggested a significant increase of stroke associated with the use of high-dose (>50 mg oestrogen/day) oestrogen-containing preparations (Gillum *et al.*, 2000). However, the association between low-dose oestrogen-containing preparations and arterial thrombosis is less certain. Two epidemiological studies in the USA found no evidence of an increased risk of stroke, while three studies in Europe found a slight increase in risk, but the difference was only statistically significant in one study (Schwartz *et al.*, 1998; Lidegaard and Kreiner, 2002). It can be concluded that there may be a slight increase in risk, but the magnitude of the increase is small. It is likely that if there is an increase in risk, it will be most evident in older women with other risk factors (e.g. smoking or hypertension), because the effect of individual

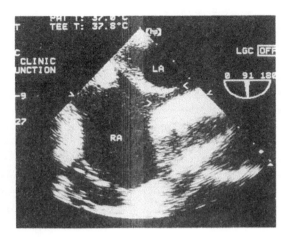

Figure 11.12 Echocardiogram showing a patent foramen ovale (fleches). LA, left atrium; RA, right atrium.

risk factors is multiplicative (Heinemann, 1999). Progesterone-only oral contraceptives do not appear to increase the risk of stroke.

PARADOXICAL EMBOLISM

Paradoxical embolism refers to embolism from the venous system, usually in the legs or pelvis, to the brain through an abnormal communication in the heart between the left and right sides. Normally, there is no direct communication between the left and right sides of the heart, and therefore embolism from deep venous thrombosis causes pulmonary embolus but not stroke. Blood is filtered in the lungs through tiny capillaries, and so any blood clots reaching the lungs from the heart do not travel any further. Emboli from the veins can only reach the brain to cause a stroke if there is either an arteriovenous fistula in the lungs or an abnormal communication between the right and left sides of the heart. This is almost invariably a congenital abnormality. During the development of a baby in utero, there is normally a communication between the right and left atria through a gap known as the foramen ovale. This normally closes completely soon after birth. However, in some people, the communication does not close completely and is then known as a patent foramen ovale (PFO)

(Figure 11.12). This is the most common persisting communication between the two atria. Where the wall between the two atria has not been properly formed, the communication is known as an atrial septal defect. Other forms of congenital heart disease, including ventricular septal defects, are also potential associations with paradoxical embolism.

Patent foramen ovale

PFO occurs in as many as 20–40% of adults and appears to be more common in young patients with idiopathic stroke than in controls. The foramen ovale is normally closed completely soon after birth by a thin tissue flap on the wall of the left atrium, which acts as a valve, closing the gap when the pressure in the left atrium rises above that of the right atrium immediately after birth. In some normal individuals, the flap does not seal completely, so that a potential communication remains between the two atria. The evidence suggests that paradoxical embolism is still a rare cause of stroke. For paradoxical embolism to occur, three coincidental conditions are required. Firstly, there must be a blood clot in the deep veins of the legs that breaks off and travels to the right side of the heart. Secondly, there must be a communication of sufficient size to allow the blood clot through the atria. Thirdly, the pressure in the right atrium must be higher than that in the left atrium. Normally, the pressure is higher on the left side than on the right side, so, even with a patent foramen ovale, the flow of blood is from left to right and paradoxical embolism does not occur even with a clot in the right atrium. However, the pressure may be increased on the right side of the heart, opening the flap closing the patent foramen ovale, and causing reversed flow from right to left, especially if the patient also has right ventricular hypertrophy. Reversed flow can occur transiently by manoeuvres that raise the intrathoracic pressure, such as straining at stool. Because all these features have to coincide, paradoxical embolism is a very rare cause of stroke. In rare cases, the coincidence of stroke with pulmonary

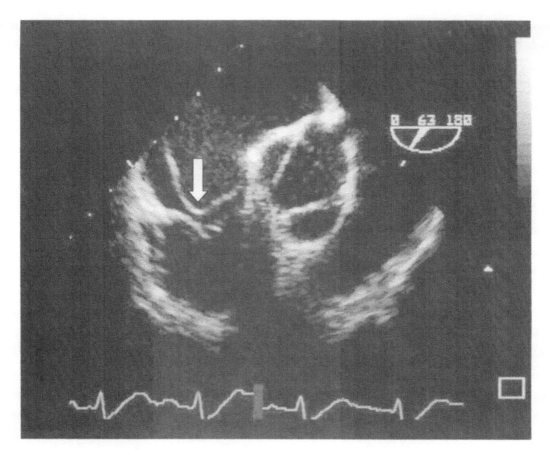

Figure 11.13   Echocardiogram showing an atrial septal aneurysm (arrow).

embolism, known deep vein thrombosis or right ventricular hypertrophy supports the diagnosis of paradoxical embolism. It is possible that the risk of embolism is determined by the size of the communication.

In some cases, the association of an atrial defect with stroke may not indicate paradoxical embolism, but another cardiac cause of stroke. For example, there is a strong association between atrial septal defects and atrial fibrillation. There is also an association between PFO and atrial septal aneurysm (Figure 11.13). Hence, stroke associated with PFO may well be the result of embolism of thrombosis formed within the PFO itself, within an associated atrial septal aneurysm or from elsewhere in the heart, rather than resulting from paradoxical embolism of thrombus formed in the deep veins. Because PFO is common in otherwise normal individuals, in many cases, the association with idiopathic stroke is likely to be a simple coincidence ('innocent PFO').

PFO can be diagnosed on echocardiography with the injection of intravenous agitated saline or ultrasonic contrast agent. Bubbles can be seen crossing the intra-atrial septum during manoeuvres that raise the right atrial pressure (e.g. Valsalva). Sensitivity is best using the more invasive transoesophageal approach. Transcranial Doppler ultrasound can also be used to make the diagnosis, with high-intensity signals due to the air bubbles being seen in the middle cerebral artery. This technique appears to be as sensitive as transthoracic echocardiography, but cannot distinguish cardiac from intrapulmonary shunts.

The optimal management of stroke in the presence of a PFO is uncertain. Where paradoxical embolism is suspected, and particularly when evidence of venous thrombosis can be found, anticoagulation with warfarin is often given. Some authorities advocate closure of the septal defect surgically, and the popularity of this is rising as it can now be performed intra-arterially. Trials are currently underway comparing percutaneous closure with anticoagulation in this patient group. However, a follow-up study has suggested that the risk of recurrence in patients with idiopathic stroke associated with isolated PFO is very low (Mas *et al.*, 2001). In this study, 581 patients aged 18–55 years with idiopathic ischaemic stroke within the preceding 3 months were treated with aspirin alone. After 4 years, the risk of recurrent stroke was only 2.3% in patients with PFO alone, compared with 4.2% in the control patients with no cardiac abnormalities. However, the risk of recurrence was significantly elevated at 15.2% in patients who had both PFO and an atrial septal aneurysm. There were no recurrences among the patients with an atrial septal aneurysm alone, but there were very few of these patients. Hence, one can conclude that the majority of patients with small isolated PFO do not require anticoagulation or closure of the defect.

PREGNANCY AND THE PUERPERIUM

Stroke complicating pregnancy is more common in underdeveloped countries. Nevertheless, in westernised countries, the incidence of stroke in women during pregnancy and the puerperium is increased compared with non-pregnant women (Mas and Lamy, 1998). Part of the slight increase in risk is due to a prothrombotic state, which most commonly presents with cerebral venous thrombosis in the puerperium. Dehydration during prolonged labour may also increase the risk of stroke. Ischaemic or haemorrhagic stroke can also occur as a result of eclampsia. There may be a slightly increased risk of bleeding from cerebral aneurysm and arteriovenous malformations, probably associated with the hyperdynamic circulation.

Ischaemic stroke and cerebral venous thrombosis are also rare complications of the *ovarian hyperstimulation syndrome* associated with *in vitro* fertility treatment (Stewart *et al.*, 1997). Possible mechanisms include the effects of high oestrogen levels, thrombosis caused by the associated endothelial abnormality, and the effects of dehydration and a prothrombotic state secondary to ascites.

SNEDDON'S SYNDROME

This condition is characterized by the association of florid skin *livedo reticularis* with ischaemic stroke, TIA or rarely vascular dementia (Wohlrab *et al.*, 2001). The aetiology is unknown. Livedo reticularis is associated with a number of autoimmune diseases, including SLE and antiphospholipid antibody syndrome (see above). Primary Sneddon's syndrome should only be diagnosed when there is no other aetiological factor present. Pathologically, small and medium-sized arteries in the skin and brain become occluded by proliferating endothelial cells. Large arteries are occasionally involved and ultrasound may rarely show thickening of the wall of the internal carotid artery. Treatment with steroids or anticoagulants has not been shown to influence the outcome.

TRAUMA

Much of the association between trauma and stroke is due to arterial dissection secondary to arterial torsion (e.g. whiplash injury) (Chapter 10). However, penetrating arterial injuries may also cause stroke. These are more likely to affect the carotid rather than the less accessible vertebral arteries. Such injuries may be complicated by acute thrombosis occluding the artery or resulting in an embolic source. After the injury, a traumatic aneurysm can occur that contains thrombus and itself acts as an embolic source, causing stroke sometimes delayed some years after the episode of trauma. Trauma may also lead to stroke via a number of other mechanisms, including cardiac contusion, fat embolism, activation of coagulation and paradoxical embolism from deep vein thrombosis.

KEY REFERENCES

CADASIL and other monogenetic causes of stroke

Desmond DW, Moroney JT, Lynch T et al. The natural history of CADASIL: a pooled analysis of previously published cases. *Stroke* 1999;**30**: 1230–1233

Hassan A, Markus HS. Genetics and ischaemic stroke. *Brain* 2000;**123**:1784–1812

Joutel A, Corpechot C, Ducros A et al. Notch 3 mutations in CADASIL, a hereditary adult-onset condition causing stroke and dementia. *Nature* 1996;**386**:707–710

Joutel A, Vahedi K, Corpechot C et al. Strong clustering and stereotyped nature of *notch 3* mutations in CADASIL patients. *Lancet* 1997;**350**:1511–1515

Singhal S, Bevan S, Barrick T et al. The influence of genetic and cardiovascular risk factors on the CADASIL phenotype. *Brain* 2004;**127**:2031–2038

Alcohol

Ben-Shlomo Y, Markowe H, Shipley M, Marmot MG. Stroke risk from alcohol consumption using different control groups. *Stroke* 1992;**23**:1093–1098

Camargo CA. Moderate alcohol consumption and stroke; the epidemiologic evidence. *Stroke* 1989; **20**:1611–1626

Street drugs

Brust JC, Richter RW. Stroke associated with addiction to heroin. *J Neurol Neurosurg Psychiatry* 1976;**39**:194–199

Kelly MA, Gorelick PB, Mirza D. The role of drugs in the etiology of stroke. *Clinical Neuropharmacology* 1992;**15**:249–275

Kernan WN, Viscoli CM, Brass LM et al. Phenylpropanolamine and the risk of hemorrhagic stroke. *N Engl J Med* 2000;**343**:1826–1832

McEvoy AW, Kitchen ND, Thomas DG. Intracerebral haemorrhage and drug abuse in young adults. *Br J Neurosurg* 2000;**14**:449–454

McGee SM, McGee DN, McGee MB. Spontaneous intracerebral hemorrhage related to methamphetamine abuse: autopsy findings and clinical correlation. *Am J Forensic Med Pathol* 2004;**25**:334–337

Neiman J, Haapaniemi HM, Hillborn M. Neurological complications of drug abuse: pathophysiological mechanisms. *Eur J Neurol* 2000;**7**:595–606

Peterson PL, Roszler M, Jacobs I, Wilner HI. Neurovascular complications of cocaine abuse. *J Neuropsychiatry Clin Neurosci* 1991;**3**:143–149

Petitti DB, Sidney S, Quesenberry C, Bernstein A. Stroke and cocaine or amphetamine use. *Epidemiology* 1998;**9**:596–600

Sloan MA, Kittner SJ, Rigamonti D, Price TR. Occurrence of stroke associated with use/abuse of drugs. *Neurology* 1991;**41**:1358–1364

Fabry's disease

Brady RO, Schiffmann R. Clinical features of and recent advances in therapy for Fabry disease. *JAMA* 2000;**284**:2771–2775

Fibromuscular dysplasia

Ortiz-Fandino J, Terre-Boliart R, Orient-Lopez F et al. Ischemic stroke, secondary to fibromuscular dysplasia: a case report. *Rev Neurol* 2004;**38**:34–37

Haematological disorders

al-Hakim M, Katirji B, Osorio I, Weisman R. Cerebral venous thrombosis in paroxysmal nocturnal hemoglobinuria: report of two cases. *Neurology* 1993;**43**:742–746

Arboix A, Besses C, Acin P et al. Ischemic stroke as first manifestation of essential thrombocythemia. Report of six cases. *Stroke* 1995;**26**:1463–1466

Baehring JM, Henchcliffe C, Ledezma CJ et al. Intravascular lymphoma: magnetic resonance imaging correlates of disease dynamics within the central nervous system. *J Neurol Neurosurg Psychiatry* 2005;**76**:540–544

Cohen YC, Djulbegovic B, Shamai-Lubovitz O, Mozes B. The bleeding risk and natural history of idiopathic thrombocytopenic purpura in patients with persistent low platelet counts. *Arch Intern Med* 2000;**160**:1630–1638

Gebreyohanns M, Adams RJ. Sickle cell disease: primary stroke prevention. *CNS Spectr* 2004;**9**: 445–449

Gruppo Italiano Studio Policitemia. Polycythemia vera: the natural history of 1213 patients followed for 20 years. *Ann Intern Med* 1995;**123**:656–664

Hankey GJ, Eikelboom JW, van Bockxmeer FM et al. Inherited thrombophilia in ischemic stroke and its pathogenic subtypes. *Stroke* 2001;**32**:1793–1799

Hart R, Kanter M. Hematologic disorders and ischemic stroke; a selective review. *Stroke* 1990; **21**:1111–1121

Keswani SC, Chauhan N. Antiphospholipid syndrome. *J R Soc Med* 2002;**95**:336–342

Kirkham FJ, DeBaun MR. Stroke in children with sickle cell disease. *Curr Treat Options Neurol* 2004;**6**:357–375

Markus HS, Hambley H. Neurology in the blood; haematological abnormalities in ischaemic stroke. *J Neurol Neurosurg Psychiatry* 1998;**64**:150–159

Yap S. Classical homocystinuria: vascular risk and its prevention. *J Inherit Metab Dis* 2003;**26**:259–265

Inflammatory vascular disorders

Berlit P, Moore PM, Bluestein HG. Vasculitis, rheumatic disease and the neurologist: the pathophysiology and diagnosis of neurologic problems in systemic disease. *Cerebrovasc Dis* 1993;**3**:139–45

Brown MM, Swash M. Systemic lupus erythematosus. In *Handbook of Clinical Neurology*, Revised Series, Volume 55. *Vascular Diseases*, Part III. Vinken PJ, Bruyn GW, Klawans HL (eds). Elsevier Science, Amsterdam, 1989:369–385

Caselli RJ, Hunder GG, Whisnant JP. Neurologic disease in biopsy-proved giant cell (temporal) arteritis. *Neurology* 1988;**38**:352–359

Hankey GJ. Isolated angiitis/angiopathy of the central nervous system. *Cerebrovas Dis* 1991;**1**:2–15

Lupi-Herrera E, Sanchez-Torres G, Marcushamer J et al. Takayasu's arteritis: clinical study of 107 cases. *Am Heart J* 1977;**93**:94–103

Shannon KM, Goetz CG. Connective tissue diseases and the nervous system. In *Neurology and General Medicine.* Aminoff MJ (ed). Churchill Livingstone, New York, 1989:389–412

Migraine

Chang CL, Donaghy M, Poulter N. Migraine and stroke in young women: case–control study. The World Health Organisation Collaborative Study of Cardiovascular Disease and Steroid Hormone Contraception. *BMJ* 1999;**318**:13–18

Hall GC, Brown MM, Mo J, MacRae KD. Triptans in migraine: the risks of stroke, cardiovascular disease and death in practice. *Neurology* 2004; **62**:563–568

Olesen J, Friberg L, Olsen TS et al. Ischaemia-induced (symptomatic) migraine attacks may be more frequent than migraine-induced ischaemic insults. *Brain* 1993;**116**:187–202

Tietjen GE. The relationship between migraine and stroke (review). *Neuroepidemiology* 2000;**19**: 13–19

Mitochondrial disease and MELAS

Ciafaloni E, Ricci E, Shanske S et al. MELAS: clinical features, biochemistry and molecular genetics. *Ann Neurol* 1992;**31**:391–398

Jackson MJ, Schaefer JA, Johnson MA et al. Presentation and clinical investigation of mitochondrial respiratory chain disease: a study of 51 patients. *Brain* 1995;**118**:339–357

Moyamoya syndrome

Chiu D, Shedden P, Bratina P, Grotta JC. Clinical features of moyamoya disease in the United States. *Stroke* 1998;**29**:1347–1351

Golby AJ, Marks MP, Thompson RC, Steinberg GK. Direct and combined revascularisation in paediatric moyamoya disease. *Neurosurgery* 1999;**45**: 50–58

Oral contraception

Gillum LA, Mamidipudi SK, Johnston SC. Ischemic stroke risk with oral contraceptives: a meta-analysis. *JAMA* 2000;**284**:72–78

Heinemann LAJ. Is the stroke risk in OC users higher in Europe than in North America? *Contraception* 1999;**60**:253–254

Lidegaard O, Kreiner S. Contraceptives and cerebral thrombosis: a five-year national case control study. *Contraception* 2002;**65**:197–205

Schwartz SM, Petitti DB, Siscovick DS et al. Stroke and use of low dose oral contraceptives in young women. A pooled analysis of two US studies. *Stroke* 1998;**29**:2277–2284

Patent foramen ovale

Mas JL, Arquizan C, Lamy C et al. Recurrent cerebrovascular events associated with patent foramen ovale, atrial septal aneurysm, or both. *N Engl J Med* 2001;**345**:1740–1746

Pregnancy and the puerperium

Mas JL, Lamy C. Stroke in pregnancy and the puerperium. *J Neurol* 1998;**245**:305–313

Stewart JA, Hamilton PJ, Murdoch AP. Thromboembolic disease associated with ovarian

stimulation assisted conception techniques. *Hum Reprod* 1997;**12**:2167–2173

Sneddon's syndrome

Wohlrab J, Fischer M, Wolter M et al. Diagnostic impact and sensitivity of skin biopsies in Sneddon's syndrome. A report of 15 cases. *Br J Dermatol* 2001;**145**:285–288

CHAPTER 12

Cerebral Venous Thrombosis

Cerebral vein and dural sinus thrombosis was first described in 1825 by Ribes in a 45-year-old man who died after a 6-month history of severe headache, epilepsy and delirium. Postmortem examination showed thrombosis of the superior sagittal sinus, left lateral sinus and a cortical vein in the parietal region. Subsequent case reports and series were also largely from autopsy material, and cerebral venous thrombosis was therefore concluded to be a rare and severe disease characterized clinically by headache, papilloedema, seizures, focal deficits, progressive coma and death, with a poor prognosis. However, more recently, with the availability of magnetic resonance imaging (MRI), it has become apparent that many cases of the disease present with a much less dramatic clinical picture and that many patients make a good clinical recovery.

EPIDEMIOLOGY

The incidence of cerebral venous thrombosis is uncertain. Most autopsy series have found a very low incidence – for example just 16 cases of straight sinus thrombosis in a series of 12 500 autopsies reported by Ehlers. Kalbag suggested that cerebral venous thrombosis was the principle cause of death in only 22 persons per year in England and Wales between 1952 and 1961. However, these are probably underestimates, as venous thrombosis is often not fatal, and recent clinical series, without giving exact estimates of incidences, suggest that it is much more common. The diagnosis is probably often missed.

AETIOLOGY

A large number of conditions have been associated with cerebral venous thrombosis, although in many cases the strength of any causal relationship is difficult to determine (Table 12.1). In most series, no identifiable aetiology is present in approximately one-quarter of cases (Bousser, 2000; Crawford et al., 1995).

There has been a dramatic reduction in the number of cases caused by infection: from approximately 40% in series in the 1960s to 10% in series in the 1980s. Nevertheless, infection is still the most common cause of cavernous sinus thrombosis and an important cause of lateral sinus thrombosis. Septic cavernous sinus thrombosis originates most frequently from haematogenous spread of infection from the medial third of the face, nose, orbital contents or paranasal sinuses, or by spread from the ethmoid or sphenoid ear cells, or through the lateral sinuses from the ear. *Staphylococcus aureus* and, less commonly, streptococci are the most important pathogens. Anaerobic and Gram-negative bacteria may be responsible, with anaerobic bacteria relatively more common when the source is sinusitis or a dental abscess. Septic thrombosis in the superior sagittal sinus may arise from spread of the infection from the nose or paranasal sinuses, or via retrograde extension from the transverse or cavernous sinus. It may also result from direct extension from osteomyelitis of the skull or from septicaemia or meningitis. In these cases, the infection is most commonly caused by Gram-positive organisms, including *S. aureus*,

Table 12.1   Causes of cerebral venous thrombosis

Septic dural sinus thrombosis
- Bacterial infections
- Fungal infections

Non-septic dural sinus thrombosis
- Haemodynamic states:
  - Diabetic ketoacidosis
  - Cardiac decompensation
- Haematological disorders and thrombophilia:
  - Activated protein C resistance–Factor V Leiden polymorphism
  - Antithrombin III deficiency
  - Protein C and S deficiency
  - Lupus anticoagulant
  - Polycythaemia rubra vera
  - Disseminated intravascular coagulation
  - Sickle cell anaemia
  - Pregnancy and puerperium
  - Combined oral contraception
- Inflammatory disorders and vasculitis
  - Behçet's syndrome
  - Inflammatory bowel disease
  - Ulcerative colitis
  - Crohn's disease
  - Systemic lupus erythematosus (SLE)
  - Polyarteritis nodosa (PAN)
- Homocystinuria
- Neoplasia
  - Usually haematological malignancies
  - Local compression (e.g. meningioma)
- Nephrotic syndrome
- Head injury
- Idiopathic

Streptococcus pneumoniae and β-haemolytic streptococci. The cavernous sinus is most frequently involved by fungal infections. *Aspergillus* can result in thrombosis by direct extension from the paranasal sinuses, meningitis or haematogenous spread from the lungs.

In infants and children, dehydration from gastroenteritis is one of the most important aetiological factors. It also appears to be a contributing cause in adults. It may account for the reported association between diabetic ketoacidosis and cerebral venous thrombosis. Congestive heart failure appears to be associated because of the increased risk of stasis

in the venous sinuses secondary to reduced cardiac output.

Venous thrombosis can be caused by a number of prothrombotic states and disorders of the clotting system (thrombophilia; see Chapter 11). The most important inherited defect accounting for systemic venous thrombosis is activated protein C resistance secondary to the factor V Leiden polymorphism. Recent studies suggest that this is also an important risk factor for cerebral venous thrombosis. Other inherited disorders include protein C resistance, protein S resistance, prothrombin gene abnormalities and antithrombin III deficiency. However protein C and S levels may be reduced secondary to systemic disease or the thrombosis itself, and it is important to retest after the acute illness and to enquire about any family history. The presence of a lupus anticoagulant and/or anticardiolipin antibodies is associated with cerebral venous thrombosis, both in the presence and absence of systemic lupus erythematosus (SLE).

Patients with Behçet's disease, which presents with a classical triad of oral and genital ulceration and uveitis, suffer neurological complications in 10–50% of cases (Chapter 11). Venous thrombosis is common and may involve intracranial veins. Cerebral venous thrombosis or benign intracranial hypertension may be the presenting features. Behçet's disease is more common in Turkish and Middle Eastern populations. A variety of other causes of vasculitis have been associated with cerebral venous thrombosis, including SLE and polyarteritis nodosa (PAN).

Direct damage to the dural sinuses or cortical veins may occur from head trauma, and reported cases include both skull fractures and non-penetrating injuries. Venous sinus thrombosis has also been reported after insertion of cardiac pacemakers and central venous lines.

As many as 5–10% of cases of cerebral venous thrombosis occur during pregnancy or the puerperium. The proportion appears to be much higher in India, where it has been reported that as many as 25% of maternal deaths may be the result of cerebral venous thrombosis. The use of combined oral contraceptives appears to be a risk factor, particularly in combination with thrombophilia from the factor V Leiden polymorphism.

A number of mechanisms may account for the association with malignancy. One of the venous sinuses can be compressed by an adjacent tumour, usually a meningioma or metastatic lesion. Glomus tumours may lead to sinus thrombosis by obstruction of the jugular bulb. Direct invasion of the sinus may occur by solid neoplasms or infiltrations by haematological malignancies (e.g. leukaemia or lymphoma). In addition, sinus thrombosis may occur without any evidence of local tumour, and in these patients hypercoagulability secondary to the malignant process is assumed to be responsible.

ANATOMY

The venous sinuses are channels that drain the blood from the brain and the bones of the skull (Figure 12.1). They are situated between the two layers of the dura mater and are lined by endothelium continuous with the veins. They contain no valves and their walls are devoid of muscular tissue. The cerebral veins are divisible into external and internal groups, which drain the surfaces or the inner regions of the hemispheres into the venous sinuses. The external cerebral veins drain the superficial part of the cerebral hemispheres, with the superior cerebral veins draining the medial aspect of the hemispheres into the superior sagittal sinus, the middle cerebral veins draining into the cavernous sinus, and the inferior cerebral veins draining into the lateral sinuses. The internal cerebral veins drain blood from the deep parts of the cerebral hemispheres into the great cerebral vein of Galen. The basal veins of Rosenthal drain part of the lower frontal lobe and the insular area. They are joined by the inferior striatal veins and proceed posteriorly around the cerebral peduncle, terminating either in the internal cerebral veins or directly into the great cerebral vein. Two internal cerebral veins drain the basal ganglia, hypothalamus, thalamus and the midbrain and unite to form the great cerebral vein of Galen, which joins the inferior sagittal sinus to form the straight sinus. Most brainstem veins

enter the inferior petrosal and basilar sinuses and the vertebral plexus. The internal and external cerebral venous systems are interconnected, which allows blood to take alternative routes if needed. Connections exist between the venous sinuses and the veins of the scalp, face, spine and neck, and the diploic veins. These provide not only an alternative route for blood to leave the cranial cavity, but also a path by which pathological processes (e.g. infection) can spread to the cerebral venous sinuses.

Superior sagittal sinus

The superior sagittal sinus occupies the attached margin of the falx cerebri. It commences in front of the crysta galli and runs posteriorly to enter one or other, usually the right, transverse sinus. It receives the superior cerebral veins. On each side of the superior sagittal sinus are venous lacunae (frontal, parietal and occipital), into which drain diploic and meningeal veins. Arachnoid granulations open into both these lacunae and into the sagittal sinus.

Inferior sagittal sinus

This lies in the posterior half or two-thirds of the free margin of the falx cerebri. It passes posteriorly and ends in the straight sinus.

Straight sinus

This lies at the junction of the falx cerebri and the tentorium. It runs posteriorly and passes into the transverse sinus of the side opposite to that into which the superior sagittal sinus continues. It is formed from the junction of the great cerebral vein of Galen and the inferior sagittal sinus.

Transverse sinuses

These begin at the internal occipital protuberance and lie in the attached margin of the tentorium cerebelli until they curve anteromedialy to become the sigmoid sinuses. The right lateral sinus is usually larger than the left and drains the superior sagittal sinus. The smaller

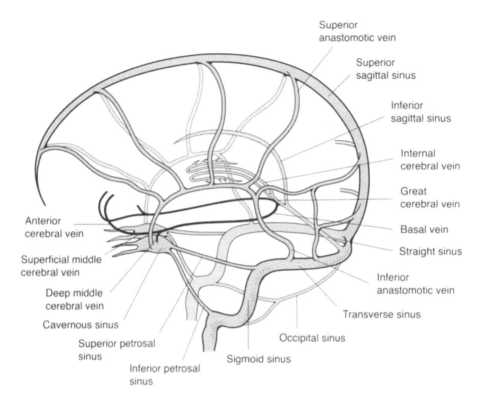

Figure 12.1   Schematic diagram of the cerebral venous sinuses, the dura mater and their connections with the cerebral veins. Adapted from *Gray's Anatomy*, 34th edn, Figure 739.

left lateral sinus usually receives blood from the straight sinus. The lateral sinuses also receive drainage from the inferior cerebral veins, which drain the temporal lobes, and from some inferior cerebellar veins. In 4% of individuals, one lateral sinus is absent and the superior sagittal and straight sinuses drain into a single lateral sinus, usually the right.

Sigmoid sinuses

These are direct continuations of the transverse sinuses and they curve downwards and medially in a deep groove on the mastoid part of the temporal bone, where only a thin plate of bone separates the upper part of the sigmoid sinus from the mastoid antrum and mastoid air cells. They become the superior bulb of the internal jugular vein in the posterior part of the jugular foramen.

Cavernous sinuses

These lie on each side of the sphenoid bone. They derive their name from their spongy structure arising from numerous interlacing filaments transversing the sinuses. They receive blood from the ophthalmic veins, several of the anterior inferior cerebral veins, the superficial middle cerebral vein, the sphenoparietal sinus and the pituitary vein. They drain through the superior petrosal sinus into the lateral sinus and through the inferior petrosal sinus into the internal jugular veins. They are transversed by a number of structures, involvement of which causes the clinical consequences of cavernous sinus thrombosis (Figure 12.2). The internal carotid artery, surrounded by a plexus of sympathetic nerves, passes through the sinus, with the abducent nerve lying inferiolaterally. The oculomotor and trochlear nerves, and the ophthalmic and maxillary divisions of the

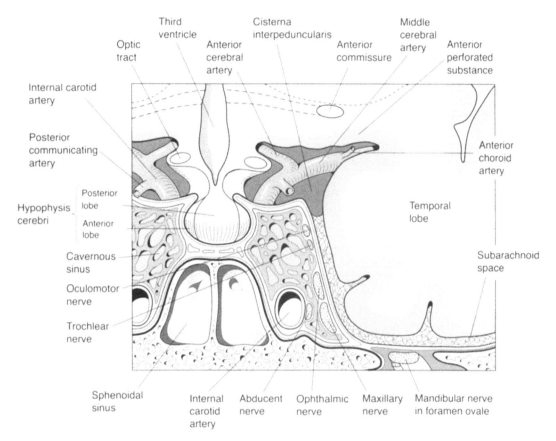

Figure 12.2   Schematic diagram of a cross-sectional view of the cavernous sinuses. The close proximity of the oculomotor nerve, the trochlear nerve, the abducent nerve and the first two divisions of the trigeminal nerve means that cavernous sinus thrombosis may present with palsies of these cranial nerves. Adapted from *Gray's Anatomy*, 34th edn, Figure 744.

trigeminal nerve, lie in the lateral wall of the sinus. The two cavernous sinuses communicate with each other with valveless connections, thus allowing flow in either direction.

CLINICAL FEATURES

Cerebral venous thrombosis may present with a variety of quite different symptoms, and a high index of clinical suspicion is required if the diagnosis is to be made without delay (Crawford *et al.*, 1995; Bousser, 2000). The symptoms may result from impaired venous drainage, intracranial hypertension, venous infarction (which may be haemorrhagic) or cerebral haemorrhage, and include the following:

- Raised intracranial pressure with headache and papilloedema. This occurs particularly when the superior sagittal sinuses are occluded due to interference with absorption of cerebrospinal fluid by the arachnoid villae.
- Isolated headache. This can occur in the absence of raised intracranial pressure and may be the result of subarachnoid haemorrhage.
- Focal neurological deficits. These may be transient and fluctuating; Hemiplegia is most frequent and, in superior sagittal sinus thrombosis, the leg may be more affected than the arm and face.
- Seizures. Both partial and generalized seizures may occur. These frequently occur

in patients with focal neurological deficits, but may occur in the absence of any deficit.

- Cranial nerve palsy. This may occur particularly in cavernous sinus thrombosis.

The mode of presentation can be divided into six temporal patterns:

- Progressive rise in intracranial pressure
- Abrupt onset of focal signs simulating an arterial occlusion
- Subacute onset of a focal deficit with or without seizures or elevated intracranial pressure
- Chronic presentations, which may be confused with a tumour
- Sudden headache resembling subarachnoid haemorrhage
- Transient focal deficits presenting like transient ischaemic attacks (TIAs)

The patient may present with the syndrome of benign intracranial hypertension, particularly with superior sagittal sinus thrombosis. Imaging is required to distinguish these cases from a similar picture occurring in the absence of cerebral venous thrombosis. In more severe cases, raised intracranial pressure, focal signs and seizures may progress to coma and death.

Cavernous sinus thrombosis

This occurs most commonly as a consequence of infection in the middle third of the face, the sphenoid, ethmoid or maxillary sinus, and, less commonly, the oropharynx, teeth, neck and ear. The symptoms and signs are related to venous obstruction, inflammation and systemic infection. Headache is common. Mechanical obstruction to venous drainage results in proptosis and oedema of the eyelids, conjunctiva and bridge of the nose and sometimes the pharynx and tonsils. Dilation of the facial veins may occur. Ophthalmoplegia may result from orbital congestion, or inflammation of the oculomotor, trochlear and abducent nerves as they pass through the sinus. The optic nerve may be involved, resulting in reduced acuity

and an afferent pupillary defect. The first two divisions of the trigeminal nerve are intracavernous, and therefore facial numbness may involve the upper two-thirds of the face. Sometimes, the thrombus or infection may spread into the inferior petrosal sinus, and the third division of the trigeminal nerve may also be affected. Papilloedema and distension of the retinal veins are frequent. The opposite cavernous sinus is often affected because of the communications across the midline through the circular or intracavernous sinuses. Meningitis and internal carotid artery thrombosis may occur rarely.

Thrombosis of the deep venous drainage

Patients with thrombosis of one or both internal cerebral veins and/or the vein of Galen may present with a short, rapidly progressive illness, characterized by headache, nausea, vomiting and reduced conscious level. Compared with dural sinus thrombosis, deep cerebral venous thrombosis is much rarer, and altered consciousness and long track signs, frequently bilateral, are more common while papilloedema and seizures are less frequent.

Lateral sinus thrombosis

Prior to antibiotics, this was a common complication of otitis media and mastoiditis. The diagnosis is suggested by a combination of high fever, acute otitis media or an aural discharge and symptoms secondary to impaired cerebrospinal fluid (CSF) dynamics. While lateral sinus thrombosis still occurs with acute ear infections, it is now more commonly associated with chronic ear infections and cholesteatomas of the petrous temporal bone in adults. It may present with headache and papilloedema, and this is more common with involvement of the right transverse sinus, which is usually the dominant one. Focal deficits rarely occur in lateral sinus thrombosis and usually signify spread to other sinuses or cortical veins, or an intracranial abscess.

Spinal venous thrombosis

Thrombosis of the spinal cord veins may result in a painful, rapidly progressing haemorrhagic infarction of the cord with both sensory, motor and sphincter disturbance. Haemorrhagic infarction tends to be more centrally located in the spinal cord than purely ischaemic infarction.

INVESTIGATIONS

Computed tomography (CT)

The posterior 6 mm of the superior sagittal sinus can be routinely visualized on CT, and the straight sinus and vein of Galen can also frequently be seen. Although CT is frequently abnormal in cerebral venous thrombosis, the findings are often non-specific and normal scans can occur, particularly early in the clinical course. The use of contrast-enhanced CT improves diagnostic yield. CT abnormalities include:

- Small ventricles.
- Generalized cerebral swelling.
- Diffuse low density, suggestive of oedema.
- Hypodensity consistent with venous infarction.
- Lesions of mixed hypodensity and increased density, corresponding to haemorrhagic infarcts.
- The thrombosed superior sagittal sinus may appear as an unusually dense triangle on an unenhanced scan (delta sign).
- Following contrast injection, the negative or empty delta sign may be seen. This consists of a central lucency ascribed to sluggish or absent blood flow within the superior sagittal sinus, surrounded by a margin of contrast enhancement.
- The 'cord sign' is considered pathognomic of cortical venous thrombosis, but occurs in a minority of cases. A rounded hyperdensity is seen on several sequential slices, due to the presence of thrombus in the lumen of a vein.

- Other patterns of abnormal enhancement may result from collateral circulation, stasis or hyperaemia within the dural venous structures, and include the presence of a dilated transcerebral medullary vein, enhancement of the tentorium, and asymmetrical meningeal enhancement overlying the cavernous sinus in cases of cavernous sinus thrombosis.

Magnetic resonance imaging and angiography

MRI, with magnetic resonance venography if required, is the first-line investigation of choice in patients suspected of having cerebral venous thrombosis (Isensee *et al.*, 1994). MRI is more sensitive than CT for detecting thrombosis and may demonstrate absence of the normal 'flow void' in the venous sinuses on T_2-weighted images (Figures 12.3 and 12.4). Intravascular thrombus may be seen within the venous sinuses. A few days after thrombosis, the clot can become clearly visible and hyperintense on both T_1- and T_2-weighted images. MRI may also show the consequences of venous thrombosis, namely infarction and haemorrhagic infarction. Magnetic resonance venography may demonstrate absent or markedly reduced venous flow at the site of thrombosis (Figure 12.5). This technique can usually clearly demonstrate thrombosis in the larger venous sinuses, but can miss thrombosis within the smaller sinuses or in thrombosis restricted to cortical veins.

Electroencephalogram (EEG)

This may be normal, show diffuse slow activity or, less frequently, show focal slow activity. Epileptic activity may be present.

Cerebrospinal fluid

Raised intracranial pressure, moderately elevated CSF protein, a mild leukocytosis

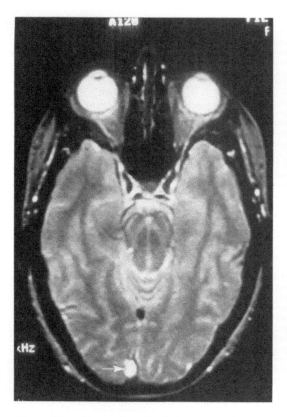

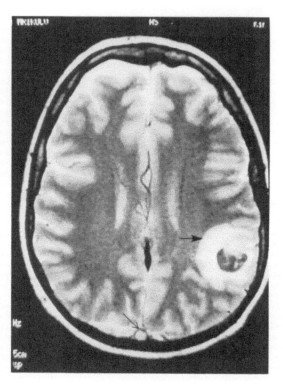

Figure 12.3 T$_2$-weighted MRI showing high signal and lack of flow void in the superior sagittal sinus indicating sagittal sinus thrombosis (arrow).

Figure 12.4 T$_2$-weighted MRI showing features of sagittal sinus thrombosis with lack of flow void in the superior sagittal sinus (open arrow head) and an area of focal haemorrhagic oedema (closed arrow head) in the left parietal lobe.

involving lymphocytes, polymorphs or a mixture, and red cells or xanthochromia may be found. However, CSF is not diagnostic, is rarely necessary and is contraindicated if there is any likelihood of significantly raised intracranial pressure.

Cerebral angiography

This remains the definitive diagnostic test, although, with the increasing use of MRI and MRA, it is frequently not necessary. It may indicate a partial or total lack of filling of one or more sinuses (Figure 12.6). Increased arteriovenous circulation time may be seen and dilation or tortuosity of collateral vessels occurs in approximately 50% of cases. Delayed venous films may be necessary to adequately visualize the occlusion.

TREATMENT

In the past, there was considerable concern that anticoagulation might exacerbate venous haemorrhagic infarction by causing additional bleeding. However, a number of retrospective analyses suggest that anticoagulation improves outcome, even in patients with haemorrhage on CT. A randomized, blinded, placebo-controlled study compared heparin therapy in 10 patients with placebo in 10 patients (Einhäupl *et al.*, 1991). After 3 months, eight of the heparin-treated patients had a complete recovery and two had slight residual neurological deficits, while in the placebo group, only one had a complete recovery, six had neurological deficits and three died. In view of this significant result, the study was terminated early despite its very small size. A second larger randomized controlled study showed better outcome in

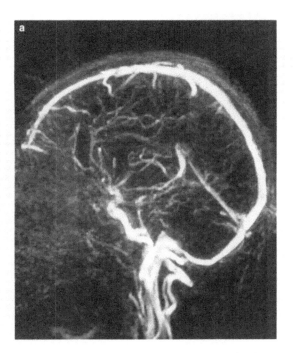 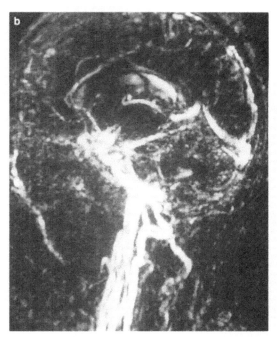

Figure 12.5 Magnetic resonance venography demonstrating (a) the normal anatomy of the venous sinuses and (b) sagittal sinus thrombosis. Note the absence of high signal most marked in the anterior and middle thirds of the sagittal sinus (partly cut off at the top of the figure).

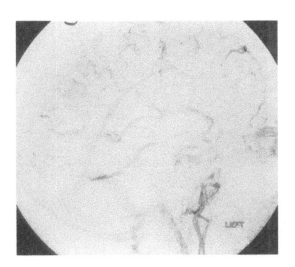

Figure 12.6 Venous phase of a digital subtraction angiogram in cerebral venous thrombosis demonstrating absence of filling of the sagittal sinus (this is the same patient as in Figure 12.4).

marked benefit for heparin. Larger studies are needed to confirm that heparin is the appropriate treatment for some or all cases of venous thrombosis. Nevertheless, anticoagulation with intravenous heparin followed by warfarin for 3–6 months is currently recommended for the majority of cases, even in the presence of mild or moderate haemorrhagic infarction. This may need to be continued for longer in some patients who have underlying prothrombotic states. Anticonvulsant drugs may also be required. Antibiotic therapy is indicated in septic cerebral venous thrombosis, and is also usually given in cavernous sinus thrombosis. Local thrombolytic therapy has been given in patients who deteriorate despite heparin, particularly those with superior sagittal sinus thrombosis, and can result in more rapid recanalization. However, there have been no controlled trials examining the efficacy or safety of thrombolysis.

PROGNOSIS

Early studies reported a very high mortality and rate of neurological disability, but with

anticoagulated patients, although this did not reach statistical significance (de Bruijn and Stam, 1999). This study was underpowered and would only have been able to show a very the increased diagnosis of less severe cases, the prognosis has improved (Ferro *et al.*, 2004). Focal neurological signs tend to recover better than after arterial ischaemic infarction. A long-term follow-up of a consecutive sample of 110 adult subjects with cerebral venous thrombosis, seen between 1975 and 1990, found that 6 patients died during the acute event, and 2 died shortly after due to underlying disease (Preter *et al.*, 1996). Of the remaining 102 subjects, 77 could be traced. Of these, 66 (86%) had no neurological sequelae, while 11 (14%) had persistent neurological impairment. Two of these had blindness due to optic atrophy secondary to intracranial hypertension, while 9, who had focal signs at the time of cerebral venous thrombosis, had a variety of cognitive and focal deficits. Four of the 28 patients who had seizures during the acute phase had recurrent seizures. One of the 51 patients with lateral sinus thrombosis developed a dural arteriovenous fistula. Nine (12%) suffered a second cerebral venous thrombosis, and all but one of these occurred within the first year. Non-cerebral thrombotic events occurred in 11 patients (14%). The finding that a second cerebral venous thrombosis or another thrombotic episode occurred in 20% of subjects emphasizes the importance of long-term anticoagulation in a subgroup of patients with identifiable haematological disorders or recurrent events. The prognosis of cases of thrombosis of the deep venous drainage of the brain is worse, with a higher mortality and disability rate.

KEY REFERENCES

Clinical features

Bousser MG. Cerebral venous thrombosis: diagnosis and management. *J Neurol* 2000;**247**:252–258

Crawford SC, Digre KB, Palmer CA et al. Thrombosis of the deep venous drainage of the brain in adults. *Arch Neurol* 1995;**52**:1101–1108

Imaging

Isensee Ch, Reul J, Thron A. Magnetic resonance imaging of thrombosed dural sinuses. *Stroke* 1994;**25**:29–34

Treatment

de Bruijn SF, Stam J. Randomized, placebo-controlled trial of anticoagulant treatment with low-molecular-weight heparin for cerebral sinus thrombosis. *Stroke* 1999;**30**:484–488

Einhäupl KM, Villringer A, Meister W et al. Heparin treatment in sinus venous thrombosis. *Lancet* 1991;**338**:597–600

Prognosis

Ferro JM, Canhão P, Stam J et al. Prognosis of cerebral vein and dural sinus thrombosis: results of the International Study on Cerebral Vein and Dural Sinus Thrombosis (ISCVT). *Stroke* 2004:**35**:664–670

Preter M, Tzourio C, Ameri A et al. Long-term prognosis in cerebral venous thrombosis: follow-up of 77 patients. *Stroke* 1996;**27**:243–246

Treatment

CHAPTER 13

Neuroprotection

This chapter reviews the theoretical basis for the acute treatment of stroke, including the physiology and biochemistry of cell injury caused by ischaemia. The practical aspects of stroke treatment are discussed in the next chapter.

There have been striking developments in our understanding of the way in which ischaemia affects the functioning of brain cells and leads to neuronal death. Neuronal metabolism is disturbed and a series of events ('the ischaemic cascade', Figure 13.1) is unleashed, which, over time, results in amplification of the intracellular response to ischaemia. These processes continue for some time after the ischaemic insult starts, and may continue even if the ischaemia resolves, to produce delayed tissue destruction. Considerable advances in our understanding of these processes have been made in animal models and are likely to be translated into real clinical benefit in the near future. A number of neuroprotective agents have been shown to prevent neuronal injury after ischaemic stroke in mammals. Unfortunately, none has yet been shown to be beneficial after human stroke. This chapter outlines the metabolic principles implicated in the pathophysiology of stroke, so that these new advances may be appreciated. The majority of work has concentrated on cerebral ischaemia and it is not known if the same principles apply to the effects of cerebral haemorrhage.

THE ISCHAEMIC PENUMBRA

The ischaemic penumbra is named after an eclipse of the Sun by the Moon, where a central region of total darkness (umbra) is surrounded by an area of less intense shadow (the penumbra) (Figure 13.2a). The pioneering studies of Astrup, Siesjo and Symon established that after experimental occlusion of the monkey middle cerebral artery, two areas could be identified: a central area of tissue necrosis surrounded by a second region of incomplete ischaemia (Astrup *et al.*, 1977). This latter area of apparently viable but uninfarcted tissue was termed the ischaemic penumbra. Astrup and colleagues showed that when cerebral blood flow (CBF) was reduced from the normal of around 50 ml/100 g/min to levels of between 10 and 20 ml/100 g/min by clamping the carotid arteries, evoked potentials and electroencephalogram (EEG) activity were silenced. This CBF corresponded to the level seen in the penumbra and was termed the flow threshold for electrical failure. At this level of blood flow, intracellular adenosine triphosphate (ATP) and energy stores were maintained, implying adequate membrane pump function, and the extracellular potassium concentration remained within the normal range. However, the tissue was functionally inert, i.e. the neurones were not active. When the CBF was reduced further to levels of below 10 ml/100 g/min, the extracellular potassium

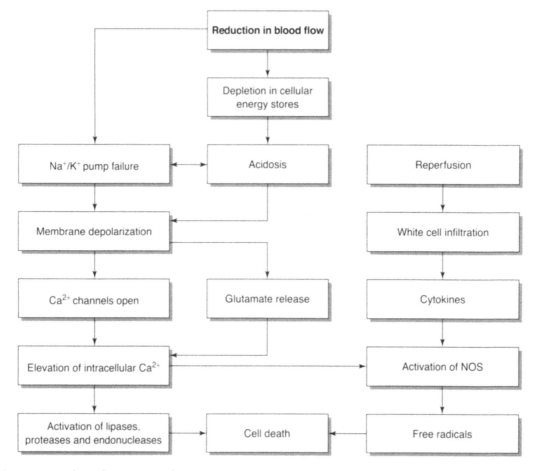

Figure 13.1   The ischaemic cascade. NOS, nitric oxide synthase.

concentration increased markedly, and there was a decrease in the energy-rich compound ATP. At these levels of cerebral ischaemia, membrane integrity could no longer be preserved due to severe energy depletion. This was termed the energy failure threshold and corresponds to the changes seen at the core of the infarct (Figure 13.2b). Tissue subjected to a CBF below the range of the energy failure threshold died and infarcted within a few minutes. However, if the CBF was reduced only to the level of electrical silence (i.e. within the range of the penumbra), the tissues recovered electrical function if the blood flow was restored to normal, even after 2–3 hours of occlusion.

The importance of these observations lies in the concept that acute occlusion of a cerebral artery may not result in complete death of all the tissue supplied by the blocked vessel. There will be a core of tissue with very little blood supply, which will survive only a few minutes before dying. However, surrounding the core may be an area with intermediate levels of blood flow ('penumbra') because of some supply from collateral vessels. Surrounding regions of compromised tissue contribute to the clinical presentation (e.g. hemiparesis) of the stroke because they are electrically silent and non-functional. Potentially, penumbral tissue is salvageable if blood flow is restored sufficiently to reverse the initial biochemical events. However, experimental evidence suggests that penumbral tissue is metabolically unstable and the continuation of events in the ischaemic cascade may convert salvageable penumbra into irreversibly infarcted tissue.

a

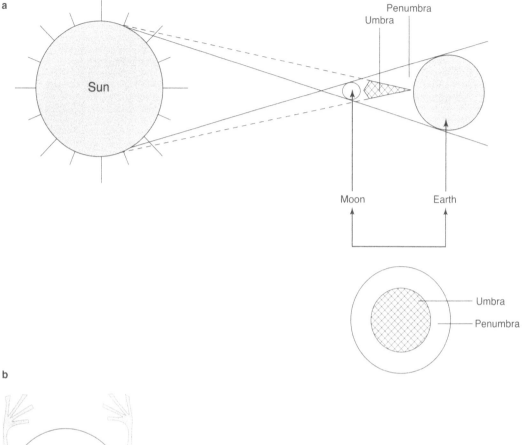

b

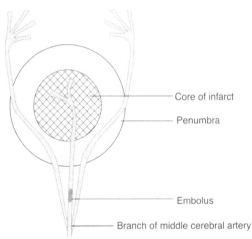

Core of infarct

Penumbra

Embolus

Branch of middle cerebral artery

Figure 13.2 (a) Diagram of a total eclipse of the Sun, showing the central dense core (umbra), surrounded by the penumbra of shadow. (b) By analogy, the ischaemic penumbra is the area in which there is partial ischaemia resulting in physiologically inert but viable tissue surrounding the more deeply ischaemic core.

The viability of the penumbra may be affected by changes in the general condition of the patient or alterations in CBF. The presence of such potentially salvageable tissue cannot be identified on clinical examination because neither core nor penumbra is functionally active and the clinical signs (e.g. hemiparesis) therefore reflect the effects of core plus penumbra.

The extent and duration of the ischaemic penumbra in humans is a matter of some uncertainty. Evidence in stroke for the existence of this border-zone region first came from non-invasive metabolic imaging, using positron emission tomography (PET) (Baron, 2001). This method employs unstable and short-lived radioisotopes of oxygen, labelling glucose and other agents to provide information about regional cerebral metabolism, pH and blood flow. The ischaemic penumbra is situated between normal tissue and infarcted tissue, the regions being defined by their blood flow and metabolic characteristics. The resolution of PET and of other non-invasive radiological imaging techniques then becomes important. In a low-resolution technique such as PET, infarcted tissue immediately adjacent to normal tissue could be incorporated into a single image that would average the CBF and metabolic characteristics. This would result in an artefact producing an area of reduced blood flow and metabolism between the dead and normal tissue with the characteristics of the penumbra. This phenomenon is termed partial volume averaging (Figure 13.3). Nonetheless, there is reasonable evidence from PET studies in favour of the existence of the penumbra as an entity. Heiss and colleagues demonstrated areas of luxury perfusion (increased CBF in the regions adjacent to the cerebral infarct) in which measures of cellular metabolism had the characteristics of the penumbra (Heiss and Graf, 1994). This cannot be explained by partial volume averaging. This tissue was identified at a mean of 23 hours after stroke onset and was not associated with MRI or CT changes. However, after 2 weeks, in many cases, the tissue progressed to show the characteristics of cerebral infarction on subsequent MRI. This occurred in the face of improvement in CBF in the peri-infarcted region. Baron and colleagues have provided persuasive evidence for the existence of a penumbra from PET studies in both humans and monkeys (Baron, 2001). Their results in patients with middle cerebral artery stroke suggest that the extent and duration of the penumbra vary considerably between individuals, although in a minority salvageable tissue might be present up to 20 hours post stroke. Further evidence for the penumbra is emerging from magnetic resonance studies using diffusion and perfusion imaging (Jansen *et al.*, 1999; Markus *et al.*, 2004). In patients imaged very early after onset, these have shown areas of reduced perfusion associated with smaller areas of

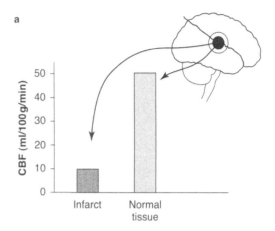

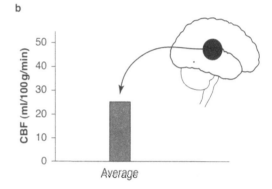

Figure 13.3 Demonstration of partial volume averaging. CBF, cerebral blood flow. (a) Measurements of CBF at high resolution; (b) measurements of CBF at lower resolution show an average of blood flow values in the infarct and the surrounding tissue.

diffusion abnormality. The areas of diffusion abnormality appear to indicate already infarcted areas, while the areas of perfusion–diffusion mismatch may indicate penumbra. The area of diffusion abnormality expand to involve the whole of the area of perfusion deficit, unless reperfusion occurs (see Colour Plate I, p. ix).

THE THERAPEUTIC WINDOW

Animal studies have shown that there is a progressive increase in the size of infarction after middle cerebral occlusion with increasing duration of ischaemia – but only for the first 2 hours or so. Beyond 2 hours, temporary occlusion produces similar deficits to permanent occlusion.

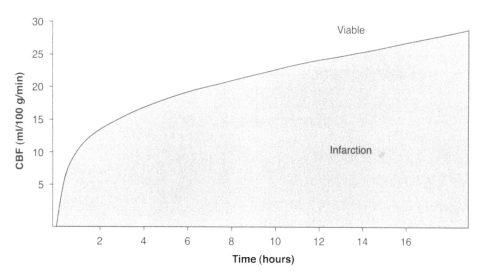

Figure 13.4 Diagram showing the duration of viability of brain tissue following arterial occlusion. CBF, cerebral blood flow.

Similarly, studies of neuroprotection in animal models have broadly shown that potential neuroprotective agents have to be given within an hour or two (sometimes less) of ischaemia to result in significant reduction of infarction size. This suggests that the ischaemic penumbra is only temporary, lasting just an hour or two before the tissue becomes permanently infarcted, although PET studies by Baron and others suggest that some potentially salvageable tissue may be present at later time points in a proportion of patients (Heiss and Graf, 1994; Baron, 2001).

Crucial issues concern the time for which the tissue in the penumbra remains alive and for how long the process of cell death can be reversed and intervention is practicable. These are not equivalent. Tissue may show the blood flow and metabolic characteristics of a penumbra for some time after stroke; however, there may be a point beyond which intervention is unable to reverse or halt the intracellular metabolic consequences of ischaemia. The cells may take some time to die after receiving a mortal injury. What is clear is that the longer ischaemia is present without reperfusion or neuroprotection, the greater the probability that the tissue will be irreversibly infarcted. The likelihood of infarction appears to be a

function both of the duration of ischaemia and of the degree of ischaemia (Figure 13.4). Evidence that this can apply to humans comes from the finding that neurological outcome after endarterectomy is determined by the level of reduction of CBF during the operation and the length of time the internal carotid artery remains clamped. Marked reductions in CBF can be tolerated without clinical deterioration, but for only very short periods of time, whereas milder reductions can be tolerated for longer.

Unfortunately, the existence of a large area of penumbra in humans appears to be uncommon, at least at the time when most PET studies have been performed, which is often many hours or even days after onset. It is certainly probable that some potentially salvageable tissue is present in the first hour or two after onset. The most compelling evidence for a limited period of salvageable brain after human stroke comes from the trials of reperfusion using recombinant tissue plasminogen activator (tPA). These suggest that the penumbra remains viable for only 3 hours after stroke onset, although there may be a small number of patients with longer-lasting penumbra up to 6 hours after onset (ATLANTIS, ECASS and NINDS, 2004). The viability of the penumbra may also depend on the general state of intracranial and extracranial vessels. Patients with multiple sites of high-grade extracranial vascular stenosis might only be able to sustain a small penumbra, if any at all, because of poor collateral supply. The extent of anatomical collateral channels, particularly via the circle of Willis plays a crucial role.

SELECTIVE VULNERABILITY

Animal studies have led to the important concept that there is selective vulnerability of brain tissue to ischaemia. In a rat global ischaemia model, Pulsinelli and colleagues showed that different regions of the hippocampus, although possessing the same blood supply, infarcted at different rates, some regions remaining viable for several days (Figure 13.5) (Pulsinelli *et al.*, 1982). The mechanism is unclear. Petito has offered preliminary evidence that this can occur in the human brain. Patients surviving for less than 18 hours after cardiac arrest (global cerebral hypoperfusion) showed little hippocampal damage. On the other hand, when patients died 24 hours or more after the arrest, the hippocampus showed severe damage.

There is some suggestion that cell death may be an active phenomenon. The neurochemical, neurotransmitter and cytokine milieu is severely altered in the vicinity of the infarction. Various agents may be generated at different times during ischaemia and possibly provide a mechanism for delayed cell death or initiation of apoptosis (see below). Of these, glutamate, nitric oxide and a variety of free radicals have received the greatest attention. Cells may have different abilities to withstand the metabolic effects of these agents, and it is likely that innate protective mechanisms underlie differential tissue susceptibility to ischaemia.

THE GLUTAMATE RECEPTOR AND EXCITOTOXICITY

A number of metabolites and neurotransmitters, which perform a signalling function in the central nervous system (CNS), can become

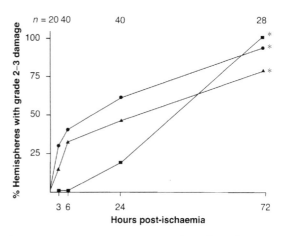

Figure 13.5 Demonstration of early selective regional vulnerability within the hippocampus in rats subjected to 30 minutes of ischaemia. The graph shows the proportion of hemispheres showing ischaemic damage to many (grade 2) or the majority (grade 3) of neurones at different times in three separate regions of the hippocampus. The asterisks indicate a statistically significant increase between 24 and 72 hours. Adapted from Pulsinelli WA *et al. Ann Neurol* 1982;**11**:491–498.

toxic under certain circumstances and are then termed excitotoxins (Benveniste, 1991). Neuronal damage may occur if the substance is released in an inappropriate location or in inappropriate amounts. The excitotoxin that has received the most attention is glutamic acid (glutamate). This is one of the principal excitatory neurotransmitters and is ubiquitous within the brain and spinal cord. When injected systemically, glutamate produces similar histological changes within the brain to those caused by global cerebral ischaemia (e.g. after cardiac arrest), following a prolonged generalized seizure or after hypoglycaemia. The receptors that mediate the effects of glutamate are classified into two major subtypes: the metabotropic receptor and the ionotropic receptor. The metabotropic receptor is linked to the phosphatidylinositol/inositol trisphosphate/diacylglycerol second-messenger complex. The role of this receptor in mediating the effects of ischaemia is unclear. The ionotropic receptor has been studied in considerable detail and

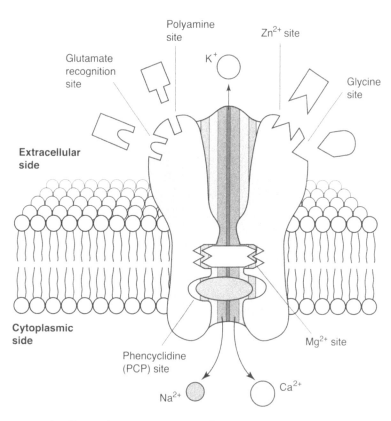

Figure 13.6 Diagram of cell membrane showing a schematic representation of the *N*-methyl-ᴅ-asparate (NMDA) receptor complex. Opening of the cerebral channel allows the influx of Na⁺ and Ca²⁺ ions and the efflux of K⁺ ions (arrows).

may be the mediator of the delayed effects of ischaemia. The distribution of these receptors may in part dictate the ischaemic vulnerability of different brain regions. In general, there are two major ionotropic glutamate receptor subtypes: the NMDA receptor (Figure 13.6), which strongly and specifically binds *N*-methyl-ᴅ-asparatate, and the AMPA receptor, which binds α-amino-3-hydroxy-5-methyl-4-isoxazolepropionate. In addition, this receptor mediates the cellular effects of kainic acid, and so is occasionally referred to as the AMPA–kainate receptor. Normally, these receptors control the entry of calcium into cells. Hyperstimulation of the receptor by excess glutamate leads to an excess of calcium flux into cells, which precipitates the cascade of events leading to cell death (Figure 13.7).

Microdialysis experiments have been performed in which a compartmentalized probe is inserted into the brain and irrigated with a solute-free solution. This is separated from brain cells by a thin membrane of selected pore size. Solutes in the extracellular fluid enter the probe along a concentration gradient and are washed into an on-line analyser for example using HPLC (high-pressure liquid chromatography). After 10 minutes of global ischaemia of the gerbil forebrain, a marked increase in the dialysate glutamate concentration occurs, which is abolished when circulation is restored (Figure 13.8). The amount of glutamate released depends both on the duration of the ischaemia and on the region under investigation. Even physiological concentrations of glutamate may become toxic in the

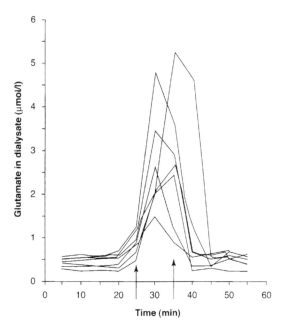

Figure 13.7 Demonstration of glutamate release within the hippocampal CA1 region using the technique of microdialysis: the period of reversible ischaemia is shown between the arrows. From Benveniste H *et al. Cerebrovasc Brain Metab Rev* 1991;**3**:213–245.

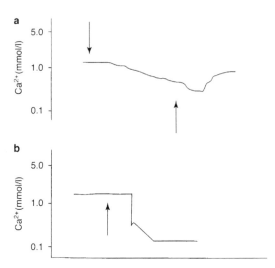

Figure 13.8 Effect of a NMDA–glutamate receptor competitive antagonist (APV) on extracellular calcium concentrations: (a) left CA1 region plus APV; (b) right CA1 region plus vehicle. The period of ischaemia is shown by the arrows. From Benveniste H. *Cerebrovasc Brain Metab Rev* 1991;**3**:213–245.

presence of ischaemia. The reduction of intracellular energy stores secondary to ischaemia disrupts membrane ionic pump activity, which may augment the excitotoxic effects of small concentrations of glutamate.

Both *in vitro* and *in vivo* evidence indicate that the metabolic and histopathological effects of ischaemia can be reduced considerably by agents that block glutamate receptors. However, there is specificity with respect to the nature of the ischaemic insult. The effects of focal ischaemia initiated by occluding the middle cerebral artery are best attenuated by NMDA antagonists. AMPA–kainate receptor antagonists have greater efficacy in models of global cerebral ischaemia. There has been some controversy as to whether the neuroprotective effects of certain NMDA antagonists are due to receptor antagonism in the ischaemic region or because they can independently lower brain temperature. In general, lowering of brain temperature itself has a neuroprotective effect.

The NMDA receptor controls a voltage-dependent ion channel. In the resting state, magnesium reversibly blocks the channel. During ischaemia, the extracellular potassium concentration rises, due in part to failure of cellular ion pumps. The resulting depolarization leads to a conformational change within the channel, allowing the extrusion of magnesium from binding sites. When the receptor is now occupied by glutamate, the channel can open completely and becomes fully permeable to sodium and calcium (Figure 13.9). In addition to glutamate, the modulator glycine must also be present for full activation of the NMDA receptor-dependent channel. The excessive increase in intracellular calcium concentration has a devastating effect on the cellular economy. A variety of proteases (e.g. calpain, which destroys cytoskeletal proteins), kinases and lipases are activated, resulting in disruption of cellular membrane integrity. A complete rundown of electrochemical and osmotic gradients can occur and produce cellular lysis. In addition, there is subsequent activation of a variety of immediate early genes that can unleash changes in the genetic structure of the

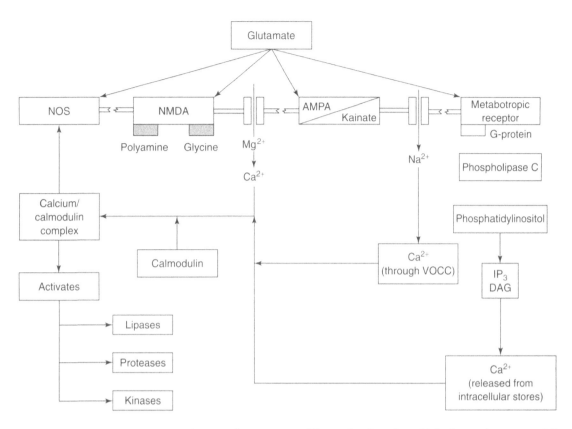

Figure 13.9 Schematic diagram showing the many possible mechanisms by which glutamate may exert its intracellular effects during cerebral ischaemia. AMPA, α-amino-3-hydroxy-5-methyl-4-isoxazolepropionate; DAG, diacylglycerol; IP$_3$, inositol triphosphate; MDMA, *N*-methyl-D-asparate; NOS, nitric oxide synthase; VOCC, voltage-operated calcium channel.

cell, including the expression of genes that terminate cellular viability, causing apoptosis (non-necrotic, programmed cell death).

The NMDA receptor can be regulated at a number of sites (Figure 13.9). These include:

- Competitive antagonism of the glutamate receptor
- Competitive antagonism of the glycine-binding site
- Non-competitive antagonism of the phen-cyclidine (PCP) site – a region within the NMDA-regulated channel to which PCA binds when the channel is open
- Antagonism of the polyamine site

The possibility of regulating these receptors has led to the concepts of cytoprotection and neuroprotection, whereby cells and neurones are protected against the metabolic effects of cerebral ischaemia.

Nitric oxide (NO)

NO is an endothelial-derived relaxation factor (EDRF) released in response to the binding of acetylcholine to blood vessels (Kumar *et al.*, 1996). In addition, it plays a role as a neuro-transmitter within the CNS. There is accumu-lating evidence that NO also partly mediates the excitotoxic effects of glutamate. Drugs that inhibit the activity of neuronal nitric oxide synthase (NOS), the enzyme that synthesizes NO from arginine, decrease infarct volume and attenuate the cytotoxic effects of glutamate. Following experimental stroke in mice, there is a marked increase in NO levels, but mice deficient in NOS have smaller infarcts when subjected to experimental cerebral arterial occlusion. The situation is complicated by the fact that NO released from the endothelium of cerebral blood vessels, resulting from production by the endothelial isoform of NOS, may play a protective role by maintaining and increasing cerebral blood flow. Knockout mice missing the gene for endothelial NOS develop smaller infarcts, while mice lacking the gene for neuronal NOS develop larger infarcts than control animals.

On formation, gaseous NO produced by neuronal NOS diffuses away from the site of production and can bind to the haem iron of guanylate cyclase, increasing the production of cyclic guanosine monophosphate (cGMP), which has a number of effects within the cell and can act as a second-messenger molecule. The precise mechanism by which the toxic effects of NO are achieved is unclear. NO may cause both necrosis (in which cell swelling vacuolation and lysis occur) and apoptosis (in which nuclear segmentation, clumping and cellular shrinkage occur without vacuolation and swelling). NO can inhibit the formation of ATP, resulting in necrotic cellular dissolution by rundown of electrochemical gradients. In addition, NO both inhibits DNA synthesis and deaminates DNA, which may cause apoptosis. NO can act as a free radical and in this way damage cellular and mitochondrial membranes as well as DNA integrity. This effect on DNA activates polyadenosine diphosphate (ADP)–ribose synthetase (PARS), causing ribosylation of nuclear proteins. Quite how this leads to cell death is unclear, but it is thought that the excessive ribosylation results in rapid reduction of neuronal nicotinamide adenine dinucleotide (NAD) levels, altering redox potentials and intracellular energy stores. PARS inhibitors block NMDA excitotoxicity in direct proportion to their inhibitory effect on this enzyme.

In summary, glutamate binding to NMDA receptors results in an increase in intraneuronal calcium, which binds to calmodulin forming an activated complex. In turn, the calcium/calmodulin complex activates NOS, with resultant NO production. In physiological situations, the gas can diffuse from the cell, activating guanylate cyclase in adjacent neurones. As an intracellular second messenger, this results in the propagation of information from one cell to another. However, under pathological situations (e.g. cerebral ischaemia), large quantities of NO are produced, which can damage not only the cell by the mechanisms detailed above, but also adjacent cells with escalation of cytotoxicity. Therefore, glutamate-induced increases in NO can rapidly and potently increase the sphere of toxicity around an activated cell. It is possible that such mechanisms lead to recruitment of surrounding tissue into the penumbra and hence to enlargement of the area of infarction.

Free radicals, reperfusion injury and white cells

Highly reactive free radicals may be generated both during ischaemia and on reperfusion. These agents will interact with cellular and mitochondrial membranes, producing irreparable damage by peroxidation of membrane lipids. Transmembrane ionic gradients are dissipated and osmotic gradients dissolved with cellular swelling, and there is a failure of the energy-generating mechanisms within the cell. Allopurinol, which inhibits xanthine oxidase and the production of free radicals, markedly decreased the volume of infarction in a rat middle cerebral artery occlusion model when administered before the experimental occlusion. In addition, there was a marked reduction in the formation of cerebral oedema in these models. Superoxide dismutase, an enzyme that scavenges the reactive hydroxyl species, converting it to hydrogen peroxide, has also been shown to decrease infarct volume in a rat model. This is associated with a significant decrease in the accumulation of intracellular calcium.

There is some evidence that free radicals are produced by endothelial cells during acute cerebral ischaemia. Other cellular sources of the increased free-radical production during cerebral ischaemia are unclear. Reperfusion itself may be harmful by providing a source of actively metabolizing cells and oxygen to feed these cells.

The role of leukocytes in stroke is controversial. It has been suggested that the infiltration of infarcted or ischaemic tissue by leukocytes may be deleterious because of the production of free radicals by these cells during activation. In this way, leukocyte recruitment which occurs within the first 24 hours of stroke could actually be harmful. Animal studies have demonstrated a reduction in infarct volume when antibodies to leukocyte adhesion molecules are infused during middle cerebral artery occlusion.

OTHER MEDIATORS OF CYTOTOXICITY

Various cytokines have been implicated in the production of ischaemic damage, and may add to the metabolic cascade unleashed by stroke.

Platelet activating factor (PAF)

This is a lipid autocoid initially identified as a product of platelets. It has since been shown to be produced by a number of cell types, including cerebellar and fetal neuronal tissue, as well as by leukocytes. Although it may possess a neuroregulatory role within the CNS, high levels of PAF have been shown to be neurotoxic *in vitro* (Yue and Feuerstein, 1994). Both *in vivo* and *in vitro* animal studies have indicated that PAF is secreted by neuronal tissue in response to cerebral ischaemia. Microdialysis techniques have determined that the release is delayed for about 2 hours and occurs after the peak of the release of other potentially neurotoxic agents (e.g. thromboxane). Use of PAF antagonists in ischaemia models *in vitro* has suggested a possible neuroprotective role for these agents. Circulating PAF has been identified in the blood of human stroke patients at higher levels when compared with healthy controls. PAF appears to be recognized by a complex receptor system and mobilizes intracellular calcium as well as activating the phosphatidylinositol system. Interestingly, PAF antagonists have also been shown to decrease the hyperperfusion, oedema and leukocyte accumulation that may occur after stroke.

Tumour necrosis factor α (TNF-α)

This is a cytokine which has a variety of actions in mediating inflammation. It may also enhance the production of leukocyte adhesion molecules. TNF-α has direct toxic effects on oligodendroglia and promotes astrocyte proliferation. This cytokine is produced by macrophages and monocytes as well as astrocytes and microglia. Following experimental middle cerebral artery occlusion in the rat, expression of neuronal TNF-α is increased within 3–6 hours (Liu *et al.*, 1994). Cytotoxic effects might occur directly or secondary to the increase in leukocyte infiltration that is a consequence of expression of this molecule. In addition, TNF-α induces PAF, which could afford another mechanism of neuronal damage. These effects suggest that TNF-α may be another possible mediator of the delayed effects of ischaemia.

Interleukins

Recent attention has focused on the role of interleukins following acute cerebral infarction. These agents mediate the inflammatory response and are produced by microglia, macrophages, astrocytes, brain endothelial cells, monocytes and other leukocytes. In experimental rat middle cerebral artery occlusion, mRNA for interleukin-1 (IL-1), an important mediator of inflammation, was identified in a time-dependent manner, peaking within 3 hours in areas that subsequently became necrotic on histological examination. In animal models, IL-1 receptor (IL-1R) antagonists markedly reduced the histological effects of cerebral ischaemia and excitotoxin-mediated damage.

Heat-shock proteins (HSPs)

These are induced in cells in response to stressors, including cerebral ischaemia (Rordorf et al., 1991). They play a role in the stabilization of molecular structures that are damaged by such stresses. Neuronal expression of HSPs is paralleled by the resistance of these cells to excitotoxin-mediated injury: prior heating of cortical cell cultures was associated with production of HSPs and a significant subsequent reduction in the cytotoxic effects of glutamate (Chopp et al., 1991). In experimental models of stroke, neurones that demonstrated production of HSP-72 were protected from ischaemic-mediated cellular necrosis; cells not expressing this HSP became necrotic. It has been suggested that regional differences in the expression of HSPs underlies the selective vulnerability of brain regions to cerebral ischaemia.

POTENTIAL NEUROPROTECTIVE AGENTS

A large number of potential neuroprotective agents that have shown considerable promise in animal studies, have been subjected to trials in human stroke, but to date none has been shown to be definitely beneficial (Lees, 2000). There are likely to be a number of reasons for these results. These include unacceptable side-effects, underpowered studies and failure to include only patients within 3 hours of stroke onset (Dyker and Lees, 1998). Furthermore, there is some evidence that many neuroprotective agents only protect cortical tissue, while the human trials have often included all sites of infarction, including subcortical strokes (Xue et al., 1992).

Nonetheless, vigorous and intensive research is still being conducted into the production of agents that could protect cells when administered after the onset of cerebral ischaemia. It is likely that different drugs will be effective according to whether ischaemia is focal or global, cortical or subcortical; different agents may also be selected according to the timing of treatment after stroke onset. It is unclear for how long such intervention may prove effective. It is likely that for many agents, intervention will only be beneficial over a limited time period of 3 hours or so after stroke. It may also be naive to expect a single agent to interrupt a complex inter-related biochemical cascade, and a 'cocktail' of multiple agents may be required. Different agents may be required, depending on whether or not occlusion is still present. The idea of combining thrombolysis with a neuroprotective agent chosen to prevent the consequences of reperfusion is attractive. On the other hand, appropriate agents may be developed that are only effective in the later stages of ischaemia, or for a longer period according to stroke location (e.g. the posterior circulation with its profuse collateral blood supply). Another intriguing possibility is prophylactic neuroprotective treatment of patients at increased risk of stroke. Such individuals, for example those with a strong family history of stroke, with numerous risk factors, or who have already had a transient ischaemic attack (TIA) or minor stroke, may be prescribed a drug that only becomes active once cerebral ischaemia occurs. Currently, no undisputed neuroprotective agents are clinically available for ischaemic stroke or primary intracerebral haemorrhage. However, intensive research is progressing and it is likely that therapeutically useful drugs will become available in the future.

Nimodipine is the only neuroprotective agent in which a clinical trial benefit has been shown in human stroke, and here the benefits seem to be limited to the treatment of subarachnoid haemorrhage, perhaps because these patients can be pretreated before vasospasm intervenes (Chapter 9). Nimodipine is a calcium-channel antagonist that blocks L-type voltage-operated calcium channels (L-VOCCs), and it is assumed that nimodipine prevents the accumulation of intracellular calcium which is so detrimental to cellular viability. However, clinical studies of nimodipine in ischaemic stroke have been disappointing, with no obvious advantage being demonstrated. In part, this may reflect the time of administration and the concentration of the drug. In addition, calcium can accumulate within ischaemic cells by mechanisms independent of L-VOCCs (e.g. by the glutamate-activated NMDA channel). Thus blockage of the L-type channel on its own may not be sufficient. Finally, nimodipine may act to vasodilate arteries in normal tissue, with less effect in the ischaemic region. This in effect would steal blood away from the ischaemic regions and decrease their supply of nutrients. It is also possible that lowering of blood pressure by nimodipine negated any beneficial effects on the penumbra.

Non-competitive NMDA antagonists have attracted much interest. These agents bind to a site within the NMDA-regulated ion channel, which must therefore be in the open state for efficacy. As mentioned earlier, ischaemia depolarizes cell membranes, overcoming the magnesium blockade. In addition, ischaemia releases glutamate, which opens these channels, allowing NMDA antagonists access. The theoretical advantage of these agents is that their maximum potency should be mainly directed to ischaemic regions and not to normal glutamatergic excitatory synapses. PCP and ketamine are examples of this group of agents. Both have anaesthetic and analgesic actions in lower doses; however, these are replaced by psychotropic responses and amnestic effects as the doses are increased. In animal stroke models, dizocilpine (MK-801) reduces infarct size when administered before as well as after experimental middle cerebral artery occlusion. However, it has a number of unpleasant psychotropic actions that prevent its use in humans. Other non-competitive antagonists of the NMDA receptor are being investigated, and it may only be a matter of time before such agents prove effective in humans, with acceptable levels of tolerability. However, to date, several large clinical trials in humans have failed to confirm the promise of NMDA receptor antagonists in stroke.

Magnesium, which blocks the NMDA-linked calcium channel, was thought to be a suitable agent for cytoprotective therapy. However, a large randomized study in which magnesium was administered within 12 hours of stroke onset has failed to show any clinical benefit (IMAGES, 2004).

CONCLUSIONS

Recent investigations have identified a series of changes in intracellular metabolism unleashed by cerebral ischaemia. Initially, some of the effects are mediated by excitotoxins (e.g. glutamate and dysregulation of NO pathways). Intracellular calcium accumulation occurs, with consequent activation of proteases and kinases and subsequent disruption of mitochondrial and cell membrane integrity. There is a resultant depletion of energy substrates. Further membrane disruption may occur during reperfusion as free radicals, including superoxide, are generated. Later mechanisms of cellular injury include the liberation of cytokines, including interleukins and PAF. Intrinsic cytoprotective mechanisms may also become activated, including HSPs, which may stabilize the protein structures damaged by ischaemia.

Understanding of these mechanisms has led to the development of various neuroprotective therapies that are undergoing evaluation. Conceptually, different agents may be effective at different times after cerebral ischaemia. Eventually, patients will be treated with a timed regimen using appropriate neuroprotective agents according to the time of presentation after stroke. The regimen may change over the ensuing days to deal with the different metabolic effects occurring at different times after stroke. Currently, we are far from achieving adequate neuroprotection. Antagonism of excitotoxic agents (e.g. glutamate) leads to a variety of behavioural and vigilance abnormalities, as the antagonists do not target ischaemic regions solely, and will interfere with general excitatory neurotransmission. Investigation is underway to identify glutamate antagonists that are effective only at ischaemic sites. Undoubtedly, the next few years will see a considerable advancement in our understanding of the metabolic and gene expression effects of cerebral ischaemia and the production of effective antagonists that are relatively free of troublesome side-effects.

KEY REFERENCES

Ischaemic penumbra and the therapeutic window

Astrup J, Symon L, Branston NM et al. Cortical evoked potential and extracellular K+ and H+ at critical levels of brain ischemia. *Stroke* 1977;**8**:51–57

ATLANTIS, ECASS, and NINDS rt-PA Study Group Investigators. Association of outcome with early stroke treatment: pooled analysis of ATLANTIS, ECASS, and NINDS rt-PA stroke trials. *Lancet* 2004;**363**:768–774

Baron JC Mapping the ischaemic penumbra with PET: a new approach. *Brain* 2001;**124**:2–4

Heiss WD, Graf R. The ischemic penumbra. *Curr Opin Neurol* 1994;**7**:11–19

Jansen O, Schellinger P, Fiebach J et al. Early recanalisation in acute ischaemic stroke saves tissue at risk defined by MRI. *Lancet* 1999;**353**:2036–2037

Markus R, Reutens DC, Kazui S et al. Hypoxic tissue in ischaemic stroke: persistence and clinical consequences of spontaneous survival. *Brain* 2004; **127**:1427–1436

Selective vulnerability

Pulsinelli WA, Brierley JB, Plum F. Temporal profile of neuronal damage in a model of transient forebrain ischemia. *Ann Neurol* 1982;**11**:491–498

Excitotoxicity and other mechanisms of ischaemic injury

Benveniste H. The excitotoxin hypothesis in relation to cerebral ischaemia. *Cerebrovasc Brain Metab Rev* 1991;**3**:213–245

Chopp M, Li Y, Dereski MO et al. Neuronal injury and expression of 72–kDa heat-shock protein after forebrain ischaemia in the rat. *Acta Neuropathol* 1991;**83**:66–71

Kumar M, Liu GJ, Floyd RA et al. Anoxic injury of endothelial cells increases production of nitric oxide and hydroxyl radicals. *Biochem Biophys Res Commun* 1996;**219**:497–501

Liu T, Clark RK, McDonnell P et al. Tumor necrosis factor-alpha expression in ischemic neurons. *Stroke* 1994;**25**:1481–1488

Rordorf G, Koroshetz WJ, Bonventre JV. Heat shock protects cultured neurons from glutamate toxicity. *Neuron* 1991;**7**:1043–1051

Yue TL, Feuerstein GZ. Platelet activating factor: a putative neuromodulator and mediator in the pathophysiology of brain injury. *Crit Rev Neurobiol* 1994;**8**:11–24

Neuroprotection

Dyker AG, Lees KR. Duration of neuroprotective treatment for ischemic stroke. *Stroke* 1998;**29**: 535–542

IMAGES: Intravenous Magnesium Efficacy in Stroke Study Investigators. Magnesium for acute stroke (Magnesium Efficacy in Stroke Trial): a randomised controlled trial. *Lancet* 2004;**363**: 439–445

Lees KR. Neuroprotection. *Br Med Bull* 2000;**56**: 401–412

Xue D, Slivka A, Buchan AM. Tirilazad reduces cortical infarction after transient but not permanent focal cerebral ischemia in rats. *Stroke* 1992; **23**:894–899.

CHAPTER 14

Acute Medical Therapy

Stroke has changed in the last few years from being a condition regarded as untreatable to being seen as a brain attack, warranting emergency treatment and active management. The management of stroke focuses on:

- Investigations to confirm diagnosis and establish cause
- Thrombolysis if indicated
- Prevention of recurrence
- Preservation of normal homeostasis
- Prevention of complications
- Rehabilitation

This chapter concentrates on the management of acute ischaemic stroke. Many of the principles apply equally to intracerebral and subarachnoid haemorrhage, which are discussed in Chapters 8 and 9. Investigation is covered in Chapters 2 and 3; prevention of recurrence is covered in Chapter 15; prevention of complications, rehabilitation and stroke unit care are discussed in Chapter 16.

SPECIFIC INTERVENTIONS IN ACUTE STROKE

Three approaches based on an understanding of the pathophysiology of ischaemia can be applied in acute stroke. Firstly, it is logical that if a stroke is due to an occluded artery then attempts should be made to reopen the artery, so long as this can be done relatively safely. Secondly, measures should be instituted to prevent early recurrence. Thirdly, metabolic

changes are initiated within cerebral tissues, which lead to the death of cells (Chapter 13). These neurotoxic processes may be exacerbated by poor management of the patient, leading to secondary brain damage, for example if the patient becomes hypotensive from dehydration. Treatment should therefore be focused on protecting traumatized tissue and limiting the consequences of the ischaemic cascade as far as possible (neuroprotection; see Chapter 13). At present, the use of specific neuroprotective agents is confined to the treatment of subarachnoid haemorrhage and research trials, but there are a number of general measures described below designed to preserve homeostasis and protect against secondary injury.

There are striking improvements in our understanding of the way in which brain tissue responds to the trauma of stroke, which have pointed the way to specific treatments in some patients (e.g. thrombolysis). Nonetheless, the very best general medical care needs to be given to all patients, in order to optimize their chances of recovery. The ischaemic penumbra (Chapter 13) is very likely to be sensitive to changes in blood pressure, blood glucose and moderate increases in temperature. These have all have been shown to be associated with worse outcome when deranged. Care of the patient must focus on the prevention of further damage to the brain as a result of a deterioration of the patient's general medical condition, which may encourage stroke extension and jeopardize the process of brain repair. Stroke should be viewed as a dynamic phenomenon in which a cascade of metabolic events is unleashed in the brain at the time of vascular injury. These may continue for several hours or days, during which appropriate care and intervention may help the injured brain to recover by limiting or terminating this cascade of events. Appropriate patient management therefore calls for expert attention to the general medical condition of the patient, as well as for the introduction of specific interventional therapies appropriate to the type and nature of the stroke. It is likely that the demonstrated benefits of stroke unit care reflect in part attention to these details, as well as the effects of early rehabilitation (Chapter 16).

To guide appropriate treatment for stroke, it is essential to establish the underlying pathology (infarction or haemorrhage), the site of the lesion (anatomy) and the mechanism of stroke (Chapters 2–4). A wide variety of different processes may lead to ischaemic stroke, and it would be naive to think that a single drug treatment will be appropriate, whatever the cause of stroke. For example, neither thrombolysis nor aspirin therapy is likely to be effective if the vessel is occluded by atheromatous debris. There is a huge difference between a large wedge of infarction secondary to middle cerebral artery occlusion and a small lacunar infarct a few millimetres across in the internal capsule, although the motor deficits may appear identical. Despite these differences, almost all the recent clinical trials have treated acute stroke as a single condition, often assuming an underlying mechanism of atherothrombosis. At present, few drug treatments are targeted at individual mechanisms, and therapy is given to a wide variety of patients, knowing that not all will necessarily benefit.

THROMBOLYSIS

The first thrombolytic agent to be tried in acute stroke was streptokinase (Mielke *et al.*, 2004). Three trials – the Multicentre Acute Stroke Trial (MAST) in Italy, MAST in Europe and the Australian Streptokinase Trial (AST) – all showed a significantly worse outcome in

streptokinase-treated patients. Each of the trials gave streptokinase intravenously within 6 hours of onset. The worse outcome in the streptokinase-treated patients was almost entirely the result of a significant excess of cerebral haemorrhage, which resulted in approximately twice as many deaths at 10 days in treated patients compared with controls. Despite the early excess of mortality, there was very little difference in the death and dependency rate at 6 months follow-up, but, nevertheless, the high rate of haemorrhage has led to the abandonment of streptokinase as a potential treatment for stroke.

In contrast, the approach to acute stroke was transformed by the results of the first trial of intravenous thrombolysis using alteplase, a recombinant tissue plasminogen activator (rtPA). The National Institute of Neurological Diseases and Stroke (NINDS) study randomized 624 patients in two parts of the study within 3 hours of stroke onset in 48 hospitals in the USA (NINDS, 1995). All the patients had neurological assessment and computed tomography (CT) scan before randomization to alteplase 0.9 mg/kg (10% given as an intravenous bolus followed by the remaining 90% as an intravenous infusion over the ensuing 1 hour) or placebo. Patients were included if they had suffered a brainstem or hemisphere ischaemic stroke, the time of onset was clearly known and they could start treatment within 180 minutes of onset. Half were randomized within 90 minutes of onset. Angiography was not performed prior to randomization. Clearly, patients were not considered appropriate for treatment if they had suffered an intracerebral haemorrhage, and there were several other exclusion criteria. It is notable that the blood pressure was carefully controlled, with intravenous agents if necessary, in all patients, which emphasizes the intensive approach required for the successful treatment of acute stroke. The patients treated with alteplase had a significantly better outcome in terms of good recovery, whatever outcome measure was used. However, as expected, there was a significant incidence of symptomatic intracranial haemorrhage of 6% in treated patients, compared with 1% in the placebo group. Those patients who

Table 14.1 Summary of the results of the major trials of thrombolysis in acute stroke using intravenous alteplase

	NINDS		ECASS–I		ECASS–II		ATLANTIS	
	Alteplase	Placebo	Alteplase	Placebo	Alteplase	Placebo	Alteplase	Placebo
Number randomized	624		620		800		613	
Dose (mg/kg)	0.9		1.1		0.9		0.9	
Time window (hours)	0–3		0–6		0–6		3–5	
Baseline NIHSS (%)	14	15	12	13	11	11	11	11
Rankin grade 0/1 (%)	39[a]	26	36	29	40	37	42	41
Symptomatic ICH (%)	6[a]	1	NR	NR	9[a]	3	7[a]	1
Mortality rate (%)	17	21	22	16	11	11	11	7

NINDS, National Institute of Neurological Disorders and Stroke Study; ECASS, European Co-operative Acute Stroke Study; ATLANTIS, Alteplase Thrombolysis for Acute Noninterventional Therapy in Ischemic Stroke Study; ICH, intracranial haemorrhage; NR, not recorded.
[a]Statistically significant.

developed intracerebral haemorrhage deteriorated clinically and also had a much higher mortality than those who did not suffer this complication. However, this did not translate into excess of deaths in treated group, which was very similar to the placebo rate (Table 14.1). Independent reanalysis of the data from the NINDS Study has confirmed the beneficial effect of alteplase treatment (Ingall *et al.*, 2004).

The positive results of the NINDS alteplase trial led to the early licensing of intravenous thrombolysis within 3 hours of stroke onset in the USA and Canada. However, two consecutive trials in Europe, the European Co-operative Acute Stroke Studies (ECASS-I and ECASS-II), and a subsequent trial in the USA (ATLANTIS) failed to show a significant benefit to alteplase on an intention-to-treat primary analysis, which examined the patients making an almost complete recovery (Rankin scale 0 or 1; Table 14.1) (Hacke *et al.*, 1995, 1998). However, there were a number of differences between these trials and the NINDS trial. All used a longer time window of up to 6 hours after onset, during which treatment could be started. ECASS-I also used a slightly higher dose of alteplase. ECASS-I also had the problem that a significant proportion of the patients were entered, despite having changes on the prerandomization CT scan indicating that more than one-third of the

middle cerebral artery territory was already severely ischaemic. These patients appear not to benefit from thrombolysis and have a high risk of haemorrhagic transformation. When post hoc analysis of the 'target' population in ECASS-I was performed on only those patients without exclusion criteria, the patients treated with alteplase had a significantly better outcome than the placebo-treated patients (Hacke *et al.*, 1995). This trial demonstrated the difficulty that inexperienced centres have interpreting the CT changes of early infarction, which can be quite subtle. The investigators therefore carried out a second trial of intravenous alteplase, ECASS-II, this time training-up the centres to read CTs beforehand. Disappointingly, ECASS-II also failed to show a significant benefit in the primary analysis, analysing patients making an almost complete recovery to Rankin grade 0 or 1 (Hacke *et al.*, 1998). However, again a post hoc analysis showed a significant benefit for alteplase, this time examining the number of patients who recovered without serious disability (Rankin grades 0, 1 or 2), which is the more usual dichotomy used in clinical trials. The ECASS trials, individually, thus suggested a benefit for thrombolysis given within 6 hours of stroke onset, but were not convincingly positive, given the failure of the primary analysis to reach statistical significance.

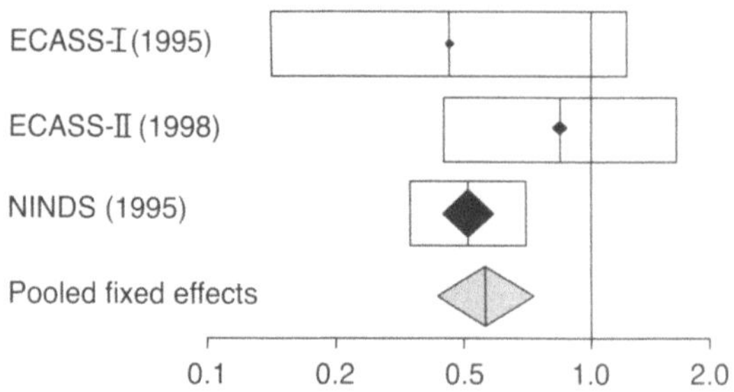

Figure 14.1 Meta-analysis of the effects of thrombolysis within 3 hours of stroke onset using intravenous alteplase: plot of odds ratio and 95% confidence intervals comparing unfavourable outcomes (alteplase versus placebo). Adapted from Ford G, Freemantle N. *Lancet* 1999;**353**:65.

The main difference between the convincingly positive NINDS trial and the less convincing ECASS trials is the longer time window in the European studies. In keeping with the importance of the time window, the ATLANTIS study of alteplase in acute stroke, which randomized patients between 3 and 5 hours after onset, had a neutral result (Clark *et al.*, 1999). It is also noticeable that the mortality rate in the placebo group of the NINDS trial was higher than the placebo group in ECASS-I and double that of the placebo group in ECASS-II. This most likely represents the randomization of more severely affected patients in NINDS. This may reflect the fact that patients with severe deficits are more likely to reach hospital within 3 hours. It is therefore relevant to examine the benefit in the ECASS trials of the patients who were randomized under 3 hours after stroke onset. When all patients treated with thrombolysis within 3 hours of onset in the three trials are combined in a meta-analysis, the reduction in unfavourable outcomes is highly significant (Figure 14.1) (Ford and Freemantle, 1999). In contrast, the meta-analysis of the patients treated between 3 and 6 hours showed only a non-significant trend towards favourable outcomes. When all the data from the trials of alteplase for acute stroke are combined and the outcomes adjusted for baseline variables, a

strong relationship between time from onset of stroke to treatment emerges, with an apparently linear relationship between time to treatment and chance of benefit (Figure 14.2) (ATLANTIS, ECASS, and NINDS, 2004). This result has led to an ongoing trial, known as ECASS-3, of alteplase 3–4 hours after stroke onset, and another trial, the Third International Stroke Trial (IST3), is testing alteplase 0–6 hours after stroke in patients in whom the investigators are uncertain about the balance of risk and benefit.

Quite why several studies have shown marked efficacy only when treatment is commenced within a few hours of symptom onset is unclear. It is possible that after several hours ischaemia of blood vessels distal to the site of occlusion results in endothelial changes, which encourage haemorrhage during reperfusion when the clot is lysed. Secondly, the metabolic cascade unleashed by ischaemia may be halted if reperfusion occurs within 3 hours but not thereafter. Reperfusion may also result in amplification of the cascade, because influx of oxygen into a previously ischaemic area results in the generation of superoxide free radicals. These highly reactive agents oxidize cell membranes, causing disruption of cellular integrity and lysis of the cell. In addition, they interfere with proton gradients and mitochondrial function. It is possible that the likelihood of generating these highly reactive species is enhanced if ischaemia persists for more than 3 hours. These considerations are conjectural rather than supported by concrete evidence, but raise the possibility that the therapeutic window for the use of alteplase might be extended by combining thrombolysis with neuroprotective agents in the future.

It is also possible that the 3-hour time window reflects the fact that salvageable penumbra is uncommon more than 3 hours after onset. An alternative approach to extending the time window for thrombolysis is therefore to select patients who have evidence of persisting penumbra on imaging (Schellinger *et al.*, 2003). One new alternative thrombolytic agent, desmoteplase, has recently been tested in a longer time window using perfusion–diffusion

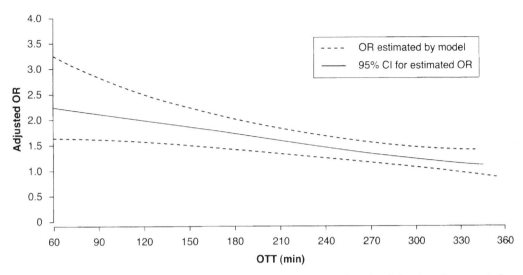

Figure 14.2 Combined analysis of the data from all of the randomized trials of alteplase for acute ischaemic stroke. The graph shows the odds ratio (OR) and 95% confidence interval (CI) comparing favourable outcome (alteplase versus placebo), after adjustment for baseline variables, plotted against time from onset of stroke to treatment (OTT). From ATLANTIS, ECASS, and NINDS rt-PA Study Group Investigators. *Lancet* 2004;**363**: 768–774.

mismatch on magnetic resonance imaging (MRI) to select patients likely to have persisting penumbra (Chapter 3). Desmoteplase is a recombinant plasminogen activator derived from *Desmodus* saliva, which has high fibrin specificity, and unlike alteplase, it is not activated by β-amyloid and shows no neurotoxic properties. The Desmoteplase In Acute Ischemic Stroke (DIAS) Trial has reported that intravenous desmoteplase administered within 3–9 hours of ischemic stroke onset in patients with perfusion–diffusion mismatch resulted in significantly greater reperfusion rates assessed on MRI after 4–8 hours compared with placebo (Hacke *et al.*, 2005). Early reperfusion correlated favourably with clinical outcome, and at lower doses desmoteplase had a low rate of symptomatic cerebral haemorrhage. These findings need to be confirmed in larger randomized trials.

A new experimental approach to improving the effectiveness of thrombolysis is to combine intravenous alteplase with ultrasound applied to the skull and focused on the site of arterial occlusion. Experimental studies have shown that ultrasound facilitates the activity of thrombolytic agents, presumably by altering the structure of fibrin clot and facilitating the access of the drug to the core of the thrombus. Earlier studies showed that kilohertz frequencies resulted in an excessive risk of intracranial haemorrhage. However, one recent randomized trial, known as CLOTBUST, showed that continuous 2 MHz transcranial Doppler ultrasonography (TCD) given for a 2-hour period after initiation of treatment of acute ischaemic stroke with intravenous alteplase, improved the rate of recanalization (Alexandrov *et al.*, 2004). Complete recanalization occurred in 49% of treated patients, compared with 30% in patients receiving alteplase and sham TCD only. However, it was notable that TCD monitoring showed that subsequent reocclusion occurred in about 20% of patients in both groups. A much larger trial is required to demonstrate that improved recanalization from the combination of ultrasound and thrombolysis results in clinical benefit. The use of TCD in this manner will be a challenge to achieve given the need to recruit centres with experienced TCD ultrasonographers available to assess and treat patients within 3 hours of onset of stroke.

In summary, the evidence strongly suggests that alteplase given within 3 hours of onset is beneficial and that the earlier the drug is given, the better. The number needed to treat to save one patient being disabled is about eight (Lees, 2000). Thrombolysis has been licensed in North America for several years and a licence for intravenous alteplase given within 3 hours of onset of stroke was granted in Europe in 2003. However, the strict protocol requirements for administering alteplase means that in parts of Europe (e.g. the UK) and even in some parts of the USA, only a small number of specialist centres currently use alteplase for acute ischaemic stroke. Trials need to continue to establish whether the time window can be extended beyond 3 hours.

Intravenous thrombolysis should only be offered to patients according to strict guidelines (Table 14.2). It is particularly important that such therapy should only be considered in patients within 3 hours of stroke onset, who have no evidence of intracerebral haemorrhage. It should be administered by experienced teams with the skills to interpret CT scans and exclude patients with early signs of a large infarct (more than one-third of the middle cerebral artery territory). Patients and carers need to be warned that thrombolysis provides a chance of benefit but also a risk of harm from cerebral haemorrhage, with a 12% absolute increase in the number of patients with minimal or no disability, compared with a 5% additional risk of significant deterioration due to intracerebral haemorrhage. It is essential that centres contemplating thrombolysis for stroke should adhere strictly to the NINDS and ECASS protocols and should audit their results.

Local arterial infusion of thrombolytic agents through an indwelling catheter may have a role to play in selected patients, particularly those with basilar artery thrombosis, in specialized neuroradiological centres, but it remains experimental. Intra-arterial thrombolysis has

the advantage that the agent can be infused exactly where it is needed, partly avoiding systemic effects. In addition, the site of occlusion can be confirmed, excluding patients who have already undergone spontaneous thrombolysis. There has been one positive randomized trial of intra-arterial thrombolysis using prourokinase, PROACT II (Furlan et al., 1999). This study showed a significant benefit for intra-arterial thrombolysis given within 6 hours of onset of symptoms. However, because of the requirement to scan the patients and perform cerebral angiography within the time window, very few patients were eligible for the study. In fact, to randomize 180 patients, an extraordinary 12 323 acute stroke patients were screened and 474 angiograms performed. The median time to randomization was 4.7 hours, demonstrating that if patients had favourable angiographic features, arterial thrombolysis can still be beneficial even beyond 3 hours.

Thrombolysis will only ever be suitable for a subgroup of eligible patients, particularly since many patients will not reach hospital within 3 hours of onset. In the NINDS study centres, only 6% of patients with acute stroke were entered into the trial. One might imagine that very few patients reach hospital in time for thrombolysis. However, an audit in accident and emergency departments at 22 hospitals in the UK before the licensing of alteplase for stroke showed that a surprising 37% of suspected stroke patients arrived within 3 hours, and 50% within 6 hours of onset of symptoms (Figure 14.3) (Harraf et al., 2002). Most of these arrived after an ambulance had been called rather than contacting a family physician, which delayed admission. Unfortunately, few patients are currently seen by a doctor immediately after they arrive in hospital except in specialized units, and a change in attitudes is needed so that acute stroke is dealt with as an emergency equivalent to an acute myocardial infarct. One way of shortening the time it takes for the patient to reach specialized services is to arrange with the ambulance service for patients with symptoms suggesting stroke to be taken directly to an acute stroke unit, bypassing the accident and emergency department (Harbison

Table 14.2 Guidelines for the use of intravenous alteplase in acute ischaemic stroke (adapted from the NINDS Protocol)

Eligibility
- Age 18 or older
- Clinical diagnosis of acute ischaemic stroke
- Assessed by experienced team
- Measurable neurological deficit
- Timing of symptom onset well established
- CT (or MRI) and blood tests results available
- CT (or MRI) scan consistent with diagnosis
- Treatment could then begin within 180 minutes of symptom onset

Exclusion criteria
- Symptoms only minor or rapidly improving
- Haemorrhage on pretreatment CT (or MRI)
- Visible changes on pretreatment CT (or MRI) of infarction > one-third of middle cerebral artery territory
- Suspected subarachnoid haemorrhage
- Active bleeding from any site
- Recent gastrointestinal or urinary tract haemorrhage within 21 days
- Platelet count less than 100×10^9/l
- Recent treatment with heparin and activated partial thromboplastin time (APTT) above normal
- Recent treatment with warfarin and International Normalized Ratio (INR) elevated
- Recent major surgery or trauma within the previous 14 days
- Recent post-myocardial infarction pericarditis
- Neurosurgery, serious head trauma or previous stroke within 3 months
- History of intracranial haemorrhage (ever)
- Known arteriovenous malformation or aneurysm
- Recent arterial puncture at non-compressible site
- Recent lumbar puncture
- Blood pressure consistently above 185 mmHg systolic or 110 mmHg diastolic
- Abnormal blood glucose (<3 or >20 mmol/l; <54 or >360 mg/100 ml)
- Suspected or known pregnancy
- Active pancreatitis
- Epileptic seizure at stroke onset

Dose of rtPA
- Total dose 0.9 mg/kg (maximum 90 mg)
- 10% of the total dose as an initial intravenous bolus over 1 minute
- Remainder infused intravenously over 60 minutes

et al., 1999). This substantially increases the number of patients treated with thrombolysis and benefiting from early stroke assessment.

MECHANICAL RECANALIZATION

Only a small proportion of ischaemic stroke patients are eligible for thrombolysis and not all patients achieve recanalization after treatment. It is therefore logical to attempt mechanical recanalization in patients ineligible for thrombolysis or in patients after failed thrombolysis who have persistent thrombotic occlusion of major arteries. Surgical thrombectomy was first reported in the 1950s, but never achieved widespread use because of the invasive nature of the surgery and lack of dramatic success, except in the occasional patient with acute carotid occlusion. The development of microcatheters and endovascular techniques

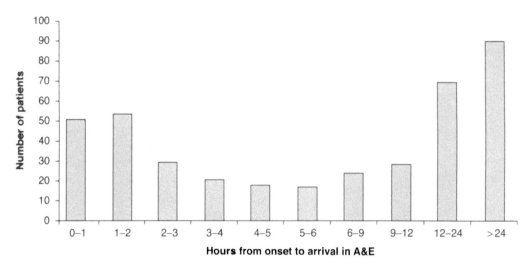

Figure 14.3   Bar graph showing the time of arrival in 14 UK Accident and Emergency (A&E) departments at set times after the onset of stroke. Graph created using data from Harraff F *et al. BMJ* 2002;**325**:17–20.

for reaching intracranial arteries has stimulated interest in using mechanical devices to extract or break up intracranial thrombosis in acute stroke. One such device specially designed for intracranial embolectomy is the Merci Retriever System. This consists of a guide catheter with a large 2.1 mm lumen and a balloon located at its tip, a microcatheter and a retriever device. The retriever is a tapered wire, made of thermal memory nitinol, with five helical loops of decreasing diameter (from 2.8 mm to 1.1 mm) at its distal end. Patients treated with this device have the guide catheter inserted in the common or internal carotid artery for anterior circulation occlusion, or the subclavian artery for posterior circulation occlusion. The microcatheter is then guided into the occluded vessel and passed beyond the thrombus. The retriever is then advanced through the microcatheter in a straight configuration and it then resumes its preimposed helical shape once it emerges from the microcatheter to ensnare the thrombus. The thrombus is then withdrawn into the guide catheter lumen. The balloon on the guide catheter is inflated during removal of the thrombus to control intracranial blood flow.

The Mechanical Embolus Removal in Cerebral Ischemia (MERCI) 1 study evaluated the safety and efficacy of mechanical embolectomy in 28 patients with acute ischaemic stroke within 8 hours from symptoms onset (Gobin *et al.*, 2004). Successful recanalization with mechanical embolectomy was only achieved in 43% of patients, but, with additional intra-arterial rtPA, recanalization was achieved in a total of 64% patients. At 1 month, 50% of the recanalized patients – but none of the 10 patients in whom recanalization was not achieved – achieved significant recovery. Although encouraging, randomized studies of mechanical recanalization in suitable patients are needed to establish the place of mechanical revascularization. However, it is likely that the use of these interventional techniques to treat acute ischaemic stroke will become more widespread in the near future.

EARLY PREVENTION OF RECURRENCE

Aspirin therapy

This is widely used to prevent recurrent stroke and myocardial infarction in patients who have recovered from a previous transient ischaemic attack (TIA) or minor stroke (Chapter 15). Until a few years ago, there was

Table 14.3   Summary of the results of the International Stroke Trial (IST) and Chinese Acute Stroke Trial (CAST), examining the benefits of aspirin given within 48 hours on acute stroke onset. (Outcomes were assessed at 28 days in CAST or at 14 days and 6 months in IST)

	CAST		IST	
	Aspirin	Control	Aspirin	Control
Number randomized	10 335	10 320	9719	9714
Death within 28/14 days (%)	3.3[a]	3.9	9.0	9.4
Recurrent ischaemic stroke (%)	1.6[b]	2.1	2.8[b]	3.9
Haemorrhagic stroke (%)	1.1	0.9	0.9	0.8
Death or dependency at 28 days/6 months (%)	30.5	31.6	61.2	63.5

[a]$p<0.01$; [b]$p<0.001$.

doubt about whether aspirin should be used in acute stroke because of concern about the risks of promoting haemorrhagic transformation of an ischaemic infarct. However, there is now good evidence about its benefits from two very large randomized trials: the International Stroke Trial (IST) and the Chinese Acute Stroke Trial (CAST) (Table 14.3) (CAST, 1997; IST, 1997). Both trials showed a small but significant reduction in recurrent ischaemic stroke of about 1 in a 100 patients treated, which was not accompanied by a significant increase in haemorrhagic stroke. There was also a small reduction in death and dependency analysed at the end of both studies, which did not reach statistical significance. However, when the two trials were combined with a small amount of data from another trial in a meta-analysis, the reduction in death and dependency from aspirin use became highly significant. Again, the number needed to prevent one patient from dying or being disabled was approximately 1 in 100. Although this benefit may seem small, it translates to a substantial cost benefit, given that stroke is common and aspirin costs little. For example, in the UK, if every patient with acute ischaemic stroke were given aspirin within 48 hours of onset then more than 1000 patients would be saved from death or disability every year.

Although there are trials suggesting that alternative antiplatelet agents, or combination antiplatelet therapy, may be more effective than aspirin alone in the prevention of stroke, no other antiplatelet regime has been tested extensively in acute stroke. There is natural concern that the newer more powerful antiplatelet agents, such as the glycoprotein IIb/IIIa (GPIIb/IIIa) receptor antagonists, may result in an increased incidence of haemorrhagic transformation.

One can therefore conclude that all ischaemic strokes should be treated with aspirin, unless contraindicated within 48 hours of onset. All patients should have a CT or MRI scan before starting aspirin to exclude haemorrhage or non-stroke pathology.

Anticoagulation

Intravenous heparin is widely used in many countries as a first-line treatment for stroke, despite the fact that almost all the randomized trial evidence is against routine anticoagulation being beneficial (Pereira and Brown, 2000). The largest trial, IST, showed no overall benefit of subcutaneous heparin with virtually identical death and dependency rates at 6 months (Table 14.4). There was a reduction in the rate of recurrent ischaemic stroke of about 1 in 100 patients treated, which was similar to that of aspirin, but, in contrast to aspirin, the rate of haemorrhagic stroke after treatment was significantly increased. This risk of haemorrhagic

Table 14.4 Summary of the results of the International Stroke Trial examining the benefits of subcutaneous heparin given within 48 hours on acute stroke onset

	Heparin	Control
Number randomized	9717	9718
Death within 14 days (%)	9.0	9.3
Recurrent ischaemic stroke (%)	2.9[a]	3.8
Haemorrhagic stroke (%)	1.2[b]	0.4
Death or dependency at 6 months (%)	62.9	62.9

[a] $p < 0.01$; [b] $p < 0.001$.

transformation was almost identical to the rate of reduction of recurrent stroke, balancing out the benefit.

There have also been several trials of low-molecular-weight heparin (LMWH). The first trial of fraxiparine in 312 patients with acute stroke in Hong Kong appeared to show a very striking benefit, but a very much larger trial of the same agent failed to confirm the initial study. Several other trials of alternative LMWHs have been equally disappointing, with no evidence of a significant overall benefit.

It can therefore be concluded that there is no place for the routine use of heparins in acute stroke. However, the low-dose subcutaneous heparin (5000 units twice daily) arm in IST was neutral, and therefore prophylactic low-dose subcutaneous heparin can be used, bearing in mind the risks, in patients who are thought to be at high risk of deep vein thrombosis. There may also be a role for the early use of intravenous heparin in patients who are at high risk of early recurrence, for example those with an obvious cardiac source or with acute vertebral or carotid artery dissection or occlusion, so long as the patient does not have a large infarct. Patients with large infarcts (more than one-third of the middle cerebral artery territory) are probably more likely to show haemorrhagic transformation. In most cases and particularly for large infarcts, anticoagulation, if indicated for stroke prevention, should probably

be delayed for 2 weeks or more (Chapter 15). This recommendation is based on consensus practice, not randomized evidence.

Prophylaxis of deep vein thrombosis and pulmonary embolism is discussed in more detail in Chapter 16.

PRESERVATION OF NORMAL HOMEOSTASIS

It is logical to attempt to maintain the brain's physiological and biochemical environment in as normal a state as possible in acute stroke to preserve the penumbra and prevent secondary deterioration (Bath, 2000). However, evidence from randomized trials that this improves outcome is currently lacking.

Blood sugar

Blood sugar levels are elevated in nearly one-quarter of all stroke admissions. In some patients (especially those with mild elevations), this represents a response to stress. Others are known diabetics. However, a significant percentage of patients (6%) are previously undiagnosed diabetics (identified by elevated glycosylated HbA_{1c} levels) and have markedly elevated random blood sugar levels (>10 mmol/l; 180 mg/100 ml). The prognosis for these patients during the first week and for those with known diabetes is poor. Mortality and infarct size are increased. Animal studies have shown that chronic or transiently elevated blood sugar is similarly disadvantageous in experimental stroke and that hyperglycaemia increases plasma viscosity and decreases cerebral blood flow. There are therefore strong arguments for instituting intravenous insulin therapy on a graded scale when blood sugar is 10 mmol/l (180 mg/100 ml) or above in an attempt to protect the ischaemic penumbra, which is poised on a metabolic knife-edge. The optimal blood sugar range should be 6–9 mmol/l (108–162 mg/100 ml). Whether lowering blood sugar within the normal range is beneficial is uncertain and is currently being investigated in clinical trials. In addition, it is probably unwise to administer intravenous glucose to stroke patients within the first 24 hours of stroke onset.

Hypertension

Approximately 80% of stroke patients are hypertensive on admission, partly because of pre-existing hypertension and also as a hormonal, stress or autonomic response to the stroke itself. It is not clear whether hypertension is harmful or beneficial in acute stages of stroke (BASC, 2001). Under normal circumstances, cerebral autoregulation ensures that cerebral blood flow remains constant over a wide range of mean arterial pressure. However, following stroke, the ability to autoregulate is lost within the environs of the infarct. Elevated blood pressure might therefore increase the risk that a bland ischaemic stroke will be transformed into a haemorrhagic infarct. However, this has not been demonstrated in clinical studies. Certainly, lowering the mean arterial pressure to a level where cerebral blood supply is compromised would be unwise. The precise level at which blood pressure therapy should be instituted remains uncertain. It should be remembered that hypertensive patients show changes in arterial structure and that they appear to autoregulate at higher levels than do their normotensive counterparts (Figure 14.4). Consequently, the lower level of blood pressure at which such patients can maintain cerebral perfusion is less than in normotensive patients, and overzealous hypotensive medication could lead to infarct extension.

High blood pressure might also have other deleterious consequences; for example, impairment of endothelial function might favour stroke progression. After cerebral haemorrhage, the risks of rebleeding might be increased. On the other hand, an increase in blood pressure might have beneficial effects by increasing flow to the penumbra (Rordorff *et al.*, 2001). Clinical trials are therefore in progress to determine the optimum management of hypertension in acute stroke.

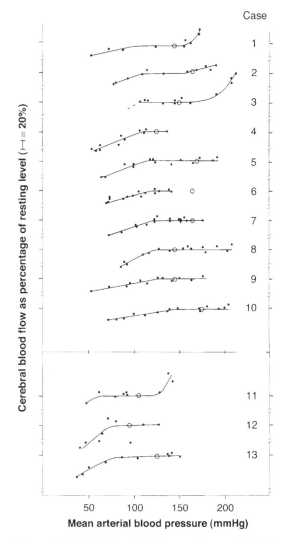

Figure 14.4   Relationship between changes in blood pressure and cerebral blood flow in 10 hypertensive patients and three non-hypertensive controls. The flat portions of the curves represent autoregulation. From Strandgaard S *et al. BMJ* 1973;i:507–510.

Currently, it is recommended that mild elevations in blood pressure do not require treatment unless they are maintained for several days after admission. Known hypertensive patients should continue their usual therapy. Additional or new anti-hypertensive treatment should not be instituted unless the blood pressure readings are maintained higher than the usual systolic threshold for treatment of 150 mmHg, especially for patients with a history of hypertension. Some guidelines only recommend immediate treatment if the patient has persistent diastolic blood pressure readings above 110 mmHg, otherwise recommending that institution of hypotensive medication should be delayed for 48 hours or more after onset to allow pressure readings to settle. Irrespective of the level of blood pressure, hypertensive encephalopathy or malignant hypertension associated with stroke should be treated as an emergency. Any treatment should be introduced cautiously. A reduction in blood pressure may lower cerebral blood flow in the regions surrounding an infarct below a critical level at which further ischaemic brain damage will occur, especially if there is a tight ipsilateral carotid stenosis. In most cases, blood pressure can be lowered using oral agents. Intramuscular agents should be avoided because of their unpredictable effect and intravenous drugs should only be used if the blood pressure can be monitored with an arterial line. In the latter case, treatment should be instituted with intravenous, rapidly metabolized agents so that the dose can be titrated against the blood pressure value without a hangover effect. Slow lowering of the blood pressure should be attempted at no more than 15 mmHg/h. Sudden precipitous falls in blood pressure should be avoided.

Hypotension

Periods of hypotension may also occur after stroke. These have not received the attention they deserve, possibly because monitoring of intra-arterial pressure in stroke patients is an exception. Such hypotensive periods may lead to decreased blood supply to the penumbra and stroke extension. Consequently, patients should be monitored for cardiac arrhythmias and hypotensive episodes over the first 3 days after stroke onset. Hypotension should be corrected by raising the foot of the bed, fluid replacement and stopping relevant hypotensive medication, and, if necessary, the administration of inotropes.

Body temperature

Recently, attention has focused on the role of body temperature and stroke prognosis. This follows the observation that the cytoprotective effects of the NMDA receptor antagonist MK 801 may be explicable in part by the 2–3°C hypothermia that the agent induces. Previously, Hindfelt showed that 44% of stroke patients were hyperthermic on admission. This was generally attributed to coincident infection (respiratory or urinary) or deep vein thrombosis rather than to the stroke itself. However, it was shown that the outcome at 3 months (as assessed by mortality and stroke score performance) was significantly worse with even mild increases of temperature (of 1°C). Animal studies have shown that a 2–3°C fall in body temperature may reduce infarct volumes by 80–100%. Hyperthermia in these animal models is associated with alterations in blood–brain barrier permeability, intracerebral acidosis, impaired cerebral energy metabolism and changes in the release of excitotoxic amino acids. These deleterious effects can be overcome by cooling. It is prudent therefore to investigate fever vigorously in the acute stroke patient and to treat underlying infections as soon as possible. Any degree of pyrexia should be treated promptly with an antipyretic agent (e.g. aspirin or paracetamol). Trials are currently underway investigating the clinical benefit of hypothermia in acute stroke.

Cardiac complications

Stroke and ischaemic heart disease frequently coexist. Notably, death from cardiac causes is predominant on long-term follow-up of stroke patients. Stroke can affect the heart independently of a cardiac ischaemic mechanism. Non-ischaemic cardiac myofibre damage (myocytolysis) and elevation of cardiac enzymes (indicative of cardiac damage) have been reported after stroke, particularly severe subarachnoid haemorrhage. There is usually no sign of acute coronary or cardiac ischaemic lesions at postmortem examination. Repolarization electrocardiogram (ECG) changes have been identified in 60–70% of cerebral haemorrhages and 5–17% of ischaemic strokes. These ECG changes are very similar to those caused by stress or infusion of catecholamines. Stroke has been shown to increase cardiac sympathetic tone if the insular cortex is involved in the lesion. The insular cortex is an important forebrain site of cardiovascular control. Conceivably, patients with insular lesions may be at greater risk of cardiovascular instability. Stroke extension or haemorrhagic conversion secondary to blood pressure lability could be more common after strokes involving this region of the brain. However, this theory awaits rigorous clinical confirmation.

Hyponatraemia

This occurs in about 10% of infarcts and 14% of cerebral haemorrhages; the aetiology may be related to inappropriate antidiuretic hormone (ADH) secretion and can be associated with stroke progression. It may initiate or exacerbate cerebral oedema. Manifestations include increasing obtundation, worsening of the clinical state and seizures. In this case, fluid restriction is required. Recently, some cases of hyponatraemia have been associated with increased secretion of atrial natriuretic factor (ANF); in such cases, patients are likely to be dehydrated. Therefore, the investigation of hyponatraemia should include measurements of plasma and urinary osmolality to differentiate this syndrome from that of inappropriate ADH secretion. Clearly, patients with hyponatraemia due to ANF increases should be rehydrated. In most cases, however, hyponatraemia is an incidental finding not associated with symptoms and requires no therapy.

Iatrogenic deterioration

Iatrogenic deterioration from therapeutic intervention is common in non-specialized units, but should be avoided as far as possible. Examples include:

- Sedation and depression induced by tranquillisers
- Pyrexia from adverse drug reactions

- Inappropriate ADH secretion caused by carbamazepine or chlorpropamide
- Hypotension from dehydration or antihypertensive therapy
- Haemorrhage from anticoagulants

CEREBRAL OEDEMA

Death is inevitable if the volume of haemorrhage or infarction is great enough or if the vital centres in the brainstem are destroyed by the stroke. However, many cases of death after stroke are avoidable, as emphasized by the reduction in mortality associated with specialized stroke unit care (Chapter 15). The causes of death differ according to time after stroke (Tables 14.5 and 14.6). During the first week, transtentorial herniation is the commonest cause of death. In these cases, there may be a stable period followed by deterioration on the second or third day, leading to progressive impairment of consciousness, coma and respiratory failure. Transtentorial herniation occurs mainly within 24 hours of cerebral haemorrhage, and at 4–5 days after infarction. The principal cause is the development of supratentorial cerebral oedema, leading to secondary brainstem compression with subsequent terminal bulbar haemorrhage or infarction. In general, cerebral oedema of this sort is unresponsive to steroid therapy. Mannitol may produce a temporal respite, by decreasing total cerebral volume, but the effects are only temporary; paralysis and hyperventilation are rarely of benefit. Decompression should be considered in the case of deteriorating cerebellar haemorrhage or infarction with progressive brainstem compression, where good recovery can be expected. In major middle cerebral artery occlusion with malignant cerebral oedema (Figure 14.5), decompressive craniectomy may be life-saving and good outcomes can be obtained in selected patients (Schwab *et al.*, 1998), particularly younger patients with non-dominant hemisphere infarction who are operated on early. However, the benefits of craniectomy have not been established by randomized trials (Brown, 2003).

Table 14.5 Causes of death after supratentorial cerebral infarction[a]

Cause of death	First week after cerebral infarction	2–4 weeks after cerebral infarction
Transtentorial herniation	78%	8%
Pulmonary embolism	0%	5%
Pneumonia	0%	35%
Septicaemia	2%	5%
Unknown	0%	15%
Cardiac complications	15%	21%
Sudden death	4%	10%

[a]Based on data obtained from the Toronto Stroke Unit in 1985.

Table 14.6 Causes of death after supratentorial cerebral haemorrhage[a]

Cause of death	First week after cerebral haemorrhage	2–4 weeks after cerebral haemorrhage
Transtentorial herniation	93%	20%
Pulmonary embolism	0%	0%
Pneumonia	2%	20%
Septicaemia	0%	0%
Unknown	2%	30%
Cardiac complications	0%	20%
Sudden death	0%	0%

[a]Based on data obtained from the Toronto Stroke Unit in 1985.

Haemorrhagic transformation

Haemorrhagic transformation of a bland infarct occurs in as many as 75% of cardioembolic strokes within 4 days and in 30% of all ischaemic strokes (Figure 14.6). It is often asymptomatic, but is associated with clinical deterioration and death in a proportion of cases. Significant clinical deterioration from haemorrhagic conversion rarely occurs in the absence of mass effect. The risk factors for haemorrhagic conversion include a large volume of infarction, a midline shift and increasing age. Hypertension and degree or extent of anticoagulation do not appear to contribute to this outcome in some studies. Possibly, the liberation of a powerful procoagulant (thromboplastin) from infarcted tissue antagonizes the effect of heparin and other anticoagulants. Despite this, anticoagulation should be either discontinued or continued very judiciously and with appropriate caution in patients who have shown haemorrhagic conversion. The treatment of haemorrhagic transformation depends on clinical status. Those deteriorating with mass effect should be considered for treatment by reducing intracranial pressure and, in some cases, by haematoma evacuation.

Acute hydrocephalus

Cerebral haemorrhage may cause acute hydrocephalus from compression of the aqueduct by blood or oedema. This may lead to deterioration or death. Management involves intraventricular shunting, treatment of cerebral oedema and haematoma evacuation. Hydrocephalus can also occur after a delay of days or weeks from obstruction to cerebrospinal fluid outflow. The management of cerebral haemorrhage is discussed in more detail in Chapter 8.

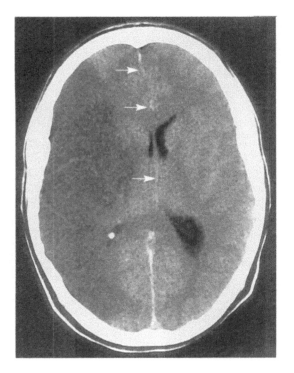

Figure 14.5 CT scan showing malignant middle cerebral artery territory infarction. Note the extensive low attenuation throughout the right middle cerebral artery territory and the mass effect shown by shift of the midline (arrows) and compression of the right lateral ventricle.

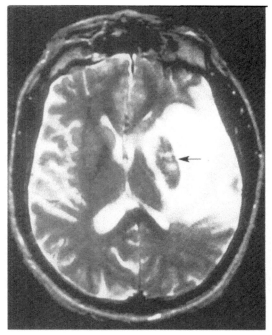

Figure 14.6 A 62-year-old patient admitted with a right hemiparesis. Her condition subsequently deteriorated 3 days later. The T_2-weighted MRI shows a large middle cerebral artery territory infarct. Within the infarct, there has been haemorrhagic conversion (seen as the dark area within the lentiform nucleus, arrow). There is also a mass effect.

Seizures

Early seizures following stroke are usually single, focal and easily controlled with mono-therapy. Seizures complicate 11% of infarcts or haemorrhages and generally indicate cortical involvement. Thirty-three percent occur within the first 2 weeks and 90% of these occur within the first day of stroke onset. There is some controversy as to whether seizures are more frequent after cardioembolic stroke. In general, early seizure onset correlates with a large stroke. Initial data suggested that seizure activity did not significantly influence morbidity or mortality, but more recent information indicates that seizures may adversely affect outcome. However, it is not clear whether this is due to the seizure itself or because of its association with a more clinically severe stroke.

Treatment of the progressing stroke patient

Stroke progression occurs in 20–40% of acute admissions (Oppenheimer and Hachinski, 1992). Several studies indicate that it is more common following vertebrobasilar than carotid territory infarction. Progression may occur at any time, but is most frequent within the first week. Associations with bilateral vertebral artery occlusion rather than basilar or branch vessel occlusion have been recorded. Likewise, progression appears to be more common following large-vessel occlusion than lacunar infarction, but is surprisingly common in the latter. Deterioration seems to be especially likely with cerebellar infarction. Understandably, the prognosis worsens in the presence of stroke progression, with a mortality rate of 27%, compared with 5% in patients who stabilized within 24 hours of admission.

The pathogenesis of progression is usually unclear. In some cases, there is progression of thrombosis by in situ accretion with subsequent blockage of perforating vessels in the brainstem or vital collateral vessels in the hemisphere. Distal embolization of friable clot may also be a mechanism. Progression of a stenotic lesion to complete occlusion may also occur, with subsequent deterioration. All of these mechanisms have been observed in angiographic investigations of the deteriorating patient, but such studies have involved small numbers and their representative nature is questionable. Other causes of deterioration include the development of cerebral oedema and haemorrhagic conversion associated with mass effect. However, in some cases, deterioration may result from expansion of the ischaemic penumbra, caused by a deterioration in the patient's general medical condition compromising collateral flow.

In the first instance, the following should be considered as soon as deterioration is noted:

- Contributing metabolic and physiological derangements, including disorders of blood sugar, cardiac output, blood pressure and cardiac rhythm (see above)
- Infections; these should be treated and pyrexia should be reduced
- Dehydration
- Hypoxia, which may result from aspiration, infection or silent pulmonary embolism
- Hyponatraemia (see above)

While metabolic factors are being sought, intracerebral causes of deterioration should be investigated by further CT or magnetic resonance imaging (MRI). These include:

- Haemorrhagic transformation
- Increasing cerebral oedema with a mass effect (see above)
- Hydrocephalus from aqueduct stenosis secondary to brainstem oedema or to subarachnoid or intraventricular haemorrhage

- Recurrent infarction or haemorrhage
- Vasospasm after subarachnoid haemorrhage

If none of these factors are present and deterioration seems likely to be caused by thrombus propagation, conventional therapy has involved anticoagulation with heparin. However, there are no convincing studies of its benefit in progressing cerebral infarction, and the trials of heparin in acute stroke argue against its use (see above). If the patient is seen within 6 hours of onset of stroke at an experienced unit, angiography and the administration of local thrombolytic therapy to the appropriate vessel in an attempt to produce reperfusion should be considered.

CONCLUSIONS

Treatment of acute stroke involves delivery of optimal medical care to the patient. This will help protect the penumbra and probably improve functional outcome. Attention to blood sugar, temperature and cardiovascular status are important, as is the prompt treatment of neurological deterioration secondary to cerebral oedema or haemorrhagic conversion of a bland cerebral infarct. These patients are best treated in specialized units, where they are in the hands of specialist physicians and nursing staff alert to the early signs of neurological compromise and motivated to provide the optimal therapy. Recently, thrombolysis and techniques for mechanical recanalization have been introduced, and the near future promises rapid advances in these approaches. Stroke unit care is discussed in more detail in Chapter 16.

KEY REFERENCES

Thrombolysis

Alexandrov AV, Molina CA, Grotta JC et al. Ultrasound-enhanced systemic thrombolysis for acute ischemic stroke. *N Engl J Med* 2004;**351**: 2170–2178

ATLANTIS, ECASS, and NINDS rt-PA Study Group Investigators. Association of outcome with early stroke treatment: pooled analysis of ATLANTIS, ECASS, and NINDS rt-PA stroke trials. *Lancet* 2004;**363**:768–774

Clark WM, Wissman S, Albers GW et al. for the ATLANTIS Study Investigators. Recombinant tissue-type plasminogen activator (alteplase) for ischaemic stroke 3 to 5 hours after symptom onset. *JAMA* 1999;**282**:2019–2026

Ford G, Freemantle N. ECASS-II: intravenous alteplase in acute ischaemic stroke. *Lancet* 1999; **353**:65

Furlan A, Higashida R, Wechsler L et al. for the PROACT Investigators. Intra-arterial Prourokinase for acute ischaemic stroke. The PROACT II Study: a randomized controlled trial. *JAMA* 1999; **282**:2003–2011

Hacke W, Kaste M, Fieshchi C et al. for the ECASS Study Group. Intravenous thrombolysis with recombinant tissue plasminogen activator for acute hemispheric stroke. *JAMA* 1995;**274**: 1017–1025

Hacke W, Kaste M, Fieschi C et al. Randomised double-blind placebo-controlled trial of thrombolytic therapy with intravenous alteplase in acute ischaemic stroke (ECASS-II). *Lancet* 1998; **352**:1245–1251

Hacke W, Albers G, Al-Rawi Y et al. The Desmoteplase in Acute Ischemic Stroke Trial (DIAS): a phase II MRI-based 9-hour window acute stroke thrombolysis trial with intravenous desmoteplase. *Stroke* 2005;**36**:66–73

Harbison J, Massey A, Barnett L et al. Rapid ambulance protocol for acute stroke. *Lancet* 1999;**353**: 1935

Harraf F, Sharma AK, Brown MM et al. A multicentre observational study of presentation and early assessment of acute stroke. *BMJ* 2002;**325**: 17–20

Ingall TJ, O'Fallon WM, Asplund K et al. Findings from the reanalysis of the NINDS tissue plasminogen activator for acute ischemic stroke treatment trial. *Stroke* 2004;**35**:2418–2424

Lees KR. Thrombolysis. *Br Med Bull* 2000;**56**: 389–400

Mielke O, Wardlaw J, Liu M. Thrombolysis (different doses, routes of administration and agents) for acute ischaemic stroke. *Cochrane Database System Rev* 2004, Issue 1

NINDS: National Institute of Neurological Disorders and Stroke rt-PA Stroke Study Group. Tissue plasminogen activator for acute ischaemic stroke. *N Engl J Med* 1995;**24**:1581–1587

Schellinger PD, Fiebach JB, Hacke W. Imaging-based decision making in thrombolytic therapy for ischemic stroke: present status. *Stroke* 2003;**34**: 575–83

Mechanical recanalization

Gobin YP, Starkman S, Duckwiler GR et al. MERCI 1: a phase 1 study of Mechanical Embolus Removal in Cerebral Ischemia. *Stroke* 2004;**35**:2848–2854

Aspirin

CAST (Chinese Acute Stroke Trial) Collaborative Group. CAST: randomised placebo-controlled trial of early aspirin use in 20,000 patients with acute ischaemic stroke. *Lancet* 1997;**349**: 1641–1649

IST: International Stroke Trial Collaborative Group. The International Stroke Trial (IST): a randomised trial of aspirin, subcutaneous heparin, both or neither among 19,435 patients with acute ischaemic stroke. *Lancet* 1997;**349**:1569–1581

Anticoagulation

Pereira AC, Brown MM. Aspirin or heparin in acute stroke. *Br Med Bull* 2000;**56**:413–421

Preservation of normal homeostasis

Bath PMW. Optimising homeostasis. *Br Med Bull* 2000;**56**:422–435

Treatment of hypertension

BASC: Blood Pressure in Acute Stroke Collaboration. Interventions for deliberately altering blood pressure in acute stroke. *Cochrane Database System Rev* 2001, Issue 2

Rordorff G, Koreshetz WJ, Ezzedine MA et al. A pilot study of drug induced hypertension for treatment of acute stroke. *Neurology* 2001;**56**:1210–3

Strandgaard S, Olesen J, Skinhoj E, Lassen NA. Autoregulation of brain circulation in severe arterial hypertension. *BMJ* 1973;**1**:507–510

Cerebral oedema

Brown MM. Surgical decompression of patients with large middle cerebral artery infarcts is effective: not proven. *Stroke* 2003;**34**:2305–2306

Schwab S, Steiner T, Aschoff A et al. Early hemicraniectomy in patients with complete middle cerebral artery infarction. *Stroke* 1998;**29**: 1888–1893

Progressive stroke

Oppenheimer SM, Hachinski V. The complications of acute stroke. *Lancet* 1992;**339**:721–724

CHAPTER 15

Prevention

APPROACHES TO STROKE PREVENTION

The main approaches to stroke prevention are:

- Avoidance of risk factors (e.g. smoking)
- Treatment of specific risk factors (e.g. hypertension)
- Treatment to reduce the coagulability of the blood (e.g. anticoagulation or antiplatelet therapy)
- Removal of focal causes of stroke (e.g. carotid stenosis)

PRIMARY PREVENTION

Primary prevention involves the prevention of stroke in individuals who have never suffered clinical cerebrovascular disease. The benefit to the individual patient may be small, but the potential benefit to the whole population is large as most strokes occur in individuals who have been previously asymptomatic. The approach of encouraging a healthy lifestyle is appropriate to the entire population. The extent to which a healthy lifestyle is adopted by the population depends primarily on education within the population as a whole via schools, media, primary care and well-person clinics.

Treatment of a specific risk factor (e.g. hypertension or atrial fibrillation) requires individuals to be screened for relevant risk factors. For screening to be cost-effective, there must be a reasonable chance of finding the risk factor of interest, screening must be relatively cheap, and proven effective treatment must be available with a risk–benefit ratio favouring treatment. In the apparently healthy population, these requirements are only satisfied for hypertension, atrial fibrillation and diabetes mellitus. The benefits of screening for hypercholesterolaemia in healthy subjects are uncertain. These risk factors only become sufficiently frequent to justify screening above a certain age, and in the UK routine health checks were at one stage only recommended above the age of 75. Nevertheless, the opportunity to check a patient's blood pressure and pulse should be taken whenever they present to the medical or nursing profession. Screening for additional risk factors, such as hypercholesterolaemia, may be of particular benefit in individuals who are already at increased risk because of known risk factors such as diabetes or a strong family history of vascular disease.

SECONDARY PREVENTION

Secondary prevention is targeted at patients who already have symptomatic cerebrovascular disease. On an individual-patient basis, there is considerably more to be gained in this patient group because they have a high risk of recurrence.

The choice of preventive treatments for individual patients should be based on evidence-based medicine and therefore supported as far as possible by the results of randomized clinical trials. Much of the relevant clinical trial data is available in the Cochrane Database of Systematic Reviews.

PREVENTION OF ISCHAEMIC STROKE

Thrombosis plays an important part in the majority of ischaemic strokes. Three main underlying pathological processes trigger thrombosis:

- Atherosclerosis
- Hypertensive small vessel disease
- Cardiac abnormalities

These mechanisms are discussed in more detail in Chapter 7.

There are several avenues to target prevention of thrombosis:

- Prevention of atheroma formation and progression (risk factor modification and statin treatment)
- Prevention of platelet aggregation (antiplatelet agents)
- Prevention of thrombosis (anticoagulants)
- Removal of stenosis (surgery or angioplasty)
- Treatment of cardiac disease (e.g. surgery for mitral stenosis)

Atherothrombosis

Patients with symptoms of atherosclerosis at one site frequently have atherosclerosis at other sites (Drouet, 2002). In keeping with this, patients with symptoms of peripheral or ischaemic heart disease are at increased risk of stroke. Similarly, patients who have survived stroke are at increased risk of ischaemic heart disease and indeed are equally likely to die from a myocardial infarct as they are to die from another stroke. The overlap between these disorders is illustrated in Figure 15.1. Measures taken to reduce risk of progression of atherosclerosis or thrombosis (e.g. stopping smoking or antiplatelet therapy) can therefore be expected to reduce the risk of any vascular event. This

reasoning has led the antiplatelet trialists to use the combination of stroke, myocardial infarction and vascular death as the primary outcome measure when assessing the value of antiplatelet agents. Measures taken to reduce the incidence of heart disease (e.g. coronary artery bypass grafting) can also be expected to reduce the incidence of stroke because there will be a reduction in cardioembolic stroke.

Lifestyle modification

Stopping smoking, healthy diet, regular exercise, light or moderate alcohol consumption, and a reduction in weight for the obese can be recommended to the population as a whole, as well as those who have had a transient ischaemic attack (TIA) or stroke. There is good evidence that a healthy lifestyle reduces the incidence of myocardial infarction. There is circumstantial evidence to suggest that it also reduces the risk of stroke.

Hormone replacement therapy (HRT)

This was originally thought to protect against the development of atherosclerosis in postmenopausal women, because case–control studies showed that women who take HRT are less likely to develop ischaemic heart disease or stroke than postmenopausal women who do not. However, it was not clear to what extent the difference was the result of other factors (e.g. socioeconomic status). One case–control study in Denmark, where socioeconomic differences are less marked than in North America, showed no difference in the risk of stroke in users compared with non-users of HRT (Pedersen *et al.*, 1997). However, a randomized study of HRT with combined oestrogen and progestogen in patients with symptomatic ischaemic heart disease suggested that the risks of myocardial infarction were slightly increased in patients randomized to combined HRT. Overall, a meta-analysis of the four existing randomized trials of HRT concluded that HRT caused a small excess of breast cancer, stroke and pulmonary

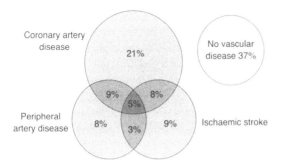

Figure 15.1 Overlapping syndromes of athero-thrombosis. The numbers are the proportion of 1866 patients in whom the various individual or combination of diseases were present. Adapted from *Am J Cardiol* 1994;**74**:64–65.

embolus amounting to 6 extra events per 1000 users aged 50–59 and 12 extra events in those aged 60–69 (Beral *et al.*, 2002). There was also a reduction in the incidence of colorectal cancer and fractured neck of the femur. However, the only randomized trial to include women with previous stroke or TIA showed no significant difference in the rate of any stroke or death over a 3-year follow-up period in patients randomized to oestrogen-only HRT (Viscoli *et al.*, 2001). Hence one can conclude that although there appears to be a small increase in the risk of vascular events, including stroke, with combined HRT, the use of oestrogen alone appears to be relatively safe in women with previous stroke or TIA. HRT should certainly not be prescribed as a treatment to prevent stroke.

Hypertension

The management of hypertension in acute stroke is discussed in Chapter 14. Here we concentrate on the treatment of hypertension when the patient has recovered from the acute stages. In TIA and minor stroke, anti-hypertensive treatment should be started as soon as the diagnosis of hypertension has been established. In more severe cases, definitive treatment may be delayed until two weeks after onset or earlier discharge if the patient has made a good recovery.

Epidemiological studies have established that hypertension is the major modifiable risk factor for stroke (Chapter 5). One of the main goals of treating hypertension is to reduce the incidence of stroke, and it has been estimated that if hypertension were abolished, the incidence of stroke would be reduced by between 50% and 80%. It is equally important to screen the healthy population, who may have no symptoms of hypertension until they have a stroke, and those with established cerebrovascular disease for hypertension. Hypertension should not be diagnosed on a single reading of blood pressure, and several readings should be performed after a period of rest on different occasions before the diagnosis of hypertension is confirmed. This is particularly important in acute stroke, when a high blood pressure may simply reflect an acute physiological response to cerebral infarction or haemorrhage. Where there is a question of 'white coat' hypertension (i.e. a physiologically mediated increase in blood pressure secondary to anxiety provoked by medical contact), 24-hour ambulatory blood pressure monitoring may be required to establish or refute the diagnosis.

Target blood pressure levels The lower the blood pressure, the better as regards stroke risk in epidemiological studies (Lawes *et al.*, 2004). The definition of levels of sustained blood pressure necessary to diagnose hypertension are therefore arbitrary (Table 15.1). Until recently, it was only recommended that patients should be treated with hypotensive drugs if their blood pressure remained above certain values, aiming to reduce the readings to target values. The 1999 British Hypertension Society Guidelines recommended always starting anti-hypertensive treatment for primary prevention if systolic blood pressure was sustained at or above 160 mmHg or if diastolic blood pressure was at or above 100 mmHg (Ramsay *et al.*, 1999). In patients at high risk because of diabetes, target organ damage (including stroke or TIA), cardiovascular disease or a 10-year coronary heart disease risk of 15% or more, it was recommended that treatment should be started at sustained blood

Table 15.1   Definition of hypertension

	Diastolic blood pressure (mmHg)
Normal blood pressure	<85
Borderline hypertension	85–89
Mild hypertension	90–104
Moderate hypertension	105–114
Severe hypertension	≥115
Systolic hypertension	Diastolic normal, systolic ≥150

At least three measurements of blood pressure should be made on separate occasions before accepting a patient as having hypertension

pressure readings above 140 mmHg systolic or 90 mmHg diastolic. Optimum treatment targets were given of below 140 mmHg for systolic blood pressure and below 85 mmHg for diastolic blood pressure. For patients with diabetes, the target was <140/<80 mmHg. It was accepted that these levels of blood pressure control may be difficult to achieve in some patients, and hence minimum levels of acceptable control were given as <150/<90 mmHg and <140/<90 mmHg for diabetic patients.

Lowering normal blood pressure after stroke
Previous trials had convincingly shown that lowering blood pressure in asymptomatic hypertensive individuals reduced the risk of stroke. Moreover, meta-analysis suggests that the degree of the risk reduction is proportional to the degree of blood pressure lowering achieved in the trials, with a reduction in risk of stroke of approximately one-third for every 10 mmHg reduction in systolic blood pressure (Lawes *et al.*, 2004). However, there had been uncertainty about the benefits and safety of blood pressure-lowering treatments in patients who had already had a stroke, particularly in patients with mildly elevated or normal blood pressure readings. PROGRESS (Perindopril Protection Against Recurrent Stroke Study) has convincingly changed this view (PROGRESS, 2001). This study randomized over 6000 patients with previous TIA or stroke between placebo and active treatment, which consisted of single therapy with an angiotensin-converting enzyme (ACE) inhibitor, perindopril (4 mg daily), or combination therapy with perindopril and a thiazide-type diuretic, indapamide. Indapamide was used because it is thought to produce less metabolic disturbance or exacerbation of diabetes. Hypertensive patients were required to have their hypertension treated without using ACE inhibitors prior to entry into the study. Only half of the participants were classified as hypertensive at the first visit (mean 159/94 mmHg) and the remainder had normal blood pressure on or off treatment. At the end of the 4-year follow-up, active treatment (single or combination therapy) had reduced the risk of stroke from 14% with placebo to 10% with treatment, a highly significant relative risk reduction of 28% (Figure 15.2). The risk of both ischaemic and haemorrhagic stroke was reduced by active treatment, with a greater relative risk reduction for cerebral haemorrhage of 50%, compared with 24% for ischaemic stroke. Active treatment also reduced the risk of non-fatal myocardial infarction by 38%. Importantly, there were similar relative risk reductions in hypertensive and non-hypertensive subgroups, although the absolute reductions were less in non-hypertensive patients, because of a lower background risk. Combination therapy with perindopril plus indapamide reduced blood pressure by a mean of 12/5 mmHg, which was about double the 5/3 mmHg effect of perindopril single-drug therapy. In the group of patients treated with combination therapy, treatment reduced the risk of stroke by a striking 43% (Figure 15.3). In contrast, treatment with perindopril alone produced only a non-significant 5% reduction in the risk of stroke, although the confidence interval was wide and consistent with the moderate effects that would be predicted for the blood pressure reduction achieved. The results suggest that 5 years' treatment with the combination of perindopril and indapamide resulted in the avoidance of one fatal or major non-fatal vascular event among every 11 treated patients.

The use of another ACE inhibitor, ramipril (10 mg daily), was also shown to benefit patients

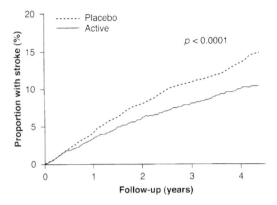

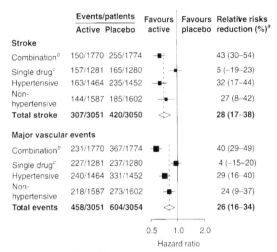

Figure 15.2   Rate of stroke during follow-up in PROGRESS. Active treatment was either perindopril or perindopril plus indapamide. From PROGRESS Collaborative Group. *Lancet* 2001;**358**:1033–1041.

Figure 15.3   Effects of treatment on stroke and major vascular events in various subgroups of patients in PROGRESS. From PROGRESS Collaborative Group. *Lancet* 2001;**358**:1033–1041.

with vascular disease irrespective of initial blood pressure in the HOPE (Heart Outcomes Prevention Evaluation) Study (Yusuf *et al.*, 2000). This trial randomized over 9000 patients at high risk of recurrent vascular events because of previous coronary artery disease, previous stroke or TIA, or diabetes plus an additional risk factor. Only half of the patients had a history of hypertension. The risk of myocardial infarction, stroke or vascular death was significantly reduced from 18% with placebo to 14% in the ramipril group. Strikingly, the relative risk of any stroke was reduced by 32% in the ramipril group compared with the placebo group, despite only a modest average reduction in blood pressure of 3.8/2.8 mmHg (Figure 15.4). However, the benefit in terms of a reduction of stroke rate was less in the 1000 or so patients randomized with a history of stroke or TIA and did not reach statistical significance, possibly because of smaller numbers of patients (Bosch *et al.*, 2002). The relative benefits of ramipril were similar at different baseline blood pressure levels, including patients randomized with a normal systolic blood pressure of <130 mmHg (Figure 15.5).

Taken together, the results of PROGRESS and HOPE suggest that all patients with stroke and TIA with significant other risk factors for recurrence should be considered for treatment with a

combination of an ACE inhibitor and a thiazide-type diuretic, irrespective of blood pressure readings. The cost–benefit ratio will depend on the risk of recurrence and hence this approach is not currently recommended for patients at low risk of recurrence (e.g. young idiopathic stroke patients with no vascular risk factors).

In general, most experts have concluded that the benefits of anti-hypertensive agents on stroke risk are caused only by lowering blood pressure and are not related to the class of drug. However, this does not necessarily mean that all classes of drugs will have the same effect. For example, the Antihypertensive and Lipid-Lowering Treatment to Prevent Heart Attack (ALLHAT) Trial showed that chlorthalidone (a thiazide diuretic) was superior to lisinopril (an ACE inhibitor) as initial therapy in preventing stroke in hypertensive subjects – probably because 5-year systolic blood pressures were lower in the patients allocated chlorthalidone (ALLHAT, 2002). However, the LIFE (Losartan Intervention For Endpoint Reduction) Study found that losartan (a selective angiotensin-II receptor antagonist) was

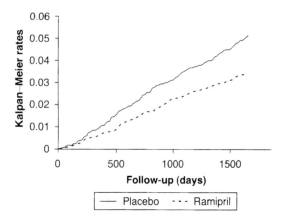

Figure 15.4   Rate of stroke during follow up in the HOPE trial. From Bosch J *et al.* *BMJ* 2002;**324**:1–5.

Diastolic blood pressure (mm Hg)	No. of patients	Relative risk with 95% CI	Placebo event rate (%)
≤79	4170		4.6
80–89	3370		4.8
≥90	1753		5.8
Systolic blood pressure (mm Hg)			
≤129	2872		4.0
130–139	2712		4.8
≥140	3710		5.6

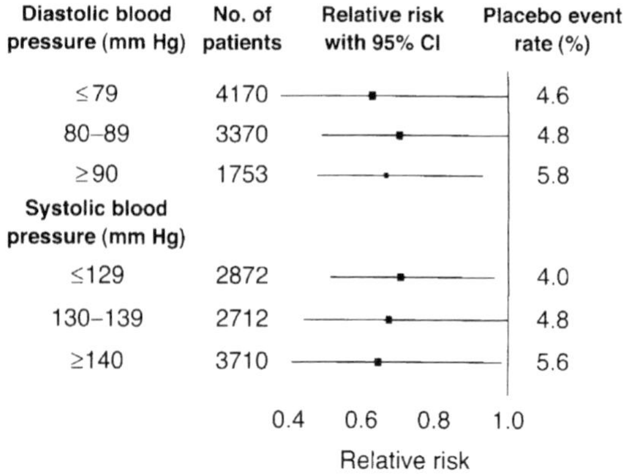

Figure 15.5   Effect of ramipril on the rate of stroke at different baseline blood pressure readings in the HOPE trial. From Bosch J *et al.* *BMJ* 2002;**324**:1–5.

significantly superior to atenolol (a β-blocker) in preventing stroke in hypertensive patients (annual rate 1.1% versus 1.5%, hazard ratio 0.75), suggesting that there are class effects independent of blood pressure effects (Dahlöf *et al.*, 2002).

The target of treatment in hypertensive individuals should be to lower the average blood pressure as low as possible and certainly to ensure a systolic blood pressure below 140 mmHg and a diastolic blood pressure below 85 mmHg, while avoiding intolerable side-effects. It might be expected that treatment of hypertension would abolish the risk of stroke or reduce it substantially. However, clinical trials of anti-hypertensive therapy compared with placebo show only an average reduction in relative risk of about 40%. Analysis of the trials also shows that, on average, the drug therapies studied in the trials only achieved 6–7 mmHg reductions in diastolic blood pressure and 10–12 mmHg reductions in systolic blood pressure compared with placebo. However, the effect is related to age, so that a 10 mmHg lower systolic blood pressure is associated with approximately 40–50%, 30–40% and 20–30% lower risk of stroke in those aged less than 60 years, 60–69 years and 70 or more respectively (Lawes *et al.*, 2004). The reduction in blood pressure and the percentage reduction in relative risk are similar in the trials recruiting patients with moderate compared with mild

hypertension, although the absolute reduction in risk in patients with moderate hypertension is higher, because the background risk is higher. The reduction in risk is similar to that predicted from epidemiological studies. The fact that better reduction in risk was not achieved in the clinical trials by treatment of blood pressure reflects a number of pharmacological factors: drug-resistant hypertension, inadequate blood pressure control over the whole of the time period between drug doses (e.g. overnight), and poor compliance. In addition, existing athero-sclerosis and small vessel disease caused by hypertension prior to starting treatment are not reversed by treatment. Outside clinical trials, the reduction in risk achieved by anti-hypertensive treatment may be less than 40%, unless accurate adherence to protocols, frequent monitoring and good compliance with therapy can be ensured. One case–control study of stroke in the northern region of England showed that the risk of stroke in known hypertensive patients was related to the average levels of blood pressure achieved by treatment in the months prior to the stroke (Du *et al.*, 1997). On the other hand, if substantial reductions in diastolic blood pressure of more than 7 mmHg can be achieved in individual patients, there will be a corresponding greater reduction in risk than achieved in the randomized trials, which usually only studied the effect of a single drug. This may require combined therapy with three or even four different hypotensive agents. Every effort should therefore be made to treat hypertensive patients as vigorously as possible.

Isolated *systolic hypertension* (i.e. systolic blood pressure greater than 150mmHg with a diastolic of less than 90mmHg) is associated with an increased risk of stroke, particularly in those aged over 60, and should therefore be treated as vigorously as other types of hypertension.

There is good evidence that the *elderly hypertensive* patients benefit from anti-hypertensive therapy and indeed have more to gain because their overall risk of stroke associated with hypertension is much greater than younger patients. Anti-hypertensive therapy should therefore not be withheld simply on the grounds of age alone. There is a common fallacy that 'normal' blood pressure rises with age and therefore there is no need to treat elderly patients until their blood pressure reaches higher levels than those indicating treatment in younger subjects. In fact the risk associated with hypertension is greater in elderly patients, and in older patients treatment should be considered at readings of 150/90 mmHg.

Malignant hypertension (also known as *accelerated hypertension*) or very severe hypertension (diastolic blood pressure greater than 140 mmHg) is an emergency and requires urgent treatment in hospital to prevent stroke from hypertensive encephalopathy. However, very rapid reduction in blood pressure by parenteral therapy should be avoided, as there is a significant risk of the sudden reduction in cerebral blood flow leading to cerebral infarction, blindness, renal failure or myocardial ischaemia. Over the first 24 hours, the diastolic blood pressure should be reduced to no less than 110 mmHg and further be reductions achieved slowly over the next few days.

Diabetes mellitus

Both type 1 and type 2 diabetes are well-recognized risk factors for stroke, mainly because of an increased incidence of hypertension and atherosclerosis. Patients with diabetes should therefore be encouraged to adopt healthy lifestyle modifications, considered for statin therapy and encouraged to control blood sugar levels as carefully as possible, particularly if they already have symptoms of cardiovascular disease or stroke. There is good evidence that vigorous control of hypertension in patients with diabetes reduces the risk of stroke (UKPDS, 1998a). For example, in patients with diabetes mellitus randomized in the Hypertension Optimal Treatment trial (HOT), there was a 51% reduction in major cardiovascular events in patients allocated to a target blood pressure of less than 80 mmHg, compared with a target of less than 90 mmHg (Hansson *et al.*, 1998). Significant reduction in cholesterol levels with atorvastatin treatment has also been shown to have a significant benefit in patients with type 2 diabetes in the primary prevention of cardiovascular events, including stroke (Colhoun *et al.*, 2004). There is less evidence that tight control of blood sugar levels reduces the risk of stroke, but it should still be recommended to reduce the risk of microvascular complications (UKPDS, 1998b).

Cholesterol lowering

Clinical trials have convincingly shown that a reduction in cholesterol reduces the risk of stroke, even though cholesterol does not appear to be an independent risk factor for stroke in epidemiological studies (Corvol *et al.*, 2003). The earlier trials of treatment for hypercholesterolaemia showed little effect on stroke incidence, but the more recent trials using 3-hydroxy-3-methylglutaryl coenzyme A (HMG-CoA) reductase inhibitors (statins) have shown a significant reduction in the incidence of stroke. The effect was initially shown in trials of patients with ischaemic heart disease, but was also shown in trials of statin therapy in the healthy population with high cholesterol levels. More recently, the Heart Protection Study (HPS) has shown that statin therapy also benefits patients with vascular disease who have a normal serum cholesterol level (HPS, 2004). HPS randomly allocated over 20 000 patients aged 40–80 years with non-fasting cholesterol levels above 3.5 mmol/l (135 mg/100 ml) and a history of coronary heart

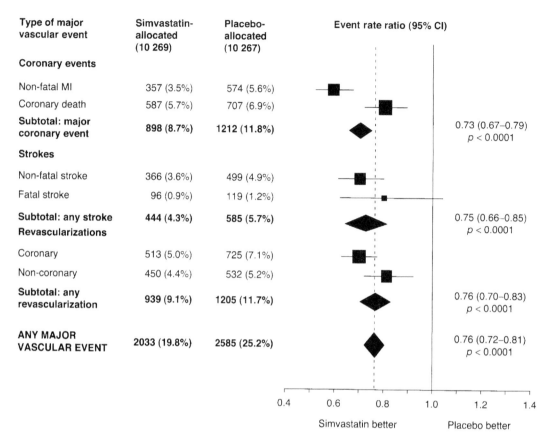

Figure 15.6   Effect of simvastatin on the number of various first vascular events in the Heart Protection Study. From MRC/BHF Heart Protection Study. *Lancet* 2002;**360**:7–22.

disease, other occlusive arterial disease or diabetes to either simvastatin (40 mg daily) or placebo. In the trial as a whole, over an average follow-up of 5 years, there were highly significant relative risk reductions in all-cause mortality of 13%, in major coronary events of 27% and in the risk of any stroke of 25% (Figure 15.6). The reduction in stroke was entirely due to a reduction in ischaemic stroke (2.8% vs 4.0%), with no apparent reduction in haemorrhagic stroke. In the subgroup of 1820 patients randomized in HPS with cerebrovascular disease and no prior history of coronary heart disease, the reduction in the rate of major vascular events (18.7% vs 23.6%) was similar to that of patients randomized with other vascular diseases (Figure 15.7). However, in this subgroup, the risk of stroke did not appear to be reduced, but this may well reflect a false-negative finding related to the relatively small number of patients

with prior cerebrovascular disease. The relative risk reduction was also similar at different levels of cholesterol and at all ages studied. These impressive benefits were achieved despite the fact that over the course of the trial, increasing numbers of patients randomized to placebo were prescribed a statin, so that the intention-to-treat figures underestimate the benefits of taking a statin by about one-third. One can calculate that 5 years' treatment will prevent about 70 patients per 1000 with stroke or TIA from suffering a recurrent major vascular event. The benefit of statins only appears after about 1 year of therapy. Other trials of statin therapy randomizing only patients with cerebrovascular disease, including SPARCL, are in progress. One can conclude that statin therapy should be considered in all patients between the ages of 40 and 80 years who present with TIA or stroke and have a cholesterol level above 3.5 mmol/l

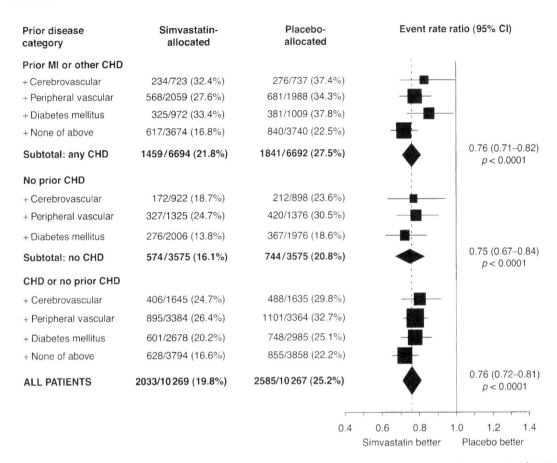

Prior disease category	Simvastatin-allocated	Placebo-allocated	Event rate ratio (95% CI)
Prior MI or other CHD			
+ Cerebrovascular	234/723 (32.4%)	276/737 (37.4%)	
+ Peripheral vascular	568/2059 (27.6%)	681/1988 (34.3%)	
+ Diabetes mellitus	325/972 (33.4%)	381/1009 (37.8%)	
+ None of above	617/3674 (16.8%)	840/3740 (22.5%)	
Subtotal: any CHD	**1459/6694 (21.8%)**	**1841/6692 (27.5%)**	0.76 (0.71–0.82) $p < 0.0001$
No prior CHD			
+ Cerebrovascular	172/922 (18.7%)	212/898 (23.6%)	
+ Peripheral vascular	327/1325 (24.7%)	420/1376 (30.5%)	
+ Diabetes mellitus	276/2006 (13.8%)	367/1976 (18.6%)	
Subtotal: no CHD	**574/3575 (16.1%)**	**744/3575 (20.8%)**	0.75 (0.67–0.84) $p < 0.0001$
CHD or no prior CHD			
+ Cerebrovascular	406/1645 (24.7%)	488/1635 (29.8%)	
+ Peripheral vascular	895/3384 (26.4%)	1101/3364 (32.7%)	
+ Diabetes mellitus	601/2678 (20.2%)	748/2985 (25.1%)	
+ None of above	628/3794 (16.6%)	855/3858 (22.2%)	
ALL PATIENTS	**2033/10 269 (19.8%)**	**2585/10 267 (25.2%)**	0.76 (0.72–0.81) $p < 0.0001$

0.4 0.6 0.8 1.0 1.2 1.4
Simvastatin better   Placebo better

Figure 15.7 Effect of simvastatin in various subgroups of prior disease categories in the Heart Protection Study: MI, myocardial infarction; CHD, coronary heart disease. From MRC/BHF Heart Protection Study. *Lancet* 2002;**360**:7–22.

(135 mg/100 ml). The benefits will be proportional to the risk of recurrence, and hence the cost–benefit ratio may argue against statin therapy in patients in low risk of recurrence. In particular, statin therapy is probably not indicated for younger patients without evidence of atherosclerosis.

ANTICOAGULATION (TABLE 15.2)

Atrial fibrillation

Atrial fibrillation accounts for about 12% of ischaemic stroke. There is good evidence that treatment of atrial fibrillation with anticoagulants prevents stroke (Hart *et al.*, 2003). Patients with recent atrial fibrillation should be cardioverted to sinus rhythm. Anticoagulation

should be considered before, and for at least 2 weeks after, cardioversion. However, cardioversion is not necessarily appropriate, particularly in long-standing cases, and is often not successful. In patients with established chronic atrial fibrillation or recurrent paroxysmal atrial fibrillation, long-term anticoagulation should therefore be considered to prevent embolic events, which are mainly stroke. It has been recognized for many years that anticoagulation was definitely indicated in patients with atrial fibrillation associated with rheumatic valvular heart disease, particularly mitral stenosis. Five separate primary prevention trials have also shown a significant benefit for anticoagulation with warfarin in the prevention of stroke in patients with non-valvular atrial fibrillation (Table 15.3) (Segal *et al.*, 2001). Patients with

Table 15.2 Indications for considering anti-coagulation in secondary stroke prevention

- Cardiac embolism:
  - Atrial fibrillation
  - Mechanical valve prosthesis
  - Recent myocardial infarction
  - Left ventricular aneurysm
  - Dilated cardiomyopathy
  - Paradoxical embolism
- Acute major vessel occlusion:
  - Internal carotid artery occlusion
  - Basilar artery occlusion
- Acute arterial dissection:
  - Internal carotid artery dissection
  - Extracranial vertebral artery dissection
- Prothrombotic states
- Severe carotid stenosis prior to surgery or stenting
- Crescendo TIA
- Recurrent TIA or stroke despite optimal antiplatelet therapy
- Cerebral venous thrombosis

Table 15.3 Stroke rate in atrial fibrillation trials (% per annum)

Trial	Control	Warfarin
AFASAK	4.6	1.9
SPAF	7.0	2.3
BAATAF	3.0	0.4
CAFA	4.3	3.0
SPINAF	4.3	0.9
Average	4.4	1.4

Overall risk reduction 68% ($p < 0.001$)

untreated atrial fibrillation who have not had a recent stroke or TIA have an average risk of embolic events (mainly stroke) of about 4.4% per annum. This is significantly reduced to about 1.4% by anticoagulation with warfarin. The benefit is greatest in patients with other risk factors, particularly hypertension, heart failure or diabetes, and less in younger patients. In patients who have had a recent TIA or stroke, the benefits of anticoagulation with warfarin are even greater than in patients with no history of embolic symptoms (Saxena and Koudstaal, 2004). For example, the European Atrial Fibrillation Trial showed that the recurrent stroke rate in control patients with recent TIA or stroke associated with atrial fibrillation who received neither warfarin nor aspirin was 12% per annum. This was dramatically reduced by warfarin to 4% per annum: a two-thirds reduction in risk.

The atrial fibrillation trials showed that aspirin was much less effective than warfarin, producing an average risk reduction of around 16%, similar to the benefit of aspirin for other vascular indications. The overall benefit of warfarin or aspirin seen in the atrial fibrillation trials takes into account haemorrhagic strokes caused by the treatment. However, extracranial haemorrhages (see below) are more likely on warfarin than on aspirin therapy. Aspirin is therefore the treatment of choice in patients with contraindications to anticoagulation (see below).

Patients with *lone atrial fibrillation* (i.e. atrial fibrillation without evidence of heart disease or other risk factors) have a very low risk of stroke, particularly below the age of 65, and the benefits of anticoagulation do not outweigh the risks. Lone atrial fibrillation should therefore be treated with aspirin rather than warfarin in most cases. All other patients with atrial fibrillation should be considered for anticoagulation with warfarin to prevent stroke, unless there are definite contraindications (see below), in which case aspirin provides a less effective alternative. There is no information about the benefits of other antiplatelet agents in atrial fibrillation, but it is reasonable to assume that the effects will be similar to those seen in other indications. Recent randomized trials suggest that a fixed dose of the oral direct thrombin inhibitor ximelagatran is at least as effective as warfarin in preventing recurrent stroke in patients with atrial fibrillation without the need to monitor the International Normalized Ratio (INR) (Olsson et al., 2003). Although major bleeding rates were similar to those with warfarin, ximelagatran was associated with an increased incidence of abnormal liver function tests. Further safety data are therefore required before the direct thrombin inhibitors can enter routine clinical practice.

Cardiac embolism

Patients who have had heart valves replaced with mechanical prostheses are routinely anticoagulated with warfarin, sometimes with the addition of aspirin or dipyridamole, to prevent cardiac embolism and stroke. Other cardiac conditions, including myocardial infarction, left-ventricular aneurysm and dilated cardiomyopathy associated with an increased risk of embolism should be anticoagulated if the patient has had a TIA or stroke, assuming that no contraindications are present. In patients with less certain cardiac sources of embolism (e.g. a patent foramen ovale or a small atrial septal aneurysm), follow-up studies show a low risk of recurrent symptoms in patients who have had a stroke treated with aspirin or TIA, and the benefits of anticoagulation are therefore much less certain (Chapter 11). The majority of these patients should therefore be treated with antiplatelet agents in the first instance and anticoagulation should only be considered for those with recurrent embolic events. Trials are in progress to determine whether patients with cardiac failure benefit from anticoagulation.

Major vessel occlusion

Anticoagulation should probably be considered in acute basilar artery thrombosis because of the high risk of propagation of the thrombosis with resulting occlusion of the brainstem perforating vessels and posterior cerebral arteries. Acute carotid occlusion also has a significant risk of recurrent stroke, and it is therefore reasonable to anticoagulate patients who have survived the acute event without major cerebral infarction with warfarin for a period of 6 months or so. These recommendations are not based on the results of clinical trials and it is possible that the risks of anticoagulation (see below) would outweigh any benefits in the prevention of recurrent events.

Dissection

The main hazard of extracranial carotid and vertebral artery dissection is stroke secondary to vessel occlusion and/or thromboembolism (Chapter 10). The majority of strokes occur in the first few days and weeks after the onset of dissection. Clinical experience suggests that anticoagulation is beneficial and is therefore recommended by most authorities to prevent recurrent stroke after dissection. Although dissection is often associated with a haematoma in the wall of the artery, this does not appear to be exacerbated by anticoagulation, and the risk of stroke appears to be primarily embolic from thrombus forming in the arterial lumen at the site of the dissection. In patients with minor degrees of dissection, aspirin therapy may be sufficient. Anticoagulation should be continued for 3–6 months after dissection. If follow-up imaging then shows recanalization, no further therapy is required. In patients with persistent stenosis or occlusion, antiplatelet therapy should be continued indefinitely after anticoagulation has been stopped. Long-term anticoagulation is indicated only for the small percentage of patients who have recurrent dissection. Surgery is hazardous for dissection, because the dissection often extends a considerable distance up the artery. In addition, most stenotic lesions secondary to dissection recanalize spontaneously. Stenting (see below) is a new alternative, which has been successfully used in a small number of patients with recurrent symptoms to correct stenosis and to seal a free intimal flap against the carotid wall.

Intracranial arterial dissection, particularly distal vertebral artery dissection, is associated with subarachnoid haemorrhage, presumably because the adventitia surrounding the intracranial arteries is relatively thin. Anticoagulation is therefore contraindicated in patients with dissection of the intracranial segments of the major vessels.

Pseudoaneurysm formation secondary to dissection rarely requires any specific treatment, because the incidence of embolism or bleeding from the aneurysm is unusual, except in the intracranial segments. In the latter cases, a surgical approach or interventional radiology techniques may be needed to obliterate the aneurysm.

Table 15.4 Complications of anticoagulant treatment

- Haemorrhage:
  - Cutaneous
  - Mucous membranes
  - Gastrointestinal
  - Intracerebral haemorrhage
  - Subarachnoid haemorrhage
  - Subdural haematoma
  - Prolonged bleeding time
- Hypersensitivity reactions
- Skin necrosis

Specific to heparins
- Thrombocytopenia
- Hyperkalaemia
- Osteoporosis

Specific to warfarin
- Alopecia
- Diarrhoea
- Nausea and vomiting
- Hepatic dysfunction
- Pancreatitis

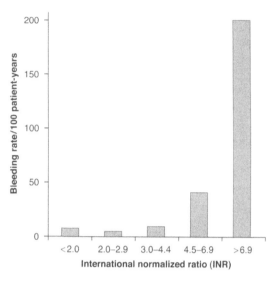

Figure 15.8 Correlation between most recent International Normalized Ratio (INR) and rate of haemorrhage complications at any site associated with anticoagulant therapy; 153 bleeds in 2011 patient-years of follow-up. From Palareti G *et al. Lancet* 1996;**348**: 423–428.

Complications of anticoagulant therapy (Table 15.4)

The main disadvantage of anticoagulant therapy is the risk of haemorrhage, which is the principal complication of anticoagulation. The bleeding can occur at any site. Spontaneous bruising and minor haematuria, epistaxis and haematuria are common. Major life-threatening haemorrhage usually occurs from the gut or intracranially. Subdural haematoma, which can occur spontaneously or after minor trauma, is the commonest neurological complication, particularly in the elderly. Any patient on anticoagulants with persistent headache, confusion or focal neurological symptoms should have a computed tomography (CT) or magnetic resonance imaging (MRI) scan to exclude subdural haemorrhage.

In the atrial fibrillation trials, the risk of major haemorrhage requiring hospital admission or transfusion was 1.6% per annum in patients on warfarin, compared with 1% on placebo. Intracranial haemorrhage was very

unusual and there were no intracerebral haemorrhages in the European Atrial Fibrillation Trial. Patients in clinical trials are likely to be highly selected because of the need for frequent follow-up and are often younger and fitter than those seen on average in clinical practice. There is therefore a danger that the haemorrhage rate will be higher in patients anticoagulated outside the context of clinical trails. An investigation in Italy examined the risks of bleeding in a prospective study of patients attending hospital anticoagulant clinics. The study included a wide range of ages and indications for anticoagulation. The rates of haemorrhage are shown in Figure 15.8. The rate of symptomatic haemorrhage associated with anticoagulation does not appear to be significantly increased in relationship to the level of anticoagulation as represented by the INR at the time of bleeding, until the level reaches a ratio of 4.5 × control or more. This may reflect the fact that anticoagulation does not cause bleeding per se, but acts to prevent stopping bleeding that has occurred for some other reason and might otherwise have

Table 15.5 Risk factors for anticoagulant-related intracranial haemorrhage

- Arterial vascular disease
- Atherosclerotic TIA and stroke
- INR > 4.5
- Age > 70 years
- First 90 days after starting oral anticoagulation
- Moderate or severe leukoaraiosis on CT

Table 15.6 Contraindications to anticoagulant therapy

- Haemophilia and other bleeding disorders
- Thrombocytopenia
- Peptic ulcer
- Cerebral haemorrhage
- Severe uncontrolled hypertension
- Severe liver disease
- Oesophageal varices
- Recent trauma
- Recent lumbar puncture
- Recent major surgery (especially ophthalmic and neurosurgery)
- Hypersensitivity
- Pregnancy[a]

[a]Avoid warfarin in the first trimester if possible and use heparins with caution in pregnancy.

been very minor or asymptomatic. In keeping with this, the risk of haemorrhage on anticoagulants is associated with a number of other risk factors (Table 15.5). Interestingly, there appears to be no correlation between the INR and the occurrence of intracerebral haemorrhage. The risk of intracranial haemorrhage is clearly increased in patients on warfarin by several-fold, but cerebral haemorrhage in patients on warfarin therapy is not always the result of the treatment and may be secondary to other factors (e.g. hypertension). However, it is possible that bleeds are larger in patients on warfarin, even if the cause is not directly related to the therapy. For example, in a middle-aged hypertensive patient on warfarin, the probability of a cerebral haemorrhage being related to warfarin is of the same order as the risks of a spontaneous hypertensive intracranial haemorrhage. One study suggested that intracranial haemorrhage resulting from warfarin therapy was distinguished from spontaneous haemorrhage by a more gradual onset of focal signs over several hours or days, as opposed to the sudden onset more common with cerebral haemorrhage. However, this study included several patients with cerebellar haemorrhage, which is known to have a gradual onset in some cases even in the absence of anticoagulation. It is therefore doubtful whether a gradual onset is specific for warfarin-related haemorrhage.

Contraindications to anticoagulant therapy are listed in Table 15.6. A history of previous haemorrhage is not necessarily a contraindication to warfarin if the risk of recurrence has been substantially reduced or abolished; for example, a previous aneurysmal subarachnoid haemorrhage is not a contraindication to anticoagulation if the aneurysm has been clipped. Similarly, a history of peptic ulceration is not a definite contraindication if the ulcer has been shown to have been healed by treatment. It may be appropriate in patients with a history of dyspepsia to cover a period of anticoagulant treatment with a proton pump inhibitor or an H_2 receptor antagonist. This has not been shown to reduce the incidence of bleeding. Appropriate therapeutics requires the risks and benefits of treatment to be assessed and balanced. In some cases, anticoagulation may still be appropriate despite contraindications – the risks of not anticoagulating may be greater than the risks of anticoagulation. For example, anticoagulation is mandatory in patients with mechanical prosthetic heart valves. In these patients, anticoagulation may need to be restarted even if the patient has had a cerebral haemorrhage once they have recovered from the haemorrhage. Similarly, the patient who has a postoperative pulmonary embolism may still need to be anticoagulated even in the presence of contraindications.

Increasing age is one of the main risk factors for serious haemorrhage on warfarin. However, the risk of stroke also rises with age and there may therefore be more to gain from anticoagulation in the elderly. The age at which anticoagulation becomes contraindicated is uncertain. Clinical trials have failed to resolve the issue. The risks arise steeply above the age of 75, and anticoagulation should only be contemplated above this age if the patient is generally fit and biologically younger than their stated years. In all patients, but particularly the elderly, the need for continued warfarin therapy should be reviewed regularly. Warfarin may need to be stopped if the patient seems likely to fall, becomes confused or cannot attend for regular blood tests.

Target INR

Warfarin therapy requires careful monitoring because of the risk of haemorrhage with overdose and the marked variation between individuals, and within individuals over time, in the dose required to achieve adequate anticoagulation. The level of anticoagulation is assessed using the INR, so that similar results can be expected from different laboratories on different occasions. A target INR should be specified. Analysis of the atrial fibrillation trials suggest that an INR of 2.0 or less is insufficient to prevent thromboembolism. In keeping with this, SPAF-4 trial showed that fixed low-dose warfarin, aiming for an INR of 1.5, was also ineffective in atrial fibrillation. There is little correlation between the INR and the risk of haemorrhage below an INR of 4.0, while the risk rises steeply with an INR of 6.0 or above. The usual target INR for treatment of atrial fibrillation is 2.5 (range 2.0–3.0), while for patients with mechanical prosthetic heart valves, a higher target of 3.5 (range 3.0–4.0) is usually chosen. A target INR of 2.5 is appropriate for most other indications.

ANTICOAGULATION FOR ATHEROTHROMBOTIC STROKE

The dangers of warfarin therapy in the elderly were emphasized by the results of the Stroke Prevention In Reversible Ischaemia Trial (SPIRIT, 1997). This trial randomized patients with recent TIA or stroke, who did not

have atrial fibrillation or cardiac embolism, between aspirin and warfarin therapy. The trial was stopped prematurely because of an excess of cerebral haemorrhage in the warfarin group. Most of the haemorrhages occurred in patients over the age of 75. The target range for warfarin therapy in SPIRIT was an INR of 3–4, which may also have increased the risk. The other important risk factor for cerebral haemorrhage on warfarin appeared to be the finding of moderate or severe leukoaraiosis on CT. Leukoaraiosis has also been shown to be a risk factor for spontaneous cerebral haemorrhage, and there are arguments for scanning all elderly or hypertensive patients before starting warfarin. Anticoagulation should then be avoided in patients with moderate or severe leukoaraiosis, unless there is a very strong indication for treatment.

The WARSS trial also examined the benefit of warfarin in non-cardiogenic atherothrombotic stroke (Mohr et al., 2001). This trial had a relatively low target INR of 2 (range 1.5–2.5) and was carefully controlled with double-blinded treatment allocation between aspirin and warfarin. At this level of anticoagulation, warfarin was remarkably safe, but there was no difference in the recurrent stroke rate in patients treated with warfarin compared with aspirin.

One can therefore conclude that, at present, the trial evidence does not support the use of warfarin in preference to aspirin in patients with TIA or stroke, except in patients with atrial fibrillation. Further trials are in progress, including ESPRIT, which is examining the benefit of aspirin plus dipyridamole versus warfarin in patients with atherothrombotic stroke or TIA using a target INR of 2.5 (range 2–3).

ANTIPLATELET AGENTS

Antiplatelet agents are the mainstay of the pharmacological prevention of ischaemic vascular events. These appear to prevent thrombosis within all the major arterial sites and it is therefore usual to analyse the benefit of treatment in terms of the percentage of relative reduction in

Table 15.7 Antiplatelet agents commonly used in stroke prevention

Antiplatelet agent	Recommended dose
Aspirin	75 mg once daily
Dipyridamole MR[a]	200 mg twice daily
Ticlopidine	250 mg twice daily
Clopidogrel	75 mg once daily

[a]Modified-release preparation.

the risk of combined outcome cluster of stroke, myocardial infarction or vascular death. The relative benefit of antiplatelet agents in reducing the risk of any of these events is similar in recently symptomatic patients, whether they have had a TIA, stroke, myocardial infarction or peripheral arterial disease. This supports the concept that the mechanism of thrombosis at different sites is linked by the common pathogenesis of platelet aggregation superimposed on atheromatous plaque (Chapter 7). Several antiplatelet agents have been shown to be effective in the prevention of vascular events in patients with TIA and stroke (Table 15.7). They have different mechanisms of action, which may be relevant when combining different agents (Figure 15.9).

Aspirin

This was first proposed as an antiplatelet agent over 40 years ago. Since then, a large number of trials of aspirin treatment for various vascular conditions have been published, including a total of 135 000 patients in whom antiplatelet therapy has been compared with placebo. The results have been pooled together by the Antiplatelet Trialists' collaboration, subsequently renamed the Anti-Thrombotic Trialists' (ATT) Collaboration (ATT, 2002). Over all indications, antiplatelet therapy (combining the effects of any antiplatelet treatment) was found to reduce the odds of the combined outcome of myocardial infarction, stroke or vascular death by 25%. When only the trials including patients

with prior TIA or stroke were analysed, antiplatelet therapy reduced the odds of recurrent vascular events by 22%, with an absolute benefit of preventing 25 non-fatal strokes per 1000 patients treated for 3 years. The majority of the patients included in this meta-analysis were taking aspirin, rather than other antiplatelet agents, but the ATT has not separately examined the effects of aspirin on stroke prevention alone. Other meta-analyses have suggested that when examining the effect of aspirin on stroke risk alone in patients treated for prior stroke or TIA, aspirin reduces the relative risk of suffering a stroke or other major vascular event by only about 13% (Algra and van Gijn, 1996). This effect appears to be highly consistent over several trials (Figure 15.10).

Aspirin is clearly effective and has the great advantage of being cheap and readily available in all parts of the world. However, it is not a panacea and only prevents less than one in six vascular events, and many recurrent events are not prevented. There is therefore considerable need for better antiplatelet agents. Aspirin also has the disadvantage of frequent side-effects, particularly in high dosage (Table 15.8). The most serious side-effects are gastrointestinal haemorrhage and intracranial haemorrhage, which have incidences of approximately 27 and 5 per 1000 patients per year, respectively. The commonest side-effect is gastric irritation with discomfort and dyspepsia. Real or perceived side-effects result in the discontinuation of aspirin treatment in as many as 25% of patients.

The optimum dose of aspirin has not been established for the prevention of stroke, but there is no evidence for a significant difference in effectiveness at different doses above 30 mg/day (Figure 15.10). The largest amount of data in patients with cerebrovascular disease comes from trials using 300 mg daily (Algra and van Gijn, 1996). Only one trial, the Swedish Low Dose Aspirin Trial (SALT), compared 75 mg of aspirin daily with placebo and showed a significant benefit, with a relative risk for a reduction of vascular events of 18%. The Dutch TIA trial compared 30 mg with 283 mg and found no significant difference in

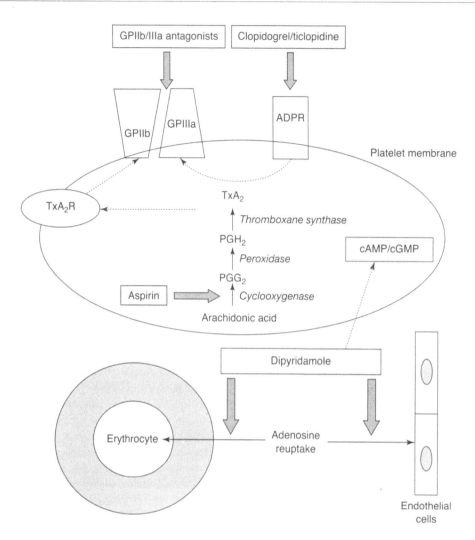

Figure 15.9　Sites of action of different antiplatelet agents. ADPR, adenosine diphosphate receptor; cAMP, cyclic adenosine monophosphate; cGMP, cyclic guanosine monophosphate; GPIIb/IIIa, glycoprotein IIb/IIIa; PGG_2, prostaglandin G_2; PGH_2, prostaglandin H_2; TxA_2, thromboxane A_2; TxA_2R, TxA_2 receptor.

effectiveness, but minor side-effects were less common at the lower dose. The European Stroke Prevention Study 2 confirmed that 50 mg of aspirin daily was significantly better than placebo at preventing stroke, with a relative risk reduction of 18% (Diener *et al.*, 1996). A dose of 300 mg probably works within 48 hours, whereas lower doses take longer to inhibit platelet function. It therefore seems prudent to start patients on a dose of 300 or 325 mg of aspirin once daily and either continue this dose or lower the dose after a few days. If aspirin in used in combination with another antiplatelet agent or an anticoagulant, it may be prudent to always use a lower dose of 75 mg daily or less.

The benefits of aspirin in primary prevention of vascular events is much less certain. Much of the benefit in healthy individuals in reducing the rate of ischaemic stroke is balanced by an increase in the rate of cerebral haemorrhage. Overall there may be a small benefit in reducing stroke in older women and myocardial infarction in men (Ridker *et al.*, 2005).

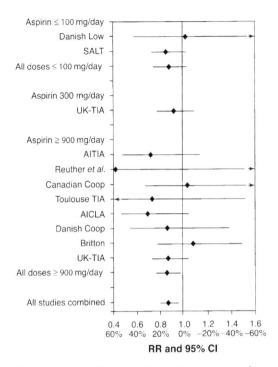

Figure 15.10 Benefit of aspirin after stroke or TIA (relative risk reduction (RR) in stroke, myocardial infarction or vascular death) in different trials of secondary stroke prevention after stroke or TIA. The combined reduction in risk was 13%. From Algra A, van Gijn J. *J Neurol Neurosurg Psychiatry* 1996;**60**:197–199.

Table 15.8 Side-effects of aspirin

- Gastrointestinal irritation
- Hypersensitivity reactions
  - Bronchospasm
  - Skin rash
  - Angioeodema
- Haemorrhage
  - Cutaneous
  - Gastrointestinal
  - Intracranial

Ticlopidine

The fact that aspirin prevents only a limited proportion of recurrent vascular events and the problem of withdrawal from aspirin therapy because of gastrointestinal side-effects mean that there is considerable scope for more effective and better-tolerated antiplatelet agents. The first single agent to be shown to be superior to aspirin in the prevention of stroke was ticlopidine. This inhibits platelet aggregation, lowers fibrinogen and prolongs the bleeding time. Two studies have demonstrated its effectiveness in the secondary prevention of stroke. The Canadian–American Ticlopidine Study (CATS) demonstrated a 23% reduction in vascular events (stroke, myocardial infarction or vascular death) in patients with a history of recent stroke compared with placebo

(Gent *et al.*, 1989). The second study, the Ticlopidine Aspirin Stroke Study (TASS), compared ticlopidine with aspirin in stroke prevention after minor stroke or TIA (Hass *et al.*, 1989). Ticlopidine reduced the rate of stroke by 21% over 3 years compared with aspirin. These trials showed a clear advantage of ticlopidine over aspirin in stroke prevention. However, ticlopidine has the disadvantage that all of the trials have shown a 1% incidence of neutropenia, which, although reversible, mandates regular haematological monitoring. There is also an increased incidence of fatal thrombocytopenic purpura. Gastrointestinal side-effects and skin rashes are common side-effects (Table 15.9). Clopidogrel (see below) is a derivative of ticlopidine that has a very similar antiplatelet effect without the propensity to cause neutropenia. Clopidogrel has therefore largely replaced ticlopidine for routine use.

Clopidogrel

This thienopyridine derivative is chemically related to ticlopidine but has a greater antiplatelet action in animal models, without bone marrow toxicity. Clopidogrel has been shown to be slightly better than aspirin in the prevention of the combined outcome of vascular events (ischaemic stroke, myocardial infarction and vascular death) in patients with recent stroke, myocardial infarction or recent ischaemic stroke in the Clopidogrel versus Aspirin in Patients at Risk of Ischaemic Events (CAPRIE) trial (CAPRIE, 1996). This trial was a landmark in antiplatelet trials, randomizing over 19 000 patients and combining three

Table 15.9   Side-effects of ticlopidine

- Bone disorders
  - Neutropenia
  - Thrombocytopenia
  - Agranulocytosis
- Nausea
- Diarrhoea
- Hepatic toxicity
- Cholestasis
- Raised serum lipid concentrations
- Hypersensitivity reactions

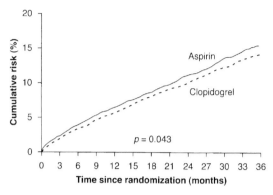

Figure 15.11   Cumulative risk of ischaemic stroke, myocardial infarction or vascular death in 19 185 patients with stroke, recent myocardial infarction or peripheral arterial disease randomized in CAPRIE between clopidogrel and aspirin. From CAPRIE Steering Committee. *Lancet* 1996;**348**:1329–1339.

subgroups of patients at risk of vascular events. There were approximately equal numbers of patients with ischaemic stroke (neurological signs persisting more than 7 days within 6 months of randomization), patients with significant peripheral arterial disease and patients with recent myocardial infarction (within 36 days of randomization). Patients entered into the trial were randomized either to aspirin (325 mg once only) or clopidogrel (75 mg once daily). On an intention-to-treat analysis, the rate of ischaemic events was significantly lower in the clopidogrel-treated group, at 5.3% per annum over 2 years, compared with 5.8% on aspirin (Figure 15.11). This equates to a relative risk reduction of 8.7% in favour of clopidogrel, but an absolute benefit of only 0.5%, which means that in patients matching the CAPRIE trial, the number needed to treat to prevent one additional event is 200. In patients at higher risk of recurrence, the absolute benefits will be greater. The relative risk reduction improved to 9.4% when an on-treatment analysis was conducted. However, when subgroup analysis was carried out, the benefit of clopidogrel compared with aspirin was only statistically significant in the subgroup of patients with peripheral arterial disease. The trend in patients with stroke was similar to the overall effect, but in the patients with ischaemic heart disease, the benefits of clopidogrel and aspirin were almost identical. It is likely that these differences in the different subgroups represent the play of chance and the fact that the trial was not powered to detect a difference in the individual disease groups. It is unlikely that there is a true

difference in the effectiveness of clopidogrel in different diseases.

Clopidogrel had a good safety profile in CAPRIE – similar to that of aspirin, but with a significantly lower incidence of gastrointestinal disturbance and haemorrhage. Rashes and diarrhoea were slightly more common (Table 15.10). Thrombotic thrombocytopenic purpura was not seen in trials or early post-marketing surveillance with clopidogrel, but has been described as a very rare complication (in most cases occurring within 14 days of initiation of therapy).

There has been considerable interest in the potential benefits of combining clopidogrel with aspirin. The CURE trial demonstrated that the combination was more effective than aspirin alone in the prevention of myocardial infarction in patients with unstable angina. However, the MATCH trial has shown that in patients with recent stroke and at high risk of recurrence, the addition of aspirin to clopidogrel was associated with an unacceptable incidence of serious haemorrhage, including intracranial haemorrhage (Diener *et al.*, 2004). Although the number of ischaemic strokes was slightly (but not significantly) less in patients treated with the combination of clopidogrel plus aspirin, this was almost exactly balanced by an increase in the rate of cerebral haemorrhage in patients

Table 15.10 Main side-effects of clopidogrel compared with aspirin in CAPRIE[a]

Side-effect	Aspirin (%)	Clopidogrel (%)
Any bleeding	9.3	9.3
Severe bleeding	1.6	1.4
Gastrointestinal haemorrhage	2.7	2.0*
Intracranial haemorrhage	0.5	0.4
Dyspepsia	17.6	15.0*
Rash	4.6	6.0*
Diarrhoea	3.4	6.0*

*$p < 0.05$.
[a]Adapted from CAPRIE Steering Committee. *Lancet* 1996;**348**: 1329–1339.

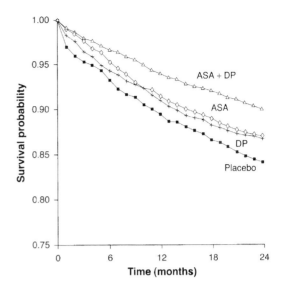

Figure 15.12 Cumulative risk of stroke in 6602 patients with recent stroke or TIA randomized to placebo, aspirin (ASA, 25 mg twice daily), dipyridamole (DP, 200 mg modified-release preparation twice daily) or the combination of dipyridamole and aspirin (DP+ASA) in ESPS-2. From Diener HC *et al.* *J Neurol Sci* 1996;**143**:1–13.

treated with the combination. Over two-thirds of the patients in MATCH had diabetes and it is possible that the high risk of cerebral haemorrhage was related to the presence of small vessel disease. Nevertheless, until further evidence becomes available with regard to the combination in other groups of patients with cerebrovascular disease, the use of aspirin plus clopidogrel in stroke patients cannot be routinely recommended.

Dipyridamole

This has only recently been accepted as being an effective antiplatelet agent in the prevention of stroke. The first European Stroke Prevention Study, published in 1987, showed that the combination of aspirin (1990 mg daily) and dipyridamole (225 mg daily) in patients with stroke and TIA reduced the rate of recurrent stroke by 38% compared with placebo (ESPS, 1987). Although this reduction was substantially greater than that shown in any of the trials of aspirin alone, the results did little to influence prescribing habits, because the trial design did not allow any individual effect of dipyridamole to be identified. However, the European Stroke Prevention Study 2 (ESPS-2) included a placebo group and separately examined the effects of aspirin (50 mg daily), dipyridamole (400 mg modified-release preparation daily) and the combination of aspirin and dipyridamole (Figure 15.12) (Diener *et al.*, 1996). The results confirmed that the very low dose of aspirin significantly reduced the relative risk of recurrent stroke compared with placebo by 18%, similar to the results of trials of higher doses. Dipyridamole alone also reduced the relative risk of stroke by 16%, which was again statistically significant. The combination of aspirin and dipyridamole was significantly better than either agent alone, with a relative reduction in stroke recurrence of 37%. However, dipyridamole was not shown to reduce myocardial infarction (perhaps because of small numbers). However, the risk reduction in the combined outcome of stroke, myocardial infarction or death compared with placebo was still significant at 15% for monotherapy and 24% for combined therapy. There has been criticism of this trial because of the low dose of aspirin used and because of irregularities at one centre that meant the patients at that centre had to be

Table 15.11 Main side-effects in ESPS-2[a]

	Placebo (%)	ASA (%)	DP (%)	ASA+DP (%)	p-Value
Any bleeding	4.5	8.2	4.7	8.7	<0.001
Severe bleeding	0.4	1.2	0.4	1.6	
Dyspepsia	16.1	17.2	16.6	17.6	
Headache	32.4	33.1	37.2	38.2	<0.001
Cessations	21.8	22.2	29.3	29.0	<0.001

ASA, aspirin (50 mg daily); DP, dipyridamole (400 mg modified-release preparation daily).
[a]Adapted from Diener HC *et al.* *J Neurol Sci* 1996;**143**:1–13.

withdrawn from the analysis. Nevertheless, the trial results provide persuasive evidence of the efficacy of dipyridamole in stroke prevention, especially in combination with aspirin. Meta-analysis of all the individual data from the randomized trials supports this conclusion (Leonardi-Bee *et al.*, 2005).

Dipyridamole is a very safe antiplatelet agent, with a lower risk of haemorrhage than aspirin alone and virtually no additional increase in the risk of haemorrhage when given with aspirin. However, it is not well tolerated by some patients because of side-effects, particularly headache (Table 15.11). The side-effects may be minimized by gradual introduction and may wear off in some patients over the course of a few weeks.

Selection of antiplatelet treatment

In choosing an antiplatelet agent, the physician needs to take into account the following factors:

- The risk of thrombosis in the individual patient
- The effectiveness of the agent (number needed to treat)
- The incidence of serious side-effects (particularly haemorrhage)
- Tolerability (minor side-effects)
- Cost (per event saved)

If cost is no object, clopidogrel or the combination of aspirin and dipyridamole would be the first-line treatment because of their superiority over aspirin in terms of effectiveness. In many countries where cost is an important consideration, aspirin will remain the first-line antiplatelet agent because of its low cost and well-established side-effect profile. In such cases, it is therefore reasonable to use aspirin as a first-line agent in the majority of patients with a relatively lower risk of recurrence and to reserve the use of the more effective, but more expensive, regimens for patients with a high risk of recurrence, or for those who have had recurrent ischaemic symptoms while taking aspirin alone. The risk of recurrence can be roughly assessed by taking into account the number of vascular risk factors present, the type of symptoms, the time elapsed since symptoms and the severity of carotid stenosis (Table 15.12).

In selecting an alternative to aspirin alone in patients with stroke, there is little to choose in terms of apparent effectiveness between clopidogrel and the combination of aspirin with dipyridamole. Both regimes appear to have a similar efficacy in the prevention of all vascular events, although they are currently being compared head to head in the PRoFESS trial. Clopidogrel appears to be better tolerated than the combination of aspirin and dipyridamole. Clopidogrel is more expensive than the combination therapy, but has the advantage of a once-daily regime. Dipyridamole has been tested in patients with TIA as well as stroke, unlike clopidogrel, but it is unlikely that clopidogrel will not be effective in TIA patients. The combination therapy should be prescribed either as a combined capsule containing 25 mg aspirin plus 200 mg modified-release dipyridamole taken twice daily or

Table 15.12   Simple stratification of risk of recurrence

Risk of stroke	Risk factors	Type of symptoms	Timing of symptoms	Severity of stenosis (ECST method)
Low	None	TMB	Distant	<70%
Moderate	Several	TIA	Within 6 months	70–80%
High	Many	Hemispheric stroke	Recent	>80%

ECST, European Carotid Surgery Trial; TIA, transient ischaemic attack; TMB, transient monocular blindness.

as separate prescriptions for aspirin 75 mg taken once daily with dipyridamole 200 mg modified-release twice daily. The latter regime is unlikely to have any different effect to the combined preparation tested in ESPS-2, but has the advantage that the patient can start the two preparations separately, allowing any side-effects to be distinguished. The combination of aspirin and dipyridamole was strongly favoured for patients with stroke and TIA over clopidogrel or aspirin alone by the UK National Institute for Clinical Effectiveness (NICE) in a report in 2005 on cost-effectiveness grounds, although they only recommended 2 years' treatment, thereafter recommending aspirin alone. NICE recommended that clopidogrel should be used in patients who are intolerant of low-dose aspirin.

Intolerance of aspirin   This is a common problem and as many as 25% of patients have withdrawn from treatment after 2 years of follow-up. Part of this may be perceived intolerance, rather than real side-effects and part may be due to poor compliance. Patients with minor side-effects should therefore be encouraged to continue with aspirin. If the patient has started on 300 mg aspirin daily, it may be helpful to reduce the dose to 150 or 75 mg daily. It is usual to prescribe a soluble preparation of aspirin, but there is probably little value in using an enteric-coated preparation, because much of the gastrointestinal side-effects are the result of systemic absorption. If the patient still complains of gastrointestinal discomfort after reducing the dose, tolerance may be improved by combining aspirin with an inhibitor of gastric acid secretion. However, it may be a cheaper option to

switch the patient to an alternative antiplatelet agent. In patients allergic or with confirmed intolerance to aspirin, clopidogrel is the next line of treatment. Dipyridamole alone appears to be less effective than clopidogrel, but provides another alternative for patients unable to take aspirin or clopidogrel, or if cost is a major factor. NICE recommended that clopidogrel should be used in preference to dipyridamole alone in patients intolerant of aspirin.

Aspirin 'failures'   Patients who have recurrent vascular symptoms while taking aspirin can be switched to clopidogrel, or dipyridamole can be added to the aspirin therapy. Because aspirin prevents less than 20% of vascular events, a patient with an annual risk of recurrence without aspirin treatment of say 5% (the risk found in patients with TIAs) will still have a risk of about 4% per annum on aspirin. Aspirin 'failures' will therefore become common over several years of follow-up. It is likely that recurrent symptoms indicate a greater risk of yet another event, and this therefore justifies the use of more effective antiplatelet therapy. *Ex vivo* platelet studies demonstrate that 'aspirin resistance' may occur and that in some patients adequate levels of inhibition of platelet aggregation may only occur with higher doses, particularly in patients who have already been on aspirin. For this reason, some authorities recommend increasing the dose of aspirin to as high as 1200 mg a day, particularly in aspirin treatment failures. There is no evidence from the aspirin trials to support this approach, and these high doses have a poor side-effect profile, but it may be reasonable to increase low doses up to 300 mg in aspirin failures.

Recurrent TIA and stroke

There is no evidence that patients with TIA or stroke benefit from anticoagulation to prevent further events, except in patients with atrial fibrillation or definite cardiac embolism. Indeed, the SPIRIT and WARSS trial results discussed above argue against using anticoagulation in atherothrombotic stroke. However, the fact that warfarin is better than aspirin in preventing recurrent events in patients with atrial fibrillation suggests that warfarin might also be superior to aspirin in other subgroups of patients at high risk of recurrent vascular events if they have a low risk of complications of anticoagulation. Trials to examine this question are in progress. One group being studied comprises patients with intracranial stenoses. In the meantime, it is important that the patients with recurrent TIA or stroke should be fully investigated to exclude other preventable causes of stroke (e.g. carotid stenosis or cardiac sources of embolism). This may require more extensive investigation, including angiography to exclude lesions missed by ultrasound. Even optimal antiplatelet therapy only prevents one-third of recurrent vascular events, and recurrent symptoms on antiplatelet therapy (aspirin failures) do not necessarily mean that anticoagulation will be beneficial. In the absence of evidence of vascular or cardiac disease, patients usually have a benign prognosis and many may sometimes have a non-vascular aetiology (e.g. migraine aura). In patients with recurrent stroke, it is reasonable to consider anticoagulation even for those in whom no possible embolic source has been identified. In such cases, anticoagulation should be limited to younger patients who do not have contraindications to anticoagulation (e.g. leukoaraiosis on CT).

Occasionally, patients who have recurrent ischaemic events on warfarin appear to respond to the combination of warfarin and low-dose aspirin (75mg daily). This combination carries an increased risk of haemorrhage and should therefore be prescribed with particular caution.

Crescendo TIAs (frequent TIAs increasing in severity or frequency) commonly progress to completed stroke. They are therefore an indication for immediate systemic anticoagulation with heparin, pending urgent investigation.

CAROTID ARTERY STENOSIS

Investigation of carotid stenosis

Ultrasound Severe internal carotid artery stenosis is one of the most important risk factors for recurrence in patients who have had ipsilateral TIA or stroke. Recent studies have shown that any delay in neurological assessment, imaging or carotid endarterectomy in patients with TIA or stroke caused by surgically treatable carotid stenosis leads to a significant rate of preventable stroke in patients while they wait for investigation and surgery. For example, in a study in Oxfordshire, England, the median times from presenting event to referral, scanning and endarterectomy were 9, 33 and 100 days respectively and the risk of stroke prior to planned endarterectomy in patients with greater than 50% stenosis was 21% at 2 weeks and 32% at 12 weeks (Fairhead *et al.*, 2005). Half of these strokes were disabling or fatal. It is therefore important that all patients with recent carotid territory symptoms who might be fit for carotid surgery should be referred, seen and investigated as soon as possible for the presence of carotid stenosis. Carotid ultrasound using duplex and colour-coded Doppler is the non-invasive investigation of choice (Figure 15.13). The severity of stenosis is most accurately graded by using a combination of duplex visualization of the stenosis with measurements of the peak and end-diastolic blood flow velocities across the stenosis using colour-coded Doppler.

The technique of carotid ultrasound requires an experienced operator for accurate results. In good hands, the sensitivity and specificity of carotid ultrasound for the presence of severe stenosis is greater than 90%. However, the severity of the stenosis may be over- or under-estimated, a very tight stenosis may be misinterpreted as occlusion and tortuosity of the carotid, or severe calcification may make the measurement of stenosis difficult. In addition, duplex ultrasound cannot insonate the distal

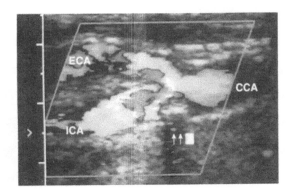

Figure 15.13 (See also Colour Plate VIII, p. xii). Colour flow Doppler and duplex ultrasonography showing severe carotid stenosis. Arrows show a large echo-dense atheromatous plaque. Turbulent flow is indicated by colour variation beyond the stenosis. ECA, external carotid artery; ICA, internal carotid artery; CCA, common carotid artery.

internal carotid artery. Distal stenosis, including stenosis of the carotid siphon, can only be detected using the Doppler modality, and this only reliably detects stenosis that results in an increased flow velocity (above approximately 60%). In patients with contralateral carotid occlusion, ipsilateral carotid flow velocities may be markedly increased and the severity of an ipsilateral stenosis overestimated. This can be overcome by calculating the ratio of peak systolic velocity in the internal carotid artery at the stenosis to the common carotid artery peak systolic velocity. If surgery is contemplated, stenosis of 60% or more suggested by ultrasound should be confirmed by an alternative imaging technique. Some vascular units that have established a very high level of reliability of their carotid ultrasound measurements are prepared to proceed directly to surgery on the basis of ultrasound measurements alone.

Magnetic resonance angiography (MRA)
Reliable MRA (Chapter 3) provides a method for confirming severe carotid stenosis after ultrasound, or it may be used as an alternative initial screening technique to ultrasound. However, it is considerably more expensive. MRA has the advantage of avoiding intra-arterial cannulation and contrast injection and is very safe. Like ultrasound, MRA requires experienced technicians and reporting to obtain reliable results and is not as accurate or detailed as conventional catheter angiography. The images tend to overestimate the severity of stenosis, especially when a flow void is present. It is important that the cross-sectional source images used to generate the angiographic images should be examined to avoid missing extremely tight stenosis (pseudo-occlusion), or overinterpreting artefact on the reconstructed angiographic images. When the results of MRA and carotid ultrasound agree with one another, there is a good correlation with conventional catheter angiography. In units with reliable ultrasound and MRA, patients can be referred to surgery without catheter angiography if both ultrasound and MRA agree about the presence of severe carotid stenosis. If the investigations are significantly discordant, catheter angiography may be needed to decide on the appropriateness of surgery. Both ultrasound and MRA are insensitive to the presence of plaque ulceration. Ultrasound does not provide information about the distal carotid, although MRA is not necessarily reliable at these sites either. The reliability of MRA may be increased by using rapid injection of an MRA paramagnetic contrast agent (contrast-enhanced MRA, CEMRA), and this may be particularly useful in estimating the severity or patency of tight stenosis.

Spiral CT Spiral CT provides an alternative method of confirming carotid stenosis, but requires a large bolus of intravenous contrast. The utility of spiral CT angiography in comparison with ultrasound or MRA has not yet been established.

Catheter angiography (see Chapter 3) This should be considered in the investigation of carotid stenosis only as follows:

- To confirm carotid stenosis suggested by ultrasound in units who do not have reliable MRA or spiral CT
- To provide a more accurate measurement of carotid stenosis when the results of non-invasive investigations conflict

- To provide accurate measurement of stenosis when the non-invasive techniques suggest that stenosis is somewhere between 60% and 80%
- To exclude distal or siphon stenosis in patients with recurrent symptoms in whom MRA is equivocal or unavailable
- When carotid dissection is suspected but not confirmed or excluded by MRA

Catheter angiography, even with digital subtraction techniques (DSA) and new non-ionic contrast media, carries a significant risk of causing a stroke and should therefore be avoided unless strictly necessary. In good hands, the risk is probably in the region of 1–2% in patients with severe carotid stenosis. In general, the risk of DSA causing a stroke is about 1%, but is less in young patients without disease and probably slightly more in patients with generalized atherosclerosis. In some units, the risks of angiography in patients with severe carotid stenosis have been reported to be as high as 5%.

Stroke occurring at the time of angiography usually occurs as a result of dislodgement and embolization of atheromatous plaque or pre-existing thrombus, mainly from the aortic arch, by the guidewire or catheter tip. Thrombus may also form in or on the catheter and then embolize. Embolic stroke, which may delayed until after the patient returns to the ward, may be also due to the dislodgement of thrombus initiated by injury or to frank dissection of the arterial wall caused by the guidewire or catheter tip. Arterial spasm may also occasionally be caused by arterial catheterization, but is rarely severe enough to result in haemodynamic compromise. Injection of contrast into the cerebral vessels may also precipitate migraine and is occasionally followed by a transient confusional state of uncertain aetiology, possibly the result of endothelial swelling. Allergic reactions, groin haematoma, embolism to the leg and contrast-related renal failure are other complications of angiography via the femoral route. The risks should be discussed with the patient in detail before obtaining consent.

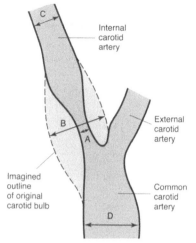

Formula for calculating percentage carotid stenosis from an angiogram film:

ECST method stenosis $= \dfrac{B-A}{B} \times 100$

NASCET method stenosis $= \dfrac{C-A}{C} \times 100$

Common carotid method stenosis $= \dfrac{D-A}{D} \times 100$

Figure 15.14 Illustration of methods for measuring carotid stenosis.

Measurement of carotid stenosis

Three methods of measuring the severity of carotid stenosis from an angiographic film have been used in different trials (Figure 15.14). The method used in the North American Symptomatic Carotid Endarterectomy Trial (NASCET) has the disadvantage that it is difficult to decide at which point to make the distal measurement (NASCET, 1991). It is recommended that the measurement should be made in the distal internal carotid several centimetres above the stenosis at a point at which the walls have become parallel to avoid post-stenotic dilation. In patients with very severe stenosis, the distal carotid artery tends to collapse and the NASCET method then underestimates the severity of stenosis, so that an arbitrary value of 95% should be applied in such cases. The method used in the European Carotid Surgery Trial (ECST) has the disadvantage that the width of the original carotid bulb has to be estimated by guesswork (ECST, 1998). Both the ECST and NASCET methods show considerable observer variability. The common carotid (CC) method is the easiest to perform and has the lowest inter- and intraobserver variability, but is not widely used. The NASCET method is the standard against which most ultrasound techniques for assessing carotid stenosis are compared, as well as being the most widely used in research publications, which argues that it should become the method of choice for angiographic measurements.

On average, measurements made using the ECST and the common carotid methods are identical. The NASCET method results in a lesser apparent degree of severity than the ECST method for any given stenosis. NASCET stenosis can be converted into ECST or CC stenosis using a simple formula:

$$\text{ECST (or CC)} = (0.6 \times \text{NASCET}) + 40$$

Scheduling investigations for carotid stenosis

Patients with severe carotid stenosis need to be operated upon as soon as possible after symptom onset, because the incidence of recurrence of stroke is highest in the first few months after symptoms. For maximum benefit, patients should therefore be investigated and treated within 2–4 weeks at the most, after the onset of symptoms, if they have made sufficient recovery to be suitable for surgery. One of the advantages of specialized neurovascular clinics is that patients with TIA and mild stroke can be rapidly assessed and investigated for carotid stenosis.

CAROTID ENDARTERECTOMY

Recently symptomatic patients

There is good evidence from NASCET and ECST that carotid endarterectomy is highly effective at preventing stroke in patients with recent ipsilateral symptoms (TIA or stroke) and severe carotid stenosis (Rothwell *et al.*, 2003).

In patients with severe stenosis, removing the stenosis surgically almost abolishes the risk of ipsilateral recurrence (Figure 15.15). The low rate of recurrent stroke after successful

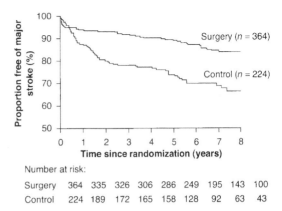

Figure 15.15 Survival curve illustrating the risks of stroke lasting more than 7 days in patients randomized in ECST with severe stenosis measuring 80–99% by the ECST method. From European Carotid Surgery Trialists' Collaborative Group. *Lancet* 1998;**351**:1379–1387.

surgery demonstrates that in almost all patients with symptoms associated with very severe stenosis, the stenosis is responsible for the episode of cerebral ischaemia. Carotid surgery is therefore a very effective operation, so long as it can be carried out without complications. Unfortunately, the operation is not without risks (Table 15.13). Carotid endarterectomy is a fairly hazardous procedure, and the risks of stroke or death within 30 days of the procedure in the clinical trials of carotid surgery, where the patients were all examined postoperatively by a neurologist, ranged from 6% to 10%.

The aim of carotid endarterectomy is to remove atheromatous plaque from the carotid artery in order to cure stenosis of the artery and remove the source of embolism. The operation is therefore only of value in preventing stroke, but does nothing to improve ongoing symptoms of the patient who has had a stroke. It might be thought that an improvement in perfusion pressure to the brain after carotid surgery would improve cognitive function, but there is no good evidence that this occurs, probably because vascular dementia is rarely the result of impaired cerebral blood flow. The occasional patient reports considerable improvement in

Table 15.13 Risks of carotid surgery

- Stroke
  Embolic
  Haemodynamic
  Haemorrhagic
- Transient ischaemic attack
- Carotid occlusion
- Unstable blood pressure
- Cranial nerve palsy
  Hypoglossal
  Facial
  Glossopharyngeal
  Spinal accessory
  Vagal
- Myocardial infarction
- Pulmonary embolus
- Deep vein thrombosis
- Pneumonia
- Wound haematoma
- Respiratory compromise
- Wound infection
- Numbness around incision
- Keloid scar formation
- Hyperperfusion syndrome
- Recurrent carotid stenosis

mental function after carotid surgery, but it is possible that this represents natural recovery after a stroke or the relief of anxiety.

Because of the hazards, carotid surgery should be limited to the treatment of patients with definite indications (Table 15.14). Surgery should only be offered to patients who have a risk of stroke treated medically considerably higher than the risk of the operation. The major determinant of recurrent events in symptomatic patients with carotid stenosis is the severity of the stenosis, whereas the risk of surgery is unrelated to the severity. There is therefore a point at which the risk of surgery outweighs the benefit of removing the stenosis in preventing recurrent events. The carotid surgery trials have shown that this point is reached in the majority of symptomatic patients at about 80% measured using the ECST method or 70% using the NASCET method (Figure 15.16). A subgroup of patients at higher risk of stroke treated medically benefit from surgery at lesser degrees of stenosis: about 70% using ECST or 50% using NASCET (see below).

All patients with carotid territory ipsilateral TIA or stroke, who have had symptoms within 6 months and have made a reasonable recovery, should therefore be investigated for carotid stenosis and considered for surgery if the stenosis is 80% or more measured using ECST or 70% or more using NASCET, so long as they are fit for operation. In patients with stenosis of

Table 15.14 Indications for carotid surgery

Definite indications (all of the following must be present)
- Severe stenosis (>70% NASCET method, excluding near-occlusion)
- History of ipsilateral carotid TIA or stroke with reasonable recovery
- Symptoms within 6 months
- Fit for surgery
- Experienced skilled surgeon available

Indications to take into account when selecting patients with moderate stenosis (50–69% NASCET method)
- Male gender
- Older age
- Recent symptoms
- Stroke rather than TIA
- Ulcerated plaque

Possible indications in selected patients
- Appropriate symptoms more than 6 months previously (stenosis >80% by NASCET method)
- Asymptomatic stenosis

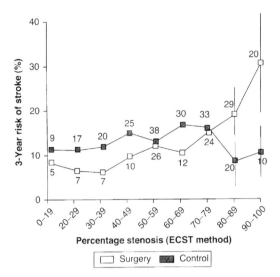

Figure 15.16 Graph illustrating the risks of any stroke lasting more than 7 days at 3 years, including operative events, according to severity of stenosis in patients randomized in ECST European Carotid Surgery Trialists' Collaborative Group. The numbers above and below the boxes are the numbers of patients with stroke. From *Lancet* 1998;**351**: 1379–87.

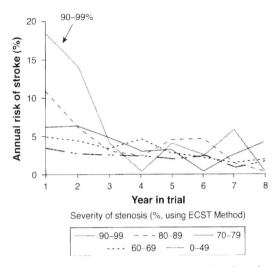

Figure 15.17 Graph illustrating the risk of stroke during follow-up over time in patients with varying degrees of carotid stenosis treated medically in ECST. From European Carotid Surgery Trialists' Collaborative Group. *Lancet* 1998;**351**:1379–1387.

between 70% and 80% measured using ECST (50–70% using NASCET), the benefits of surgery are less certain, because the risks and benefits are more evenly balanced. However, it is reasonable to treat these patients if other factors are favourable (see below). Patients with less than 70% stenosis using ECST (less than 50% using NASCET) should not be offered surgery. Even if there is ulceration, these patients do not benefit, because the risk of surgery is much greater than the risks when treated medically.

Timing of surgery

The chances of a recurrence of stroke are greatest a few weeks after an ischaemic event, and much of the potential benefit of surgery is lost if surgery is delayed (Fairhead *et al.*, 2005). However, surgery should probably be delayed for 4 weeks in patients who have had a major stroke with cerebral infarction on imaging because of the risk of reperfusion injury and haemorrhage into a fresh infarct after reopening

a stenosed carotid artery. The symptomatic trials only provide evidence that surgery is beneficial in patients who have had symptoms within 4–6 months at the most, and surgery should not routinely be considered in patients whose symptoms are more distant. Moreover, the benefits of surgery decline with the passage of time from most recent symptom to treatment (Rothwell *et al.*, 2004). However, if they are high risk (e.g. have more than 80% stenosis using the NASCET method) and have had symptoms for between 6 and 12 months, it may be reasonable to consider surgery in patients who are also at low risk from surgery. Patients with more distant symptoms should be treated as though they were asymptomatic (see below). The risks of recurrent symptoms in patients with severe stenosis treated medically declines with time, and in the ECST reached a similar level of risks to patients with lesser degrees of stenosis 3 years after the last symptom (Figure 15.17).

One consistently high risk factor for surgery is a history of crescendo TIA (frequent TIAs increasing in frequency or severity). These patients should probably be stabilized by a period of anticoagulation with heparin before surgery is performed. But none of the adverse factors for surgery are absolute contraindications, because these factors also increase the risk of stroke in patients who are treated medically.

Stratification of risk

Analysis combining the data from NASCET and ECST has shown that patients with near-occlusion (sometimes known as pseudo-occlusion, or string sign on angiography) of the internal carotid artery do not benefit from endarterectomy, because of a low risk of stroke when treated medically (Rothwell *et al.*, 2003). Endarterectomy for complete carotid occlusion is a hazardous operation because the thrombus usually extends right up into the first branch of the internal carotid artery, which is the ophthalmic artery. Carotid artery occlusion and near-occlusion should therefore in most cases be treated conservatively.

A number of factors influence the risks of recurrence on medical treatment. Ocular TIA (amaurosis fugax) has a relatively benign prognosis and is less likely to be followed by stroke than hemispheric symptoms. Not surprisingly, the more risk factors, the higher the risk of recurrent stroke. In patients treated surgically, the risks of the operation are greater in women than men and are increased by the presence of uncontrolled hypertension and peripheral arterial disease. In the combined analysis of the NASCET, ECST and VA trials, the benefits of surgery were present in all subgroups of patients with carotid stenosis over 69% (NASCET method) (Rothwell *et al.*, 2003, 2004). Between 50% and 69% stenosis, the benefits were less and were greater in men, older patients, patients with prior stroke compared with prior TIA, and patients with ulceration on angiography. These factors should be taken into account when considering surgery and discussing the risks and benefits with the patient. For example, a female elderly patient with only one episode of amaurosis fugax several months ago and 65% carotid stenosis has much less to gain from surgery than the young male patient with recent recurrent hemispheric symptoms

and more than 80% carotid stenosis. The first patient should have the risks and benefits presented as fairly even, while the second patient can be strongly encouraged to have surgery as soon as possible. The majority of patients with symptomatic carotid stenosis are elderly, and age by itself is not a contraindication to surgery. However, the risks of surgery increase with age, and patients need to have an expectation of a good-quality life of at least 2 years to stand a reasonable chance of benefiting from surgery. However, analysis of the trials has shown that older patients actually benefit more from surgery than younger patients (Alamowitch *et al.*, 2001). It is therefore reasonable to investigate with carotid ultrasound and consider surgery in older patients up to the age of 80 and in selected patients who appear 'biologically' younger up to the age of 85. Patients with recent symptoms who have also had symptoms attributable to the severe stenosis more than 6 months previously have about twice the risk of stroke if treated medically than patients who are only recently symptomatic.

RISKS OF CAROTID SURGERY (TABLE 15.15)

Major morbidity

The most important complication of carotid surgery is stroke at the time of the procedure or in the first few days after surgery. A number of mechanisms may be responsible for surgical stroke, including:

- Dislodgement of embolic material (thrombus or atheromatous debris) during carotid manipulation or dissection
- Haemodynamic ischaemia during clamping of the carotid artery
- Emboli from shunt insertion, if used
- Perioperative thrombosis, which may result in vessel occlusion and/or distal embolism
- Cerebral haemorrhage and/or seizures after reperfusion (see Chapter 8)
- Preoperative or postoperative thrombosis in other diseased arteries (e.g. the contralateral internal carotid artery)

Table 15.15   The risks of stroke or death from the two largest trials of carotid surgery compared with best medical care in patients with severe stenosis

	NASCET		ECST	
	Medicine	*Surgery*	*Medicine*	*Surgery*
Stroke and death rate in the 30 days after surgery (%)	—	5.8	—	7.5
Total rate of stroke (and perioperative death) after 2 years of follow-up (3 years in ECST) (%)	32.3	15.8	21.9	12.3

The differences between medical care alone and surgery were highly significant. The greater rate of stroke in the medical patients in NASCET is explained by inclusion of patients in this table with a greater severity of stenosis than in ECST

NASCET, North American Symptomatic Carotid Endarterectomy Trial; ECST, European Carotid Surgery Trial.

- Residual stenosis because of poor operative technique or failure to remove all of the distal or proximal atheroma

Most strokes after carotid endarterectomy are not disabling: however, there are still a significant percentage of disabling strokes. A stroke is the major cause of fatality after carotid surgery, but death can also occur as a result of myocardial infarction, pulmonary embolism or respiratory failure. Table 15.15 gives the risks of stroke or death from the two largest trials of carotid surgery compared with best medical care. Because surgical stroke can be delayed in up to one-third of cases, it is usual to count any strokes occurring within 30 days of surgery as surgical complications. The benefits of carotid endarterectomy depend on a low surgical complication rate, and these benefits will disappear rapidly if the stroke or death rate rises much above 10%. It is therefore essential that carotid surgery should be limited to units and surgeons who carry out carotid surgery regularly, and these units should audit their results with the aim of minimizing complications. It is important to bear in mind that an individual surgeon's complication rate may depend as much on the case mix of patients operated as

on the surgeon's skills. When neurologists examine patients after carotid surgery, significantly higher complication rates are recorded than when surgeons audit their own results. This should be kept in mind when assessing the results reported by surgical units or individual surgeons.

Despite efforts to improve the safety of surgery, recent trials have not demonstrated a dramatic improvement in stroke rate over the last few years. Surgeons vary in their use of shunts during the operation, but this has not been demonstrated to improve the rate of stroke during the procedure. The use of preoperative angiography or ultrasound may reduce the risk of leaving a residual stenosis or intra-arterial thrombus, and the use of vein patches to increase the diameter of the artery at the site of endarterectomy may reduce the risk of recurrent stenosis. Some surgeons are enthusiastic about the use of monitoring procedures (e.g. transcranial Doppler) during the procedure, but trials have not been performed to evaluate the effect of these on outcome. If ischaemic symptoms develop in the immediate postoperative period and an immediate ultrasound shows carotid thrombus or occlusion, immediate reoperation to remove the thrombus can result in dramatic resolution of clinical deficit. Reoperating on the patient is more likely to be harmful than beneficial if more than a few hours have elapsed.

To reduce the risks of stroke, patients are usually anticoagulated with heparin during carotid endarterectomy, but this is usually reversed at the end of the procedure. Patients should be treated with an antiplatelet agent before the operation and should continue the agent after the procedure. A randomized clinical trial has shown that medium- or low-dose aspirin (325 mg or less) is more effective than higher doses at preventing stroke during the operation (Taylor *et al.*, 1999). It is probable that some of the complications of surgery may be avoided by using local anaesthesia. However, many centres still favour general anaesthesia. Clearly, other vascular risks factors (e.g. hypertension and hypercholesterolaemia) should not be neglected.

Patients considered for carotid surgery need to be fit for the operation, but with modern anaesthetic techniques this excludes very few patients, except for those with recent myocardial infarction, unstable angina, cardiac failure or severe respiratory disease. A number of factors increase the risk of stroke or death at the time of surgery in patients who are otherwise considered fit for surgery (Table 15.16). There is considerable uncertainty regarding how best to treat patients with recent neurological symptoms who need both carotid surgery and coronary artery bypass graft (CABG) surgery. The options are simultaneous CABG and carotid endarterectomy at one operation or staged procedures (carotid endarterectomy then CABG after an interval) or even reversed staged procedures (CABG then carotid endarterectomy). The evidence suggests that the staged procedure is the least risky.

Minor morbidity

The major disadvantage of carotid surgery other than the risk of stroke or death is the need for an incision in the neck. The postoperative period may be complicated by wound haematoma, which can compress the trachea

Table 15.16 Clinical characteristics associated with an increase in the risk of carotid surgery in patients otherwise considered fit for surgery

- Female gender
- Cerebral versus ocular symptoms
- Age >75 years
- Systolic hypertension
- Peripheral arterial disease
- Contralateral internal carotid artery occlusion
- Ipsilateral carotid syphon stenosis
- Ipsilateral external carotid artery stenosis

causing respiratory distress, and wound infection. An unsightly scar may result. The interruption of cutaneous nerves leads to numbness on the neck, which may spread up onto the angle of the jaw and is occasionally permanent. The incision and retraction can injure the cranial nerves in the neck – most commonly the hypoglossal nerve, resulting in tongue weakness. Occasionally, the facial nerve and rarely the spinal accessory nerve are injured. Usually, cranial nerve injury recovers and is rarely disabling. These minor complications affect about 10% of patients undergoing carotid surgery.

ASYMPTOMATIC CAROTID STENOSIS

The risk of stroke in patients found to have carotid stenosis but who have never had ipsilateral symptoms is surprisingly low. Long-term follow-up studies have shown that the annual risk of stroke in patients with severe carotid stenosis who have not had previous symptoms is around 2% per annum (Benavente *et al.*, 1998; Halliday *et al.*, 2004). Surgery is therefore not considered to be warranted by many neurologists in the majority of asymptomatic patients, because it takes several years for the benefits of surgery in reducing the risk of recurrence to outweigh the risk of stroke or death at the time of the operation. It may be better to educate patients with asymptomatic stenosis to report the symptoms of TIA or stroke, so that they can then be referred for carotid surgery urgently if they become symptomatic. However, in some centres (particularly in North America) that can demonstrate very low rates of perioperative stroke, surgery is routinely offered to asymptomatic patients.

Patients with asymptomatic stenosis should have vigorous control of other vascular risk factors and should probably be treated with an antiplatelet agent, particularly if they have other vascular risk factors. It would be useful to identify a subgroup of asymptomatic patients who have a higher risk of developing symptoms treated medically, which would allow surgery to be targeted at a higher-risk group. In some patients with asymptomatic carotid stenosis, micro-emboli can be detected using transcranial Doppler in the middle cerebral artery. The significance of these micro-emboli is uncertain, but it is possible that monitoring for micro-emboli using transcranial Doppler may allow the selection of patients at high risk of future stroke. The technique has not been sufficiently validated to enter routine clinical practice.

Screening for asymptomatic carotid stenosis

Most early trials of surgery for asymptomatic surgery failed to show a benefit of surgery (Benavente *et al.*, 1998). However, more recent trials have demonstrated a small overall benefit to carotid endarterectomy. The Asymptomatic Carotid Atherosclerosis Study (ACAS), based in North America, reported a significant benefit for surgery compared with medical treatment in patients with severe stenosis (ACAS, 1995). This trial suggested that at best carotid surgery for asymptomatic stenosis reduced the risk of stroke from 11% over 5 years to about 5% per year – that is, a reduction in the absolute risk of stroke or death of only about 1% per annum. It can be calculated from the ACAS results that it would be necessary to operate on about 85 patients every year to prevent one ipsilateral stroke per annum. Recently, the Asymptomatic Carotid Surgery Trial (ACST) has reported similar results in mainly European centres (Halliday *et al.*, 2004). A policy of immediate operation on asymptomatic stenosis reduced the 5-year risk of any stroke or perioperative death to

6.4% from 11.8% in patients in whom surgery was deferred until a more definite indication appeared (e.g. the stenosis became symptomatic) (Figure 15.18). Subgroup analysis suggested that patients over the age of 75 did not benefit from surgery. There is also no clear evidence that women benefit from surgery, perhaps because insufficient numbers were included in the randomized trials. These results imply that screening for asymptomatic stenosis is not cost-effective or clinically appropriate. Moreover, any benefit of surgery relies on a low rate of perioperative stroke or death, which in ACST was just less than 3%. However, the trials provide justification for surgery at centres with a proven low complication rate, in selected patients who are prepared to take a small immediate risk in exchange for a small longer-term benefit.

If patients are known to have asymptomatic carotid stenosis, the risks and benefits of early surgery and delaying surgery until symptoms occur should be explained to the patient. Most patients are reassured by the low risk of symptoms when treated medically and choose not to have surgery. A small percentage of patients dislike the anxiety of knowing that they have a potential source of stroke, which could be removed, and elect for surgery knowing the risks at the time of the operation. Although the presence of asymptomatic carotid stenosis increases the risks of CABG surgery, there is no good evidence that this justifies carotid surgery prior to CABG in neurologically asymptomatic patients. There is no value in following known carotid stenosis with regular ultrasound examinations to detect progression. In most cases, the rate of progression of stenosis is very low and does not justify regular surveillance even if surgery is regarded as beneficial.

CAROTID ANGIOPLASTY AND STENTING

Percutaneous transluminal angioplasty (PTA) and stenting (endovascular treatment) are rapidly developing as alternatives to carotid endarterectomy for the treatment of carotid stenosis (Figure 15.19) (Brown, 2004). The

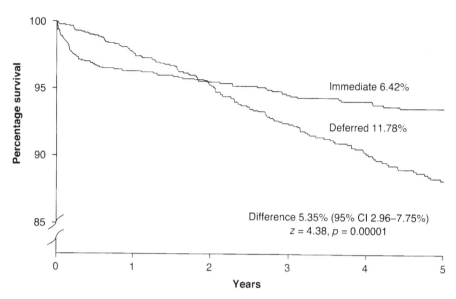

Figure 15.18   Survival curve showing risk of any stroke or perioperative death in ACST over 5 years. From Halliday A *et al. Lancet* 2004;**363**:1491–1502.

techniques of interventional radiology have become standard for the treatment of ischaemic heart disease and peripheral arterial stenosis, but until recently have not been considered safe in the carotid arteries because of concern about the risks of cerebral embolism. However, endovascular treatment has the great advantage in comparison with surgery of always being carried out under local anaesthetic and avoiding the trauma from the surgical incision. If all goes well, endovascular treatment is less invasive than surgery and from the patient's point of view is very little different to an angiographic procedure. The patient can be discharged home within 24 hours. The cost of angioplasty is usually less than surgery because of a shorter hospital stay, although if stents are used, the costs of the devices may cancel out any savings.

The major risks of angioplasty and stenting causing stroke or death from the procedure appear to be similar to those of carotid endarterectomy (Coward *et al.*, 2005). The Carotid and Vertebral Artery Transluminal Angioplasty Study (CAVATAS), showed almost identical risks and long-term effectiveness of endovascular treatment compared with

surgery for carotid stenosis (CAVATAS, 2001). CAVATAS confirmed that endovascular treatment avoids many of the less serious complications of surgery, particularly cranial nerve injury and wound problems (Figure 15.20). Two smaller trials of carotid stenting were stopped early because of poor early results in the stented patients. In contrast, the SAPPHIRE (Stenting and Angioplasty with Protection in Patients at High Risk for Endarterectomy) trial has reported 1-year results favouring stenting in patients at high risk with surgery (Yadav *et al.*, 2004). Further randomized trials are in progress to compare carotid stenting with surgery. Until these have been completed, carotid angioplasty and stenting will be regarded by many as an experimental treatment.

Complications of carotid angioplasty and stenting (Table 15.17)

The main hazard of carotid angioplasty is intimal dissection caused by balloon dilation and cracking of the atheromatous plaque or by trauma from the insertion of a guidewire across the stenosis. Dissection can lead to acute thrombosis and occlusion of the carotid artery, with

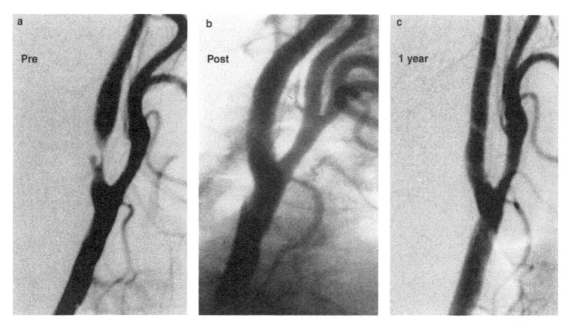

Figure 15.19 Carotid angiography showing results of simple balloon angioplasty in a patient with severe ulcerated internal carotid artery stenosis: (a) immediately before angioplasty; (b) immediately after angioplasty; (c) 1 year after angioplasty.

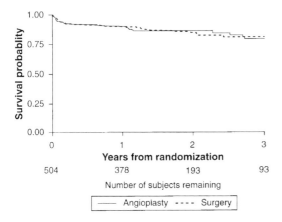

Figure 15.20 Comparison of surgery and angioplasty in patients with carotid stenosis randomized in CAVATAS, showing number of patients free of death or disabling stroke in any territory during follow-up from the time of randomization. From CAVATAS Investigators. *Lancet* 2001;**357**:1729–1737.

subsequent stroke. Embolization may also occur as a result of dislodgement of atheromatous material or thrombus in the plaque during the procedure. Stents have therefore been

developed for use in the carotid artery that are flexible and non-collapsing and have a narrow meshwork, the assumption being that such stents will reduce the incidence of dissection. In the technique of primary stenting, a self-expanding or balloon-expandable stent is inserted and expanded across the stenosis as a primary procedure without (or with only minimal) initial balloon dilation. Primary stenting has the advantage that the adverse consequences of any dissection, including acute carotid occlusion, initiated by dilation of the artery are minimized, because the stent maintains good flow across the stenosis and seals the site of dissection, preventing a free intimal flap. In addition, the stent mesh limits the size of any thrombus or atheromatous debris that may be dislodged from the atheromatous plaque at the time of balloon dilation. The combination of aspirin and clopidogrel is usually prescribed before and for 4–6 weeks after stenting, to further reduce the risk of stent thrombosis. The initial results of carotid stenting are often superior to those obtained with simple balloon angioplasty (Figure 15.21), and stenting has therefore

Table 15.17 Complications of carotid angioplasty and stenting

Acute complications

Mechanical
- Intimal dissection
- Aneurysm formation
- Carotid sinus stimulation
- Bradycardia and asystole
- Hypotension
- Arterial spasm
- Vessel rupture
- Balloon rupture

Neurological
- Haemodynamic ischaemia
- Cerebral embolism
- Vessel occlusion

Angiographic
- Groin haematoma
- Puncture site pain
- Contrast reactions
- Haemorrhage from anticoagulation
- Femoral artery thromboembolism

Delayed complications
- Cerebral embolism
- Vessel occlusion
- Cerebral haemorrhage
- Hyperperfusion syndrome
- Restenosis
- Stent collapse

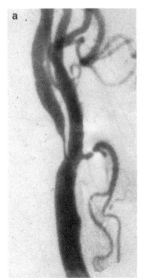
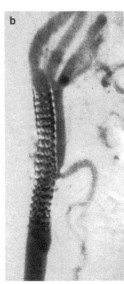

Figure 15.21 Carotid angiogram: (a) immediately before stenting; (b) immediately after stenting.

become the technique of choice for endovascular treatment of carotid and vertebral stenosis.

Concern about the risk of embolization to the brain during deployment of a carotid stent has led to the development of endovascular protection devices. The most widely used protection devices are filters or distal occlusion balloons, which are placed distal to the stenosis to catch debris dislodged during stent deployment. The disadvantages of these devices are that they have to be passed across the stenosis (which itself may dislodge emboli to the brain) before the protection device is in place, and that the protection device may cause additional complications as a result of injury to the wall or difficulty extracting the device. An alternative is to use a proximal protection technique, in which occlusion balloons are placed in the external carotid artery and common carotid artery. This results in retrograde blood flow down the internal carotid artery, which protects the brain during the critical phase of stent insertion. No protection device can be expected to protect against angiographic stroke during initial catheterization or stroke in the postprocedural period, which in CAVATAS accounted for one-third of events occurring within 30 days of treatment. Most case series suggest that protection devices reduce the overall rate of stroke, but one very large registry in Germany showed little difference between the rates of stroke between protected and non-protected patients (Kastrup *et al.*, 2003; Theiss *et al.*, 2004).

The long-term results of carotid angioplasty and stenting have yet to be established, but preliminary data from CAVATAS suggest that endovascular treatment is as effective as surgery at preventing long-term recurrence. Restenosis is less of a problem after carotid angioplasty and stenting in the carotid artery than is seen in the coronary artery. Restenosis after carotid angioplasty occurs in about 20% of patients at 1 year, but is rarely symptomatic. This is probably because restenosis is usually the result of fibrointimal hyperplasia, and this may be less likely to embolize. Haemodynamic symptoms due to a reduction in flow are rarely significant in carotid disease, in comparison with coronary artery disease, where recurrence of flow-related angina is relatively common after angioplasty. When a recurrence of symptoms is associated with restenosis after carotid angioplasty or stenting, angioplasty can be repeated or the patient can be offered surgery as an alternative.

Because of its advantages, carotid stenting may in the future replace carotid surgery in many patients with bifurcation stenosis, if the safety and durability of stenting is confirmed by ongoing trials. Carotid stenting also has the advantage that it is suitable for the treatment of carotid stenosis in patients who are not fit for surgery or who have distal stenosis of the carotid at a site inaccessible to surgery. Decisions about the most appropriate method of treating carotid stenosis require close collaboration between neurologists, interventional radiologists and surgeons with an interest in carotid disease.

Stenting for dissection

Carotid stenting provides an option for the treatment of dissection, particularly where there is a free flap and an obvious true lumen. However, because the treatment is unproven, stenting should probably be reserved for patients who have had an unsuccessful trial of anticoagulation.

Stenting for vertebral artery stenosis

Vertebral angioplasty without stenting is frequently followed by restenosis at the origin of the vertebral artery. However, vertebral artery stenosis can be more successfully treated by stenting, but the benefits in comparison with medical treatment are uncertain. Vertebral artery stenting can therefore be considered as an option for patients with recurrent vertebrobasilar TIAs or definite vertebrobasilar infarction associated with severe stenosis of

the origin of one vertebral artery. PTA has also been used to treat basilar artery stenosis, but the hazards of causing stroke from occlusion of the perforating branches of the basilar artery are considerable.

EXTRACRANIAL–INTRACRANIAL BYPASS SURGERY

Extracranial–intracranial (EC–IC) bypass surgery is an operation in which an anastomosis is made between the superficial temporal branch of the external carotid artery and an intracranial branch of the internal carotid on the surface of the brain through a burr hole in the skull. At one time, the operation was very popular for the treatment of internal carotid artery occlusion, and stenosis or occlusion of the middle cerebral artery. However, the EC–IC Bypass Trial convincingly demonstrated that the operation failed to prevent stroke (Figure 15.22), mainly because of a high risk of stroke at the time of the procedure (EC/IC Bypass Study Group, 1985). The operation is therefore no longer routinely performed for carotid occlusion, although it is still performed in some units for specific indications (e.g. moyamoya disease), without any definite evidence of benefit. It has been argued that only patients with haemodynamic compromise are likely to benefit from EC–IC bypass. Measures of cerebral blood flow were not required in the EC–IC Bypass Trial, and further trials are therefore underway to test the benefit of the operation in selected patients with clear evidence of impaired cerebrovascular reserve.

TREATMENT OF VASCULITIS

Patients with temporal arteritis and cerebral vasculitis require urgent immunosuppression to prevent recurrent stroke. Temporal arteritis usually responds rapidly to oral prednisolone. Patients with other forms of vasculitis (e.g. systemic lupus erythematosus, SLE) may require intravenous methylprednisolone in high doses to induce remission. Consideration should then be given in consultation with an expert in vasculitis to maintenance therapy with

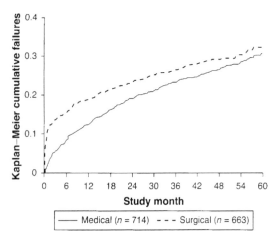

Figure 15.22 Results of the EC–IC Bypass Trial showing the rate of any stroke after randomization. Modified from EC/IC Bypass Study Group. *N Engl J Med* 1985;**313**:1191–1200.

cyclophosphamide, azathioprine or other immunosuppressive agents, with the aim of reducing the dose of steroid therapy.

PREVENTION OF HAEMORRHAGIC STROKE

The avoidance of vascular risk factors discussed above, particularly avoidance of smoking and heavy alcohol intake, and the effective treatment of hypertension will reduce the risk of subarachnoid haemorrhage and intracerebral haemorrhage, as well as the risk of cerebral infarction. In patients with haemorrhage resulting from arterial venous malformations or aneurysms, neurosurgical or interventional radiological treatment is the mainstay of prevention; this is discussed in Chapter 9. Many patients who have had a cerebral haemorrhage are also at increased risk of cerebral infarction, but in general antiplatelet therapy and anticoagulation are contraindicated for life after any form of non-traumatic intracranial haemorrhage. An exception is made for patients with prosthetic heart values, in whom anticoagulation should be restarted 4–6 weeks after the bleed.

KEY REFERENCES

Atherothrombosis

Drouet L. Atherothrombosis as a systemic disease. *Cerebrovasc Dis* 2002;**13**(Suppl):1–6

Hormone replacement therapy

Beral V, Banks E, Reeves G. Evidence from randomised trials on the long-term effects of hormone replacement therapy. *Lancet* 2002;**360**:942–944

Pedersen AT, Lidegaard O, Kreiner S, Ottesen B. Hormone replacement therapy and risk of non-fatal stroke. *Lancet* 1997;**350**:1277–1283

Viscoli CM, Brass LM, Kernan WN et al. A clinical trial of estrogen-replacement therapy after ischemic stroke. *N Engl J Med* 2001;**345**:1243–1249

Hypertension

ALLHAT Officers and Coordinators. Major outcomes in high-risk hypertensive patients randomized to angiotensin-converting enzyme inhibitor or calcium channel blocker vs diuretic: The Antihypertensive and Lipid-Lowering Treatment to Prevent Heart Attack Trial (ALLHAT). *JAMA* 2002;**288**:2981–2997

Bosch J, Yusuf S, Pogue J et al. Heart outcomes prevention evaluation. Use of ramipril in preventing stroke: double blind randomised trial. *BMJ* 2002;**324**:1–5

Dahlöf B, Devereux RB, Kjeldsen SE et al. Cardiovascular morbidity and mortality in the Losartan Intervention For Endpoint reduction in hypertension study (LIFE): a randomised trial against atenolol. *Lancet* 2002;**359**:995–1003

Du X, Cruickshank K, McNamee R et al. Case–control study of stroke and the quality of hypertension control in north west England. *BMJ* 1997; **314**:272–276

Lawes CMM, Bennett DA, Feigin VL, Rodgers A. Blood pressure and stroke: An overview of published studies. *Stroke* 2004;**35**:1024–1033

PROGRESS Collaborative Group. Randomised trial of a perindopril-based blood-pressure-lowering regimen among 6105 individuals with previous stroke or transient ischaemic attack. *Lancet* 2001; **358**:1033–1041

Ramsay LE, Williams B, Johnston DG et al. Guidelines for management of hypertension: report of the Third Working Party of the British

Hypertension Society. *J Hum Hypertension* 1999; **13**:569–592

Yusuf S, Sleight P, Pogue J et al. Effects of an angiotensin-converting-enzyme inhibitor, ramipril, on cardiovascular events in high-risk patients. The Heart Outcomes Prevention Evaluation Study Investigators. *N Engl J Med* 2000;**342**:145–153

Diabetes mellitus

Colhoun HM, Betteridge DJ, Durrington PN et al. Primary prevention of cardiovascular disease with atorvastatin in type 2 diabetes in the Collaborative Atorvastatin Diabetes Study (CARDS): multicentre randomised placebo-controlled trial. *Lancet* 2004; **364**:685–696

Hansson L, Zanchetti A, Carruthers SG et al. Effects of intensive blood-pressure lowering and low-dose aspirin in patients with hypertension: principal results of the Hypertension Optimal Treatment (HOT) randomised trial. *Lancet* 1998; **351**:1755–1762

UKPDS: UK Prospective Diabetes Study Group. Tight blood pressure control and risk of macrovascular and microvascular complications in type 2 diabetes. *BMJ* 1998a;**317**:703–713

UKPDS: UK Prospective Diabetes Study Group. Intensive blood-glucose control with sulphony-lureas or insulin compared with conventional treatment and risk of complications in patients with type 2 diabetes. *Lancet* 1998b;**352**: 837–853

Cholesterol lowering

Corvol JC, Bouzamondo A, Sirol M et al. Differential effects of lipid-lowering therapies on stroke pre-vention: a meta analysis of randomized trials. *Arch Intern Med* 2003;**24**:669–676

HPS: Heart Protection Study Collaborative Group. Effects of cholesterol-lowering with simvastatin on stroke and other major vascular events in 20 536 people with cerebrovascular disease or other high-risk conditions. *Lancet* 2004;**363**: 757–766

Atrial fibrillation

Hart RG, Halperin JL, Pearce LA et al. Lessons from the stroke prevention in atrial fibrillation trials. *Ann Intern Med* 2003;**138**:831–838

Olsson SB, Executive Steering Committee on behalf of the SPORTIF III Investigators. Stroke preven-tion with the oral direct thrombin inhibitor xime-lagatran compared with warfarin in patients with non-valvular atrial fibrillation (SPORTIF III): randomised controlled trial. *Lancet* 2003;**362**: 1691–1698

Saxena R, Koudstaal PJ. Anticoagulants for prevent-ing stroke in patients with nonrheumatic atrial fibrillation and a history of stroke or transient ischaemic attack. *Cochrane Database System Rev* 2004, Issue 1

Segal JB, McNamara RL, Miller MR et al. Anticoagu-lants or antiplatelet therapy for non-rheumatic atrial fibrillation and flutter. *Cochrane Database System Rev* 2001, Issue 1

Anticoagulation for atherothrombotic stroke

Mohr J, Thompson JLP, Lazar RM et al. A compari-son of warfarin and aspirin for the prevention of recurrent ischemic stroke. *N Engl J Med* 2001; **345**:1444–1451

SPIRIT: Stroke Prevention in Reversible Ischaemia Trial Study Group. A randomized trial of antico-agulants versus aspirin after cerebral ischaemia of presumed arterial origin. *Ann Neurol* 1997;**42**: 857–865

Antiplatelet agents

Algra A, van Gijn J. Aspirin at any dose above 30 mg offers only modest protection after cerebral ischaemia. *J Neurol Neurosurg Psychiatry* 1996; **60**:197–199

ATT: Antithrombotic Trialists' Collaboration. Collaborative meta-analysis of randomised trials of antiplatelet therapy for prevention of death, myocardial infarction, and stroke in high risk patients. *BMJ* 2002;**324**:71–86

CAPRIE Steering Committee. A randomised, blinded, trial of clopidogrel versus aspirin in patients at risk of ischaemic events (CAPRIE). *Lancet* 1996; **348**:1329–1339

Diener HC, Cunha L, Forbes C et al. European Stroke Prevention Study 2: Dipyridamole and acetylsal-icylic acid in the secondary prevention of stroke. *J Neurol Sci* 1996;**143**:1–13

Diener HC, Bogousslavsky J, Brass LM et al. Aspirin and clopidogrel compared with clopidogrel alone after recent ischaemic stroke or transient ischaemic attack in high-risk patients (MATCH): randomised, double-blind, placebo-controlled trial. *Lancet* 2004;**364**:331–337

European Stroke Prevention Study (ESPS). Principal end-points. The ESPS Group. *Lancet* 1987;**ii**: 1351–1354

Gent M, Blakely JA, Easton JD et al. The Canadian American Ticlopidine Study (CATS) in thromboembolic stroke. *Lancet* 1989;**i**:1215–1220

Hass WK, Easton JD, Adams HP Jr et al. A randomized trial comparing ticlopidine hydrochloride with aspirin for the prevention of stroke in high-risk patients. Ticlopidine Aspirin Stroke Study Group. *N Engl J Med* 1989;**321**:501–507

Leonardi-Bee J, Bath PM, Bousser MG et al. Dipyridamole for preventing recurrent ischemic stroke and other vascular events: a meta-analysis of individual patient data from randomized controlled trials. *Stroke* 2005;**36**:162–168

Ridker PM, Cook NR, I-Min L et al. A randomized trial of low-dose aspirin in the primary prevention of cardiovascular disease in women. *N Engl J Med* 2005;**352**:1293–1304

Carotid artery stenosis

ACAS: Executive Committee for the Asymptomatic Carotid Atherosclerosis Study. Endarterectomy for asymptomatic carotid artery stenosis. *JAMA* 1995;**273**:1421–1428

Alamowitch S, Eliasziw M, Algra A et al. Risk, causes, and prevention of ischaemic stroke in elderly patients with symptomatic internal-carotid-artery stenosis. *Lancet* 2001;**357**:1154–1160

Benavente O, Moher D, Pham B. Carotid endarterectomy for asymptomatic carotid stenosis: a meta-analysis. *BMJ* 1998;**317**:1477–1480

ECST: European Carotid Surgery Trialists' Collaborative Group. Randomised trial of endarterectomy for recently symptomatic carotid stenosis: final results of the MRC European Carotid Surgery Trial (ECST). *Lancet* 1998;**351**:1379–1387

Fairhead JF, Mehta Z, Rothwell PM. Population-based study of delays in carotid imaging and surgery and the risk of recurrent stroke. *Neurology* 2005;**65**:371–375

Halliday A, Mansfield A, Marro J et al. Prevention of disabling and fatal strokes by successful carotid endarterectomy in patients without recent neurological symptoms: randomised controlled trial. *Lancet* 2004;**363**:1491–1502

NASCET: North American Symptomatic Carotid Endarterectomy Trial Collaborators. Beneficial effect of carotid endarterectomy in symptomatic patients with highgrade carotid stenosis. *N Engl J Med* 1991;**325**:445–453

Rothwell PM, Eliasziw M, Gutnikov SA et al. Analysis of pooled data from the randomised controlled trials of endarterectomy for symptomatic carotid stenosis. *Lancet* 2003;**361**:107–116

Rothwell PM, Eliasziw M, Gutnikov SA et al. Endarterectomy for symptomatic carotid stenosis in relation to clinical subgroups and timing of surgery. *Lancet* 2004;**363**:915–924

Taylor DW, Barnett HJ, Haynes RB et al. Low-dose and high-dose acetylsalicylic acid for patients undergoing carotid endarterectomy: a randomised controlled trial. ASA and Carotid Endarterectomy (ACE) Trial Collaborators. *Lancet* 1999;**353**: 2179–2184

Carotid angioplasty and stenting

Brown MM. Carotid artery stenting – evolution of a technique to rival carotid endarterectomy. *Am J Med* 2004;**116**:273–275

CAVATAS Investigators. Endovascular versus surgical treatment in patients with carotid stenosis in the Carotid and Vertebral Artery Transluminal Angioplasty study (CAVATAS): a randomised trial. *Lancet* 2001;**357**:1729–1737

Coward LJ, Featherstone RL, Brown MM. Safety and efficacy of endovascular treatment of carotid artery stenosis compared with carotid endarterectomy: a Cochrane systematic review of the randomized evidence. *Stroke* 2005;**36**:905–911

Kastrup A, Groschel K, Krapf H et al. Early outcome of carotid angioplasty and stenting with or without cerebral protection devices. A systematic review of the literature. *Stroke* 2003; **34**:813–819

Theiss W, Hermanek P, Mathias K et al. Pro-CAS: a prospective registry of carotid angioplasty and stenting. *Stroke* 2004;**35**:2134–2139

Yadav JS, Wholey MH, Kuntz RE et al. Protected carotid-artery stenting versus endarterectomy in high-risk patients. *N Engl J Med* 2004;**351**: 1493–1501

Extracranial–intracranial bypass surgery

EC/IC Bypass Study Group. Failure of extracranial–intracranial arterial bypass to reduce the risk of ischemic stroke. Results of an international randomized trial. *N Engl J Med* 1985;**313**:1191–1200

CHAPTER 16

Rehabilitation

Rehabilitation is an important part of the management of all but the mildest of strokes. The aim of rehabilitation is to return the patient to the normal activities of daily life as far as possible. Where this is not possible, rehabilitation aims to adjust the individual's physical and social environment to maximise the patient's independence and participation in society while reducing the stress on the carer and family. Rehabilitation also needs to provide information, psychological support and sometimes psychiatric treatment, to enable the patient to come to terms with their illness and its consequences. The patient may need to undergo a period of grieving for loss of previous cognitive and physical function. Many patients report that the losses of status, employment and independence are the most distressing features of stroke and are much worse than the direct physical consequences. Dependence on others is for many patients both distressing and demeaning. The burden on carers can be equally important, especially if the patient is incontinent, has cognitive impairment or lacks insight.

In general, rehabilitation concentrates on restoring function, not necessarily curing disability. For example, restoration of mobility may be addressed by providing the patient with a stick, Zimmer frame or wheelchair. This approach is epitomized by viewing a paralysed patient, not as confined to a wheelchair, but as freed by the wheelchair to mobilize.

Effective rehabilitation requires a multidisciplinary approach with input from a variety of professionals, depending on the needs of the patient. Regular multidisciplinary team meetings, on at least a weekly basis, are needed to ensure a consistent approach, set realistic goals for therapy, review progress and plan appropriate discharge arrangements. Involvement of the patient and any close carers is essential. Rehabilitation is an active problem-solving approach that involves assessment, education and goal-setting, as well as therapy and the provision of aids.

THE MULTIDISCIPLINARY TEAM

The professional disciplines included in a multidisciplinary stroke rehabilitation team are listed in Table 16.1. Occasionally, help from other departments will be required: for example orthotic appliances, pain experts and information technology. Input may be needed from other medical disciplines: for example gastroenterology for the insertion of endoscopic gastrostomy feeding tubes or urology for advice about the management of bladder problems. The organization of stroke services requires the involvement of a large number of agencies, depending on the needs of the patient, which are enormously varied.

Rehabilitation requires the therapy programme to be tailored to the patient's disability and needs on a very individual basis, unlike many medical treatments for stroke. Hence, good communication and planning within the multidisciplinary team, involving the patient

Table 16.1 Disciplines represented in the multidisciplinary stroke rehabilitation team

- Specialist physicians:
  - Neurologist
  - Stroke physician
  - Care-of-the-elderly physician
  - Rehabilitation specialist
  - Pyschiatrist
- Specialist trained nurses
- Physiotherapist
- Occupational therapist
- Speech and language therapist
- Neuropsychologist
- Social worker
- Dietician

Table 16.2 Domains requiring assessment

- Swallowing
- Speech and communication
- Hydration and nutrition
- Risk of complications, including:
  - Pressure sores
  - Shoulder pain
  - Contractures
  - Deep vein thrombosis
  - Pneumonia
- Memory and visuospatial skills
- Conscious level, orientation and attention
- Upper limb function
- Lower limb function and gait
- Disorders of muscle tone and spasticity
- Mobility indoors and outdoors
- Ability to climb stairs
- Bladder and bowel function
- Pain relief
- Rest and sleep requirements
- Personal appearance (e.g. hair and nails)
- Ability to carry out activities required for daily living, for example:
  - Dressing
  - Washing
  - Taking a bath or shower
  - Brushing or combing hair
  - Cooking
  - Performing household chores
- Aids required (e.g. stick, frame or wheelchair; special utensils)
- Orthotic requirements (e.g. ankle splint)
- Adaptations required to home or work environment, for example:
  - Non-slip mats
  - Grab rails
  - Commode
  - Disabled shower
- Employment requirements
- Driving and vehicle modifications
- Mood (depression and anxiety)
- Motivation
- Sexual function and needs
- Socialization
- Carers' needs

and carer as necessary, are essential components of successful rehabilitation.

REHABILITATION GOALS

The process of stroke rehabilitation involves assessment in a number of fields, so that appropriate education, treatment, provision of aids or environmental adaptation can be initiated (Table 16.2) (Rice-Oxley, 1999). A number of scales are available to assess some of these functions. The most widely used as global indicators are the Barthel Index and the Modified Rankin Scale, although these emphasize predominantly motor function (see Chapter 1). The assessments may need to be repeated at regular intervals to guide therapy and assess progress.

STROKE UNIT CARE

It is now well established that patients with a recent stroke benefit substantially from admission to a dedicated stroke unit (Indredavik *et al.*, 1999). Rehabilitation is provided by a multidisciplinary team devoted to stroke care. Meta-analysis of randomized clinical trials has shown that management of patients with stroke by an organized unit significantly reduces mortality and disability in comparison with standard care on a general medical ward, even when the latter includes therapy input (Figure 16.1) (Stroke Unit Trialists' Collaboration, 1997).

More patients are discharged from stroke units to their own homes than are discharged home from general medical wards. The average length of stay on a stroke unit is similar to, or even less

Study	Treatment (n/N)	Control (n/N)	Peto odds ratio and 95% CI	Weight (%)	Peto odds ratio [95% CI]
Stroke ward versus General medical ward					
Akershus	103/271	110/279		15.4	0.94 [0.67, 1.33]
Dover	54/98	50/89		5.5	0.96 [0.54, 1.70]
Edinburgh	93/155	94/156		8.8	0.99 [0.63, 1.56]
Gšteborg–Sahlgren	108/166	54/83		6.0	1.00 [0.58, 1.74]
Nottingham	63/98	52/76		4.6	0.83 [0.44, 1.56]
Orpington, 1993	38/53	39/48		2.2	0.59 [0.24, 1.48]
Orpington, 1995	36/36	37/37		0.0	Not estimable
Perth	10/29	14/30		1.7	0.61 [0.22, 1.71]
Trondheim	54/110	81/110		6.2	0.36 [0.21, 0.61]
Umea	52/110	102/183		8.1	0.71 [0.44, 1.14]
Subtotal (95% CI)	1126	1091		58.5	0.80 [0.67, 0.95]

Total events: 611 (treatment), 633 (control)

Test for heterogeneity chi-square = 12.18, df = 8,
$p = 0.14$, $I^2 = 34.3\%$

Test for overall effects $z = 2.51$, $p = 0.01$

Mixed rehabilitation ward versus General medical ward					
Birmingham	8/29	9/23		1.4	0.60 [0.19, 1.90]
Helsinki	47/121	65/122		7.2	0.56 [0.34, 0.93]
Illinois	20/56	17/35		2.5	0.59 [0.25, 1.39]
Kuopio	31/50	31/45		2.6	0.74 [0.32, 1.72]
New York	23/42	23/40		2.4	0.90 [0.38, 2.13]
Newcastle	26/34	28/33		1.3	0.59 [0.18, 1.96]
Subtotal (95% CI)	332	298		17.2	0.63 [0.46, 0.88]

Total events: 155 (treatment), 173 (control)

Test for heterogeneity chi-square = 1.02, df = 5, $p = 0.96$, $I^2 = 0.0\%$

Test for overall effects $z = 2.75$, $p = 0.006$

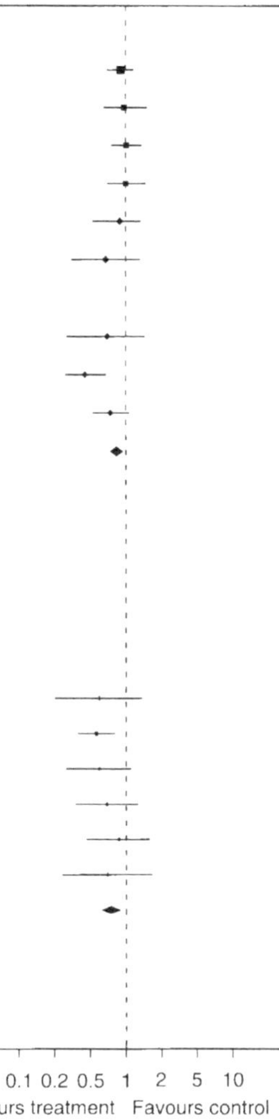

```
        0.1 0.2 0.5  1   2   5  10
      Favours treatment   Favours control
```

Figure 16.1 Meta-analysis showing the odds ratio for death and dependency at the end of follow-up, comparing organized inpatient stroke unit care with routine care in a medical ward (control). From Stroke Unit Trialists' Collaboration. *Cochrane Database System Rev* 2001, Issue 3: CD000197.

than, on general medical wards. These benefits are achieved by organizing stroke care within a single environment, usually on a single ward. Stroke units are not necessarily more expensive than standard care, because the patient is already admitted to hospital and stroke units are not necessarily staffed with a greater number of therapists. However, nursing and therapy time may well be used more efficiently because the patients are located on a single unit with adjacent space for therapy to take place. Stroke units provide other benefits, including:

- Improvements in patient and staff morale
- Provision of information on stroke for patients and carers
- Enhancement of teaching and research on stroke

The characteristics of stroke units that distinguish them from non-specialized wards include:

- Nurses interested in stroke care
- Multidisciplinary team meetings
- Physicians interested in stroke
- Early-onset rehabilitation
- Regular staff training
- Carers involved in the rehabilitation

The exact components of stroke unit care responsible for the improvements in outcome have not been established by research, but it is likely that all of these have important roles to play (Langhorne *et al.*, 2002). One of the most important components is the provision of specialized nurses, trained and experienced in stroke care. Good stroke nurses are able to apply the principles of rehabilitation throughout 24 hours of a patient's care and will continue the patient's programme of therapy outside the context of organized sessions with therapists. Nurses have an important role to play in understanding the needs of stroke patients, including positioning, hydration and feeding, neurological observation, and the provision of information to patients and carers. It is likely that knowledge and enthusiasm, combined with a positive approach to stroke care from the stroke unit staff, and active early provision of medical therapy, all contribute to the improved outcome (Evans *et al.*, 2001). One randomized trial showed that better outcomes were obtained in patients admitted to an organized stroke unit in a discrete location than were obtained by attempting to provide organized care using a 'roving' team of dedicated staff who visited patients on other wards (Kalra *et al.*, 2000).

Multidisciplinary meetings provide the opportunity for communication between stroke unit doctors, nurses and therapists, which ensures that everyone looking after the patient has a consistent approach and ensures that the programme of rehabilitation is properly organized. In addition, plans for appropriate timely discharge to home or another facility need to be made as soon as the patient's prognosis is clear. This will often require close liaison with the patient and carer, as well as between the multidisciplinary team and community services, including district-based nurses, social workers, therapists and the patient's general practitioner. Early supported discharge with continued rehabilitation provided in the community has been shown to reduce long-term dependency, especially in patients with mild or moderate disability (Langhorne *et al.*, 2005).

Who should be admitted to a stroke unit?

Analysis of the randomized trials shows that the benefits of stroke unit care apply to a similar extent to elderly and younger patients, both sexes, and irrespective of whether the stroke is mild, moderate or severe. Patients should not therefore be selected for admission to a stroke unit on the grounds of age, gender or clinical severity. The earlier the patient is admitted to a stroke unit, the more likely they are to benefit. The concept that patients should only be selected for rehabilitation if they remain moderately disabled a week or more after onset is not appropriate to stroke unit care. Even mild patients benefit from the facilities on the stroke unit (e.g. planned investigation). At the other end of the scale, the severely disabled patient benefits particularly from the specialized nursing, even if they are too sick to collaborate much in therapy sessions. All patients with stroke should therefore be admitted to a stroke unit as early as possible. The only possible exceptions are patients with rapidly recovering stroke, so long as they can be seen urgently in a neurovascular clinic, and patients with severe comorbidity (e.g. advanced cancer or dementia). Unfortunately, the provision of stroke units even in the developed world is lamentably poor. In areas lacking a stroke unit, physicians, nurses and therapists should attempt to apply the principles of rehabilitation as outlined in this chapter, meanwhile pressing for organized services to be set up for stroke patients as soon as possible.

It is not possible to achieve the benefits of stroke unit care by managing the patient at home from the start of their illness, even if therapy is provided. However, the organization of local community stroke services can facilitate the early discharge of patients to their homes with definite psychological benefits and cost savings within the acute hospital sector. Clinical trials have suggested that the outcome in patients discharged early is similar to the outcome in those who remain in hospital, so long as appropriate therapy is provided in the patient's home or at a community centre.

When should the patient be admitted to the stroke unit?

Most trials of stroke unit care have admitted patients within a week or so of onset. However, it makes sense that the earlier the patient is admitted to the unit, the more likely the they are to benefit. Modern stroke units are therefore often organized to take patients directly from the accident and emergency department (A&E). The time to treatment can be reduced by liaison with local ambulance services to ensure that suitable patients with suspected stroke are rapidly transferred directly to the stroke unit, bypassing A&E assessment (Harbison *et al.*, 1999). This may be particularly valuable in units using thrombolysis to treat appropriate patients within the first few hours after onset. Stroke units require facilities for intensive monitoring of patients if thrombolysis is used, but the benefits of routine intensive monitoring for other patients is currently uncertain.

How long should the patient stay on the unit?

Unlike coronary care units, the patient will not benefit from stroke unit care if they only stay on the unit for a few days, unless they have made a good recovery by then. Patients with more severe stroke have an ongoing need for medical input for up to 4 weeks after onset, which implies that stroke units taking patients acutely should plan to keep them for up to 4 weeks or more if necessary. The length of stay of stroke patients varies considerably

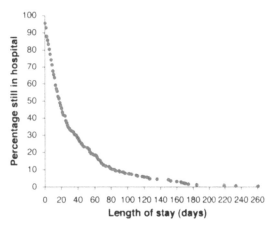

Figure 16.2   Length of stay of consecutive patients with stroke admitted to a teaching hospital in the UK over a 12-month period (*n* = 316).

according to severity. The average length of stay is about 14 days, but the distribution around the mean is not even (Figure 16.2). The majority of patients are discharged within 4 weeks of admission, but there is a small tail of patients who need to stay for up to 6 months. To facilitate discharge from a stroke unit, close liaison needs to be developed with other rehabilitation services, including specialized neurological rehabilitation centres and, for elderly patients who require slower stream rehabilitation, care-of-the-elderly services (Figure 16.3).

INDIVIDUAL COMPONENTS OF STROKE REHABILITATION

Physiotherapy

Physiotherapy has an important role to play in the rehabilitation of physical disabilities. Physiotherapists pay particular attention to improving posture, balance, upper limb function and gait. Graded exercises are used to prevent contracture, improve muscle tone, encourage and strengthen the use of appropriate muscle groups, and enhance motor recovery. Evidence is accumulating that various focused intensive physiotherapy approaches, including

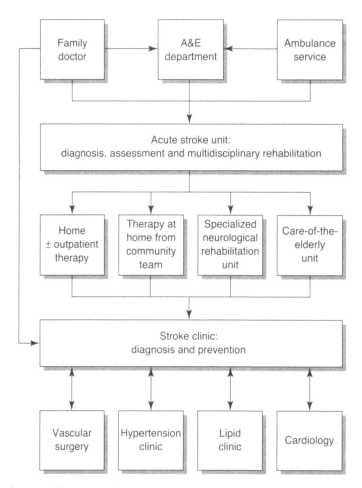

Figure 16.3   Flow diagram illustrating the components of a comprehensive stroke service.

constraint-induced therapy, improve functional outcome in selected patients (Kwakkel *et al.*, 1999; Miltner *et al.*, 1999; Woldag and Hummelsheim, 2002). Physiotherapists may also use prostheses (e.g. an ankle splint for foot drop) or walking aids (e.g. a stick or frame to improve functional outcome).

Occupational therapy

Occupational therapy concentrates on the assessment and treatment of impairment of the ability to carry out the main activities of daily life (e.g. the preparation and cooking of a meal). Occupational therapists are responsible for organizing the provision of aids to improve functional ability (e.g. the provision of large

handed eating utensils) and are involved in the provision of wheelchairs. They play an important part in visits to the patient's home and will recommend improvements or adaptations to their environment to enable the patient to return home or improve their safety (e.g. non-slip mats, bath seats, grab rails or the provision of a stairlift).

Speech and language therapists (SALT or SLT)

Speech and language therapists play an important role in the assessment and treatment not only of dysphasia and dysarthria after stroke, but also of swallowing disorders (see below). Therapy for dysphasia and dysarthria concentrates on improving communication skills. In a severely anarthric patient, this may involve the provision of communication aids.

Psychology and psychiatry

Psychologists have a particularly important role to play in the treatment of patients with cognitive impairment, particularly memory impairment. Cognitive assessment is also useful to other members of the team and may help to guide rehabilitation and discharge planning. Depression is common after stroke, and psychiatric input may be beneficial in appropriate patients.

Social workers

Social workers have a major role to play in organizing community support and appropriate placement for patients who cannot return to their own home because of severe disabilities. They are also able to advise patients about their entitlement to state benefits.

PREVENTION AND TREATMENT OF COMPLICATIONS

Swallowing and nutrition

Impairment of swallowing is common in the early stages of stroke. Nearly 30% of unilateral hemispheric stroke patients and 67% of those with brainstem involvement suffer impairment of swallowing or silent aspiration. Attempts to swallow may then result in aspiration pneumonia, which may impede recovery or prove fatal. Pneumonia can lead to further stroke or to deterioration from hypoxia and pyrexia. Prevention of aspiration is therefore an important part of stroke care. All patients should have their swallowing assessed as soon as possible after admission and should be kept nil-by-mouth until this has been completed and swallowing assessed as safe. Wards caring for stroke patients should therefore have a protocol for swallowing assessment at the bedside.

In general, patients should be fed in an upright position with food of appropriate consistency and small boluses. They should be encouraged to cough gently after each swallow and to swallow several times after each bolus. In addition, obtunded patients and those with impairment of consciousness should not be permitted to take oral fluids or nutrition. In cases where there is doubt about the safety of swallowing, video fluoroscopy during swallowing may establish whether or not aspiration takes place.

Malnutrition is common in stroke patients (Dennis, 2000). It is essential that patients who are not able to swallow safely or in whom intake is inadequate for other reasons should have fluids and nutrition by an alternative route. In the early stages of stroke, dehydration is likely to be harmful, and fluid replacement should commence as soon as the patient is admitted, if swallowing is not safe. Feeding should probably also start within 24 hours of admission. Even if a patient can swallow safely, the spontaneous intake of food and liquid is often inadequate because of poor appetite, cognitive impairment, neglect or physical difficulties in feeding. Nurses or carers will therefore need to allocate adequate time to encouraging or helping the patient to eat and drink. However, the routine use of oral nutritional supplements does not appear to benefit patients substantially (Dennis *et al.*, 2005a).

When the oral route is not safe or practical, it is essential to establish other routes. In the short term, it is often convenient to replace fluids via an intravenous route, but this has the disadvantage of immobilizing the patient's limb and limits general mobilization. A nasogastric tube is therefore preferred and has the advantage of allowing feeding as well as fluid replacement. There is also less risk of cardiac overload or infection. If oral intake is likely to be unsafe or inadequate for more than 2 weeks, consideration should be given to using feeding directly into the stomach via an endoscopically inserted gastric tube (percutaneous endoscopic gastrostomy (PEG) feeding) (Figure 16.4). This has the advantage that a larger tube can be used and is less unsightly and usually more comfortable than a nasal tube. Surveys have shown that patients usually prefer PEG feeding to a nasogastric tube, but risks associated with PEG

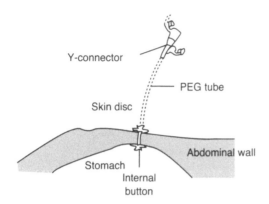

Figure 16.4 Drawing to illustrate percutaneous endoscopic gastrostomy (PEG) tube feeding. Adapted from Dennis M. *Br Med Bull* 2000;**56**:466–475.

insertion include peritonitis. The recently published Feed or Ordinary Diet (FOOD) trials assessed the benefits on outcome of the early initiation of tube feeding after stroke, and also compared early PEG feeding with nasogastric tube feeding (Dennis *et al.*, 2005b). Early tube feeding was associated with a reduction in the risk of death, but not in poor outcome. There was no outcome advantage of PEG feeding compared with a nasogastric tube.

Deep vein thrombosis (DVT) and pulmonary embolism

DVT is a recognized complication of immobility and is usually seen in severely hemiparetic limbs. Radiographic studies show that subclinical DVT is common after stroke. However, DVT is only very occasionally complicated by pulmonary embolus. Nevertheless, it is important to institute a policy for the prevention of DVT. The routine use of subcutaneous heparin has not been shown to improve outcome following stroke, despite the potential benefits of preventing pulmonary embolism, and may cause haemorrhagic transformation of an infarct. There is therefore no indication for the routine use of subcutaneous heparin, but it should be considered in patients with ischaemic stroke with severe immobility or in patients with a past history of DVT or known thrombophilia. Probably the most important measure for preventing DVT is

early mobilization. On an active stroke unit, all conscious patients will be sat up and out of bed within a day of admission, which is a great contrast to traditional management. The regular use of TED stockings is often recommended, but has not been proven to prevent DVT after stroke.

Pressure sores

Immobilized patients require frequent turning to prevent pressure sores and may need special bedding, such as fleeces and occasionally special mattresses. The prevention of pressure sores is an important component of good nursing care. Pressure sores should very rarely be seen in any patient with stroke.

Shoulder pain

Pain in the paralysed shoulder used to be a common complication of stroke, but is largely preventable by good positioning of the shoulder and early physiotherapy (Walsh, 2001; Gamble *et al.*, 2002). It is important to prevent a paralysed limb from hanging unsupported at the side of the patient, because the weight of the limb leads to subluxation of the shoulder joint. This in turn leads to a painful frozen shoulder and in extreme cases to the shoulder–hand syndrome. Shoulder pain is not only distressing for the patient, but may limit the use of the limb and impair recovery. The correct positioning of a patient in bed or chair is very important to prevent complications and minimize increase in tone. The paralysed or weak limb should be supported at all times in bed or a chair to maintain a symmetrical position of the shoulder (Figure 16.5). Patients who already have shoulder pain may benefit from standard rheumatological treatments for shoulder pain, including non-steroidal anti-inflammatory agents (NSAIDs) and local articular steroid injections.

Limb swelling

Swelling of the hand or foot of a hemiparetic limb is quite common. The cause is poorly understood, but physiological studies suggest

a

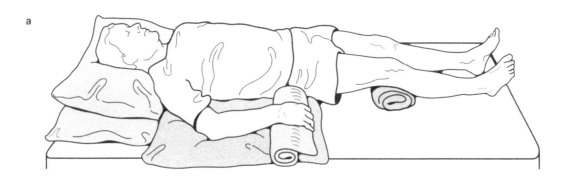

b

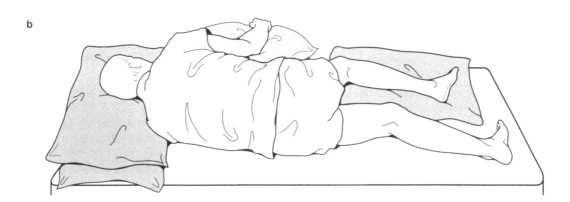

c

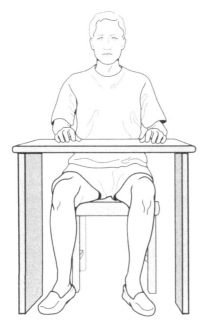

Figure 16.5 Drawing to illustrate correct position-ing of the hemiparetic limb when supine (a), lying on the unaffected side (b) and sitting (c). If the patient is sitting without a table, or the table is too low, a pillow should be used to support the limb.

that excessive sympathetic activity with peripheral vasodilation is partly responsible. The patient often complains that the limb is cold, because the vasodilation results in heat loss, even though the limb may feel warm to observers' touch. Treatment is difficult, but diuretics are not indicated. Elevation of the limb may help. This type of oedema should be distinguished from unilateral limb oedema secondary to DVT.

Spasticity

Spasticity is a common, but not universal, feature of upper motor neurone lesions resulting from stroke. Increase in tone often develops several days or weeks after the onset of the stroke and varies considerably in extent and severity. In the upper limb, the pattern of spasticity leads to flexion at each joint, and in the lower limb to extension. The muscle weakness is often more severe in the antagonist group of muscles in a pyramidal distribution. Spasticity is therefore often seen as inhibiting recovery, for example extension of the fingers or dorsiflexion of the foot. However, relief of spasticity rarely improves strength, and function does not often improve, unless the spasticity is very severe in the presence of preserved power. Occasionally, severe spasticity results in painful muscle cramps, and then treatment may relieve pain. Early mobilization and appropriate physiotherapy are the mainstay of treatment, and limit the development of spasticity and contractures.

A number of drugs are available to treat spasticity (Table 16.3). The dose of muscle relaxants has to be built up slowly. Tolerability is often limited by side-effects, particularly sedation and muscle weakness. The latter often limits the benefit of antispasticity drugs. Moreover, reducing spasticity is not always helpful. In the lower limb, increased extensor tone may actually be beneficial in allowing a patient to stand and bear weight on the limb. Reduction in tone may impair weight-bearing, and in this situation measures to reduce spasticity should be approached with caution.

Table 16.3   Drugs used to treat spasticity

Drug	Recommended dose (mg/day)
Baclofen	15–100
Dantrolene	25–400
Diazepam	2–60
Tizanidine[a]	2–36
Botulinum toxin[b]	Local injection

The dose should be started at the lower range indicated, divided over the course of the day, and then increased gradually according to response and side-effects

[a]Not licensed for stroke.
[b]Specialist use only.

Local injections of botulinum toxin into spastic muscles may have some benefit in patients in whom spasticity is causing focal problems (Brashear *et al.*, 2002). For example, injections into the long flexor muscles of the fingers may allow toileting of the hand in the rare patient in whom severe spasticity has resulted in a clenched fist in which extension of the fingers is impossible.

Depression

Depression is very common after stroke and is often multifactorial in origin (Berg *et al.*, 2003; Bogousslavsky, 2003). There is no relationship to the level of physical disability, suggesting a direct neurophysiological cause, possibly due to involvement of central monoaminergic pathways. Significant improvement in the Barthel Index of depressed patients treated with antidepressants over a control group suggests that depression adds significantly to stroke disability. Attention to psychiatric disorders attending stroke may improve function. Depression should therefore be treated routinely and expert psychiatric advice sought if necessary.

Post-stroke pain

Post-stroke pain of central neurogenic origin is unusual, but when it occurs it can be extremely distressing (Andersen *et al.*, 1995). In most cases, the patient has had ischaemia or haemorrhage involving the thalamus (Bowsher *et al.*, 1998). The pain is characteristically described as a deep burning pain felt throughout one limb or the whole of one side of the body. Unlike the other symptoms of stroke, which tend to improve with time, post-stroke pain often develops days, weeks or even months after the onset of stroke. The pain may be made worse by movement or touch, and the pressure of clothing or bed covers may be unbearable at times. The pain often limits the patient's activities and may lead to severe depression. Treatment is difficult, but some relief may be achieved with tricyclic anti-depressant therapy, particularly amitriptyline taken at night (Lampl *et al.*, 2002). Carbamazepine or gabapentin can also be tried. Local measures (e.g. transcutaneous nerve stimulation) are rarely helpful. Patients with post-stroke pain should be encouraged to carry on with as many activities as possible to try and direct attention away from the painful limbs.

KEY REFERENCES

Rehabilitation goals

Rice-Oxley M. Effectiveness of brain injury rehabilitation. *Clinical Rehabilitation* 1999;**13**(Suppl 1): 7–24

Stroke unit care

Evans A, Perez I, Harraf F et al. Can differences in management processes explain different outcomes between stroke unit and stroke-team care? *Lancet* 2001;**358**:1586–1592

Harbison J, Massey A, Barnett L et al. Rapid ambulance protocol for acute stroke. *Lancet* 1999;**353**: 1935

Indredavik B, Bakke F, Slørdal SA et al. Stroke unit treatment. 10 year follow-up. *Stroke* 1999;**30**: 1524–1527

Kalra A, Evans I, Perez M et al. Alternative strategies for stroke care: a prospective randomised controlled trial. *Lancet* 2000;**356**:894–899

Langhorne P, Pollock A, in conjunction with The Stroke Unit Trialists' Collaboration. What are the components of effective stroke unit care? *Age Ageing* 2002;**31**:365–371

Langhorne P, Taylor G, Murray G et al. Early supported discharge services for stroke patients: a meta-analysis of individual patients' data. *Lancet* 2005;**365**:501–506

Phillips SJ, Eskes GA, Gubitz GJ. Description and evaluation of an acute stroke unit. *CMAJ* 2002; **167**:655–660

Stroke Unit Trialists' Collaboration. Collaborative systematic review of the randomised trials of organised inpatient (stroke unit) care after stroke. *BMJ* 1997;**314**:1151–1159

Stroke Unit Trialists' Collaboration. Organised inpatient (stroke unit) care for stroke. *Cochrane Database System Rev* 2001, Issue 3

Physiotherapy

Kwakkel G, Wagenaar RC, Twisk JWR et al. Intensity of leg and arm training after primary middle-cerebral-artery stroke: a randomised trial. *Lancet* 1999;**354**:191–196

Miltner WHR, Bauder H, Sommer M et al. Effects of constraint-induced movement therapy on patients with chronic motor deficits after stroke. *Stroke* 1999;**30**:586–592

Woldag H, Hummelsheim H. Evidence-based physiotherapeutic concepts for improving arm and hand function in stroke patients: a review. *J Neurol* 2002;**249**:518–528

Swallowing and nutrition

Dennis M. Nutrition after stroke. *Br Med Bull* 2000; **56**:466–475

Dennis MS, Lewis SC, Warlow C. FOOD Trial Collaboration. Routine oral nutritional supplementation for stroke patients in hospital (FOOD): a multicentre randomised controlled trial. *Lancet* 2005a;**365**:755–763

Dennis MS, Lewis SC, Warlow C. FOOD Trial Collaboration. Effect of timing and method of enteral tube feeding for dysphagic stroke patients (FOOD): a multicentre randomised controlled trial. *Lancet* 2005b;**365**:764–772

Shoulder pain

Gamble GE, Barberan E, Laasch HU et al. Poststroke shoulder pain: a prospective study of the association and risk factors in 152 patients with consecutive cohort of 205 patients presenting with stroke. *Eur J Pain* 2002;**6**:467–474

Walsh K. Management of shoulder pain in patients with stroke. *Postgrad Med J* 2001;**77**:645–649

Spasticity

Brashear A, Gordon MF, Elovic E et al. Intramuscular injection of botulinum toxin for the treatment of wrist and finger spasticity after a stroke. *N Engl J Med* 2002;**347**:395–400

Depression

Berg A, Palomaki H, Lehtihalmes M et al. Poststroke depression: an 18-month follow up. *Stroke* 2003; **34**:138–143

Bogousslavsky J. William Feinberg Lecture 2002: Emotions, mood, and behavior after stroke. *Stroke* 2003;**34**:1046–1050

Post-stroke pain

Andersen G, Vestergaard K, Ingeman-Nielsen M et al. Incidence of central post-stroke pain. *Pain* 1995;**61**:187–193

Bowsher D, Leijon G, Thuomas KA. Central poststroke pain: correlation of MRI with clinical pain characteristics and sensory abnormalities. *Neurology* 1998;**51**:1352–1358

Lampl C, Yazdi K, Roper C. Amitriptyline in the prophylaxis of central poststroke pain. Preliminary results of 39 patients in a placebo-controlled, long-term study. *Stroke* 2002;**33**:3030–3032

Index

T - #0623 - 071024 - C287 - 254/178/16 [18] - CB - 9780415385350 - Gloss Lamination